THREE-DIMENSIONAL TREATMENT
FOR SCOLIOSIS:
A PHYSIOTHERAPEUTIC METHOD
FOR DEFORMITIES OF THE SPINE

By Christa Lehnert-Schroth, P.T.

Christa Lehnert-Schroth, P.T.

THREE-DIMENSIONAL TREATMENT FOR SCOLIOSIS

A PHYSIOTHERAPEUTIC METHOD FOR DEFORMITIES OF THE SPINE

The Martindale Press
Palo Alto, California

Published by The Martindale Press
Palo Alto, California
www.schrothmethod.com

Originally published in German as *Dreidimensionale Skoliose-Behandlung* (Stuttgart: G. Fischer, 1973). 7th edition 2007 by Urban & Fischer Verlag, Elsevier GmbH, Munich, as *Dreidimensionale Skoliosebehandlung: Eine physiotherapeutische Spezialmethode zur Verbesserung von Rückgratverkrümmungen. Atmungs-Orthopädie System Schroth*. The translation is based upon the 7th edition.

Lehnert-Schroth, Christa
Three-Dimensional Treatment for Scoliosis:
A Physiotherapeutic Method for Deformities of the Spine

First edition in English.
Translated by Christiane Mohr, Alistair Reeves, and Douglas A. Smith.
276 pages. 679 illustrations.
Includes bibliographical references.
ISBN 978-0-914959-02-1
I. Scoliosis. II. Physiotherapy.

Christa Lehnert-Schroth (1924-)
www.scoliosistreatment-schroth.com

Notice: The pictures presented in this book are amateur photographs taken over the past 60 years. They have been preserved to document this book.

Dedicated with admiration to my mother
Katharina Schroth by

Christa Lehnert-Schroth

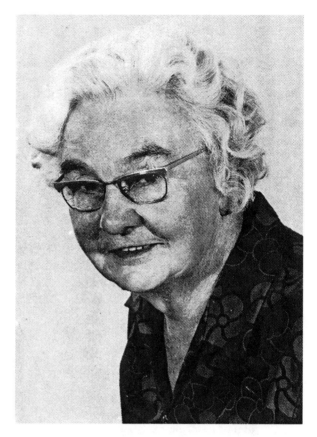

Katharina Schroth (22 February 1894 – 19 February 1985)

Katharina Schroth was awarded the *Bundesverdienst-kreuz* ("Federal Cross of Merit" of the Order of Merit of the Federal Republic of Germany) for the introduction and development of her treatment for scoliosis, because this system was unique in its intensity, effect, and results.

From among all the people
Whom you meet in the course of your life
You are the only one
Whom you will neither leave nor lose.
You are the only answer to
That Question of the meaning of life.
You are the only solution
To the problem of life.

Maynard

Table of contents

Foreword to the English edition

I am very pleased that this textbook is now available in the English language. This means that English-speaking physiotherapists who wish to treat patients suffering from scoliosis now have a very broad range of exercises at their disposal for all cases and shapes of scoliotic bodies.

For fifty years I worked as a physiotherapist with patients suffering from scoliosis, introducing the specific system of treatment that bears the name of my mother, Katharina Schroth, to therapists and patients.

Because she suffered from scoliosis herself during her youth, she developed the program now known in Germany as 'The Three-Dimensional Scoliosis Treatment' or 'Three-Dimensional Scoliosis Physiotherapy'. This is a conservative method of treatment, which works among other things with exercises that elongate the trunk, correct the imbalance of the body, and fill the concavities of the trunk using a special breathing technique which she called 'rotational breathing'.

Katharina Schroth's approach to treatment was far ahead of her time. Many patients are helped by the treatment we give and by the courses we offer for physiotherapists, who come from many countries, at our Katharina Schroth Spinal Deformities Rehabilitation Centre. In 1981, on the occasion of Katharina Schroth's 60th professional anniversary, Professor Friedrich Brussatis, M.D., said in his address:

"I am myself a member of the research society of the American Orthopedic Society, which has designated itself specifically as the 'Scoliosis Research Society'. The fact alone that such a society exists may indicate to you what extraordinarily great, only partly solved problems still exist today in the diagnosis and treatment of scoliosis.

"Precisely because of so many failures and great attempts and disappointments over the centuries, it constitutes an extraordinarily important landmark to have recognized the three-dimensional flow of motion and deformation of the spine, and above all to have applied it extensively in practice. I believe the most important part of your treatment method is the fact that you proceed from a given situation of malposture, whose faulty form in itself we cannot alter much. But we can proceed into a situation, in which you apply everything functionally available for better conditioning of the body, particularly the breathing function, in order to help the patient and to motivate him psychologically despite a sometimes extraordinarily great handicap.

"When we once again observe this combination of thought processes in connection with your life work passing before us, we know what we have to thank you for. And we also know exactly where the path in the future will lead us: precisely to the three-dimensional treatment of scoliosis".

The book is a description of the techniques of the Schroth method. It describes almost all trunk deviations and their treatment, thus it is a wonderful source of information for therapists who wish to treat scoliotic patients.

The book is strongly practice-related. It should be possible for therapists who treat their patients following the book's guidelines to achieve successful results. The Schroth method has long been regarded as the gold standard in German physiotherapy.

I am very pleased that this method of treatment has already been the subject of repeated scientific investigations and has now been described in several books at large. My mother's basic three-dimensional idea is also incorporated into the current bracing concept in Central Europe that has been shown to be effective.

May this book help many physiotherapists and ease the burden of all young children, adolescents and adults suffering from scoliosis.

Bad Sobernheim, Spring, 2007,
Christa Lehnert-Schroth, P.T.

Foreword

The problems of treating scoliosis have hitherto remained unsolved either by surgical or non-surgical methods. Years of research and the development of more and more complicated procedures have not changed the substance of this development. The goal is still correction of the deformity and maintenance of the correction. This would certainly be possible with an outrageously elaborate set of pre-operative, operative, and post-operative procedures. However, is fusion of a large part of the spine after correction desirable? Do we know whether the satisfaction of scoliosis patients following such surgery – beyond the very expensive, partly cosmetic correction for the patient, who now has a reduced scoliosis but also a stiff spine – is greater than it would have been if he had not been operated upon?

Judging by the remarks after successful surgery, we know this. Yet no large-scale and long-term follow-up studies exist to prove whether it would be true in view of the patient's capacity to withstand future physical stress and cope with professional life.

In the final analysis, not just the objective physical condition but rather motivation is the decisive factor, once the patient has returned from the Procrustean bed or surgery to his or her familiar environment. This is why any proposals for treatment that not only have a physical but also a psychological impact on the scoliotic patient should be welcomed.

Katharina Schroth, who suffered from scoliosis herself, developed exactly sixty years ago a treatment method that was unique both in terms of intensity and success rate. This admirable system is practiced nowhere else on the Continent in this manner, intensity, and with these successes. It consists of a logical series of exercises based upon fixing the pelvis, as the foundation of scoliosis, in an actively corrected position, and subsequently performing trunk-elongating exercises. This process also addresses derotation of the ribs and flattening the rib hump, which have a positive secondary effect on breathing. However, we are primarily dealing with a functional treatment method that helps patients to preserve their own well-being.

Continuing the tradition of her mother, Christa Lehnert-Schroth has directed the clinic in Sobernheim for the past twenty years and developed it into an internationally recognized centre for the conservative treatment of scoliosis. The first edition of this monograph was published in 1973. In the meantime, the treatment has been refined further. The method was initially relegated to the field of complementary medicine, primarily because it was labelled an 'orthopaedic breathing method', but today its principles have long been recognized and embraced by experts and authorities on scoliosis. The formula of 'three-dimensional treatment' referred to the medico-mechanical aspect of the Schroth exercises, which was later incorporated into traditional medicine by the recognized expert Dr. Cotrel and his treatment based on the principle of EDF (extension, derotation, flexion).

Katharina Schroth developed her method that could be suited to each patient using active measures and corrections with simple aids, and Cotrel later continued with the help of straps on the extension table. Subsequently he fixed the correction using plaster casts, in which he left windows to enable breathing movements to assist in reversing the thoracic deformations.

Throughout its entire history, physicians have been intimately involved in the development of Katharina Schroth's methods, currently Public Health Officer Otto Hundt, M.D., and Karl Gross, M.D. In his preface to the first edition, Dr. Hundt expressed the wish that: "this book shall serve its purpose and give patients support in exercises and life, as well as providing medical experts with critical insight into a proven system".

This new edition has been revised by the author and expanded with new text and more illustrations. Some cases are documented not only photographically but also radiologically.

Naturally even the Schroth method is not the philosopher's stone as far as treating scoliosis is concerned. However, again and again therapists observe that it creates a better feeling for posture and partially actively corrects the secondary factors which make a scoliosis appear larger. Of course the method has its limits. In a growing body, the maximum that can be treated is a scoliosis of 50°. Yet even severe scoliosis in an older patient reacts positively to intensive treatment at the clinic. Group interaction and becoming familiar with the visual image of one's own scoliosis result in a cooperative patient-partner, which is a prerequisite for the success of all further medical treatment, be it conservative, physiotherapeutic with or without apparatus, or even surgical.

In this regard, we wish for a broader adoption of the principle of three-dimensional treatment of scoliosis, further success for this ingenious concept of Katharina Schroth and its intensive development by mother and daughter, and therefore for this book.

March, 1981
K. F. Schlegel, M.D.
Professor and Director of the Orthopaedic Clinic,
University of Essen, Germany

Foreword to the sixth edition

I am delighted that this book has met with such lively interest that again a reprint is necessary.

This 6th edition has again been revised carefully and a number of important sections have been added. To compensate for this, I have deleted some of the X-ray material and shortened some of the other chapters radically. The fact that the last edition sold out so quickly shows that a new edition is necessary. This book has become a real reference work and textbook for therapists treating scoliosis.

I am also very pleased that we receive such positive feedback from participants in our physiotherapists' training program, who report that they are able to achieve improvements in their patients that are demonstrable even by X-rays. They are themselves delighted that they are able to teach their patients to help themselves. They have found enjoyment and confidence in the treatment of scoliosis, which is very important.

Very special, heartfelt thanks are due to my son, Hans-Rudolf Weiss, M.D., orthopaedic specialist and current medical director of our clinic, for his unrelenting efforts to consolidate the scientific basis for the Schroth method. The results of the research he has published are given in the bibliography of this book.

My greatest wish is that this book should serve as an aid and support for therapists and for their patients.

Bad Sobernheim, Winter, 1999
Christa Lehnert-Schroth, P.T.

Foreword to the first edition

This book is about the practical experience of treating scoliosis for half a century. The author herself has thirty years of professional experience in the treatment of scoliosis.

The aim of this book is to explain the basics of the treatment method. However, it is often difficult to explain details of the method in writing, since written explanations become complicated, whereas during actual treatment the ideas flow together and are simplified. Participation in one of our training courses is therefore recommended.

I hope that this rotational breathing method will be spread with the help of interested physicians and physiotherapists, since after it is learned, the method is also a successful tool for patient self-treatment. I would be happy if this book became the basis for discussion, and motivation for a precise scientific corroboration of the method.

I am grateful particularly to Hede Teirich-Leube, M.D., F. Baumann M.D., Otto Hundt, M.D., and all others who have supported this book project.

Bad Sobernheim, 1972
Christa Lehnert-Schroth, Physiotherapist

About this book

This book explains functional treatment of scoliosis using the method developed by Katharina Schroth. This method differs from previous therapies in its completely new approach to structural correction of the spine. Two basic concepts mark this principle. First, activation of inactive muscles in the concavities. Second, correction of vertebral distortion and scoliosis using breathing movement, employing the ribs as levers.

The book serves as a guide to scoliosis treatment and as a stimulus for physiotherapists.

Spring, 1973
Baumann, M.D.

This new edition shows that the Schroth method has received widespread acknowledgement that must be considered astonishing, since the method itself is not being taught as part of physiotherapy training at our physical therapist schools. In spite of this, many physicians such as ourselves, especially orthopaedists, have recognized the often astounding effects of this treatment on their patients.

In our years of work at the Schroth Clinic, we often found it a deeply moving experience to see how young people who arrived frustrated and depressed because of their faulty posture, returned after a few weeks for their final physician examination self-confident and radiant, with changed facial expression. The feeling and knowledge that they could influence their faulty development with their own energy and effort gave them hope, which often made more positive the whole person in her relation to herself and her environment.

This is a treatment method which has been developed and explained empirically. Some aspects still remain to be proven scientifically. Documentation of success using X-rays is difficult, since X-rays from both before and after in-patient treatment are seldom available to us.

The success of this conservative physiotherapeutic treatment depends on duration and intensity of daily application at home. This is a non-controllable risk factor which is easily charged against the method. We are aware that scientific facts are still missing which would support our empirical practice. We would therefore be grateful for any help and comments, in particular any usable and comparable X-ray documentation.

The Schroth method will continue to forge ahead. The best evidence is the necessity for this new edition, expanded with resistance-band exercises and exercises to correct lumbosacral curvature. This book is meant to be an advisor to physicians, physiotherapists and patients. Its basic format has therefore been retained. We intend to remain active as medical advisors for the Schroth method.

Spring 1981,
O. Hundt, M.D. Surgeon / K. Gross M.D. Orthopaedist

Development of the Schroth Rotational Breathing System

Katharina Schroth was born in Dresden, Germany, on February 22, 1894. In her youth, she had scoliosis herself. She suffered mentally because of her deformity, and more so since she had to wear a brace. This orthopaedic support device did not bring about the desired result because it hindered physical activity. At that time there was no adequate treatment for scoliosis. All she wanted was to be able to 'stand straight up' and live without the brace.

A rubber ball with a depression that could be pressed out by air gave her the original idea for self-treatment and the firm resolve to work on her body according to this principle. The depression seemed to her like the concave side of her body. She started to breathe into her concave side in order to fill it with air. Creativity, methodical thinking, and continuous working at it soon brought the first successes. By practising between mirrors, she was able to follow visually what was happening to her body. In the middle of her right side was the rib hump, and she saw how it flattened out when she directed her breath into her left side. She realized: **this is actually not a rib hump – the ribs are just twisted**! These twisted ribs could be turned back into their normal position. Scoliosis lost its fateful power and became simply a disorder to be corrected, if not completely cured.

One realization led to another. For instance, there was a flat area on the front of the rib cage – exactly opposite the rib hump on the back. She succeeded in pushing out this part by breathing into it. She felt the rib hump flat-tening accordingly. This meant that correcting the front simultaneously resulted in correction of the back.

The left front part of her rib cage also had a rib hump. She could not simply push it in. But it lowered and flattened when she breathed into the indentation of the left side of her back. In this way, the 'rotational breathing' method was conceived. When correct changes were happening in one place, other body parts were forced to correct themselves as well.

She then recognized that the trunk was formed of three body segments: pelvic girdle, rib cage, and shoulder girdle, and that in her body these three parts were rotated against each other (which she later noticed in her patients). It was necessary to derotate these three segments and to use the ribs as lever arms. What followed was elimination and flattening of the three high parts on the back and the frontal rib hump, while the low areas were built up. At the time, Katharina Schroth was a teacher at the Rackow Business School in Dresden. Her colleagues noticed the positive physical change. She was asked to deliver speeches, and prepared for them by studying anatomy intensively. She was tested by Sentkowsky, M.D., in Dresden. These speeches were followed by courses which she gave all over Germany.

In 1921, she married and moved to Meissen on the Elbe. After a short while she was treating patients from Germany and foreign countries. She worked hard on her patients with unceasing idealism. Year after year, she gained new insights and created a mosaic piece by piece.

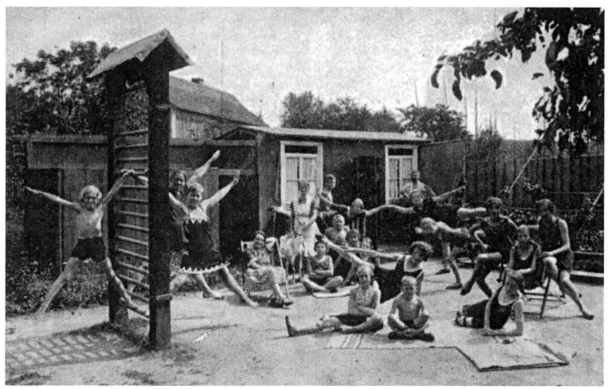

Fig. 2: Open-air exercises in Meissen, in 1924

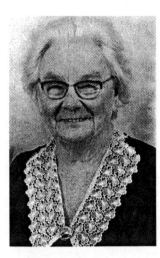

Fig. 3: Mrs. Katharina Schroth
at age eighty-five

The rotational breathing method was continuously improved. Each new case perfected her knowledge further. Soon she was called upon to speak at conferences. As early as 1925, the journal *Medizinalpolitische Rundschau* commented that the Schroth method was epoch-making in the treatment of scoliosis.

In 1927, Katharina Schroth completed training at the Erna Graf Klotz School for Functional Gymnastics and Movement in Dresden, where she earned her diploma with the highest marks. During her training, she had learned about all the different systems of gymnastics, such as Laban, Klapp, Medau, Hellerau-Lachsenburg, Surén, Gindler, and Kallmeyer. She took dancing lessons with Mary Wigman and Palucca. She also studied Swedish Gymnastics at the 'Königliches Palais' in Dresden. She became convinced that these methods represented a good basis, but that they were not specific enough for treating scoliosis. None of these methods included targeted methods to help people specifically with spinal deformities. These circumstances forced her to observe closely her own body and those of her patients in order to discern principles behind the exercise effects. She sought the principles according to which a posture-dependent scoliosis developed, and she sought, in its turnaround by pertinent exercises, conditions that could influence a scoliosis to traverse its same developmental path in reverse.

The method had already enjoyed considerable success before World War II. After a large-scale comparison of various methods during a controlled experiment in Hindenburg, a commission of experts noted that the Schroth system's results far outstripped other methods. The gap between Schroth treatment results and those of the other systems was so great that they began to retrain the instructors at the other schools in the Schroth method.

In 1934, Prof. Gebhardt of Hohenlychen and Prof. Wilhelm of Freiburg confirmed the success of the Schroth method. After the war, the Ministry of Internal Affairs in East Germany ordered a three-year investigation of the method. Afterwards the Schroth house was nationalized on the grounds that "the method must be open to a larger circle of sick people". In 1955, Katharina Schroth moved to West Germany. In 1961 she founded her clinic

in Bad Sobernheim, where it has remained ever since, treating patients from all over the world.

Katharina Schroth received the *Bundesverdienstkreuz* (Federal Cross of Merit) from the government of the Federal Republic of Germany.

Physicians and orthopaedic clinics, as well as health insurance companies and the Social Security Office, were quite cooperative with our clinic, which was and is fruitful for its further development. The author is grateful for their support and encouragement.

In 1976, Johannes Heitland and Erhard Schulte wrote their diploma thesis on the following topic: "Sozialpsychologische Beobachtungen an jugendlichen Skoliosepatienten aus der Sicht des Sozialpädagogen" (Socio-psychological observations of young scoliotic patients from the viewpoint of the social worker). Over a treatment period of four weeks at our clinic in Sobernheim, both men interviewed patients in groups and individually, and presented the essence of these discussions in detail.

In 1979, Andreas Prager completed his doctoral dissertation in dentistry at the University of Mainz, writing on "Untersuchungen über die Zusammenhänge zwischen Deformitäten der Wirbelsäule und Kieferanomalien" (Research into the correlation between deformities of the spine and anomalies of the jaw). The greater part of his research was done at our clinic. Groups of 80, 100, 120 and 130 patients were examined. Results: almost all had pathological findings. There were malocclusions that suggested a connection between the spine and jaw. We also observed that children with anomalies of the jaws usually breathe through the mouth.

In 1983, Angela Blume wrote her diploma at the University of Brussels on "De Schroth Methode". She had also done measurements on patients during their exercises and demonstrated that these exercises corrected the position of the spine.

On May 17, 1981, a ceremony honoured the 60th anniversary of Katharina Schroth's professional career. The clinic's orthopaedist, Dr. Karl Gross, described the many attempts to treat scoliosis during the 19th Century: "Many exercise tools were developed, and there were already orthopaedic gymnastics systems. However, methods propagated in those days did not adequately consider the aetio-pathological processes of spinal distortion. Despite great efforts, the success rate was almost zero. This is the point where Frau Schroth and her secure intuition began when she included spinal derotation, which is always a consequence of sideways bending, in her physiotherapeutic efforts".

On this occasion, the designated president of the German Society for Orthopaedics and Traumatology, Professor Brussatis, also a member of the American Scoliosis Research Society, gave the speech excerpted above in my Foreword to the English Edition.

In February 1983, the clinic was named "Katharina Schroth Klinik" in honour of the founder's method. Katharina Schroth died on February 19, 1985.

Sample of early brochures and booklets

Katharina Schroth's first booklet was published in 1924: *Die Atmungskur, Leitfaden zur Lungengymnastik* (The Breathing Cure: a Guide to Exercises for the Lungs). It contained exercises for the breathing system and important tips for patients with scoliosis. The third edition of this booklet was issued in 1930, with an excellent foreword by Dr. L. Grewers of Essen. At that time, other systems were practiced in Germany and elsewhere on the Continent, often counterproductively.
(See pages 144-152 for some of the faulty exercises they recommended.)

Fig. 4: 1928: The garden in which the exercises were performed.

a) The group is exercising to strengthen the weak lumbar musculature below the rib hump.
b) A very unsuitable Swedish exercise for reversal of curvature, as was practised in those days.
c) Practising 'Rotational Angular Breathing' (RAB), sitting cross legged.
d) Strengthening the weak lumbar musculature (at wall bars outdoors).
e) RAB practised with tactile stimulation by the partner.
f) 'Rotational sitting' in front of a mirror.

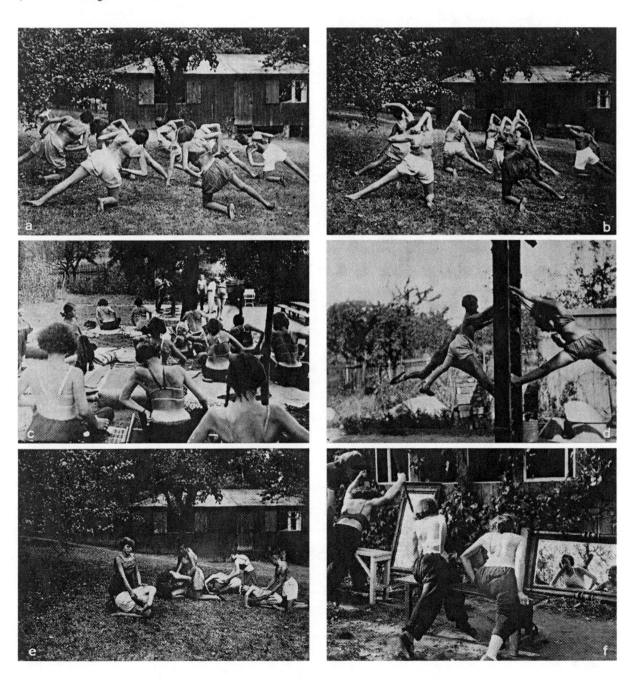

Fig. 5: First Schroth prospectus in 1925: "The New Breathing Orthopaedic System, Original Schroth, Meissen, Boselweg 52"

Frames 1 – 4 (top row): Rib hump made smaller by breathing exercises in 3 months. Previously treated for about 10 years unsuccessfully, using specialist orthopaedic techniques (all original photographs).

Frames 5 – 8 (middle row): Six weeks of rotational breathing, original Schroth system, Meissen, 16-year-old patient. Individual training for the skeleton.

Frames 9 and 10 (bottom row, left): Three months of breathing correction. Previously treated for 5½ years by 4 experts, with progressive deterioration from first-degree scoliosis.

Frames 11 and 12 (bottom row, right): 2½ months of rotational breathing, 33-year-old patient. Treated by orthopaedic specialists from the age of 1 year. No longer needed brace and was able to resume work because major pain ceased

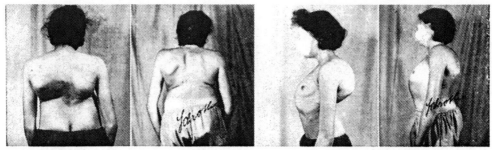

Rippenbuckel in 3 Monaten kleingeatmet, 19 Jahre alt. Vorher ca. 10 Jahre lang Behandlung mit f a c h orthopädischen Mitteln. **(Durchweg Original-Photos)**

Freiluftarbeit. Sonne an die kranken Knochen!

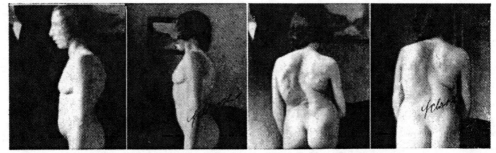

6 Wochen Atmungsorthopädie Original Schroth, Meißen, 16 Jahre alt.

Individuelle Skelett-Erziehung!

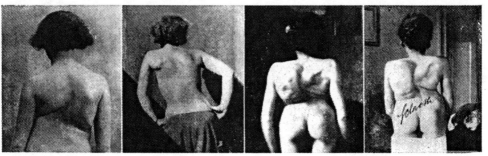

3 Jahre Atmungs-Korrektur, vorher 5½ Jahre von 4 Kapazitäten behandelt, vom 1. Grade aus sich verschlimmernd.

2½ Monate Atmungsorthopädie, 33 Jahre alt, seit dem 1. Lebensjahre f a c h orthopädische Behandlung. Wurde Korsett los und wieder arbeitsfähig durch Wegfall großer Schmerzen.

1 Monat Kur 100 Mk.
1 Woche Kur 35 Mk.

Pension
monatlich ab 90 Mk.

Die neue
Atmungs-Orthopädie Original Schroth
Meißen, Boselweg 52

Reviews and comments (imprinted in the first prospectus in 1925):
"Her approach is quite revolutionary and the effect of rotational breathing is inspired!" ...."a born doctor"......"has earned an immortal reputation"..... "Anyone with eyes to see must inevitably reach the irrefutable conclusion that this is a good thing for a condition for which previously there was no remedy at all" ..... "My parents were astonished that such an improvement was possible in just 3 months" ..... "This success in our son's case is so splendid: it doesn't just meet but far exceeds all expectations" ..... "Absolutely amazed at the development of little Kurt's body" ..... " It's just the thing"

Fig. 6 a: Second prospectus in 1929. We have printed it in this book because the content is still valid today.

Gefahren
bei Behandlung seitlicher Rückgratverkrümmungen.

Von Frau **Käthe Schroth-Meißen,**

Schöpferin der neuen Atmungs-Orthopädie

Die jedem Lebewesen, sei es Pflanze, Tier, Mensch, eingeborene Wachstumsenergie hat das Bestreben, jedem Körperorgan, jedem Körperteil und zusammenfassend jedem Ganzkörper die ihm bestimmte harmonische Form anzuschaffen.

Diejenige Form, die den göttlichen Schöpfergedanken am reinsten zur Darstellung bringt, ist auch stets die beste

---

Translation (abbreviated form):

Dangers in the treatment of scoliotic curves

by Katharina Schroth, Meissen, author of the New Breathing Orthopaedic System

The intrinsic growth energy inborn in every living plant, animal, or human strives to create the harmonious form predestined for its every bodily organ, body part, and finally complete body. That form which most purely realizes the divine creative thought is always the best, the one that allows all organs and parts of this body to function most completely.

Curvature of the spine, or scoliosis, is a precarious formal defect in terms of health, appearance, and the spiritual-psychological aspect. When attempting to help a scoliotic with this defect, we must not view the matter primarily from the mechanical standpoint, namely the malfunctioning body. For we have before us not a mechanical structure of bony levers and the muscles that move them, but rather an unfortunate person who has lost the form originally created for her and who cannot restore it by herself. With all scoliotic people, the cause probably lies partly in the mental realm. Envision what the expression "not in good form" means. Imagine the mental state of a child scolded by his mother. The psychic depression and loss of equilibrium are immediately visible in his abnormal bodily form. How wonderful the form of a little child's body is! What a victorious, natural, matter-of-fact nature he has in the representation of his Self, and in every movement and in all of his life statements.

However, let us observe a school class three or four years later. What has happened to these children? Almost all are missing their original sense of complete, untroubled comfort within. Many children have pronounced signs of suffering in their faces, and their depressed mental state finds expression in their bodies.

Why do gymnastic attempts to erect such a troubled child often fail completely? It is because they approach the child much too mechanically, much too much in the form of exercises, without first becoming familiar with his life difficulties, his unfulfilled needs, which to the adult may seem trivial. Straightening of the external person will only succeed when we can erect the inner person, open an avenue of hope, and allow him to breathe a sigh of relief

Externally we can say that for those individuals who suffer from constitutional weakness, the loss of inner balance necessarily leads to formal defects and thus to a defect in physical function. Exterior assistance consists therefore in great measure of constitutional treatment, which often must reverse the mistakes of generations.

---

und Funktionsverbesserung des deformierten Körpers gestellt werden. Der normal-gesunde Zustand des lebenden Körpers hat von sich aus schon das innere Streben, zu ordnen, normale Funktionsverhältnisse, also auch

Fig. 6 b (translated captions)

normale Form anzunehmen. Die lokalen Hilfen, nämlich zielsichere Zweckarbeit am Körper, müssen da

The normal, healthy condition of the living body has a natural, inner aspiration to ensure that normal functional relationships assume a normal form. Local assistance, namely goal-directed work on the body, must support this natural striving for order, the drive to assume a normal structure.

This constitutional therapy will not only induce inner bodily harmony, but also a surplus of strength, which then directly serves rebuilding of the external person as well as the load-bearing capacity, as it were, of the person with regard to life's adversities and defeats.

This latter element is important, because the work on the inner person must go hand in hand with assistance to the externals. We must readjust the thought life of the sufferer and help her give up wasting time on useless protests against fate or making her environment responsible for her condition. Our job is to help her orient herself such that difficulties disappear, that she is adaptable and productive enough to work on turning her disability into an advantage – on freeing her strength to work on improving her fate.

Only when the therapist has helped the patient learn that she cannot avoid the consequences of her posture, "that she must bear the consequences of flight from the consequences", can local help – healing gymnastics exercises – bear fruit.

weiß, wenn er sich also seiner Eigenverantwortlichkeit gar nicht bewußt sein kann, sehe der **Heiler**, der Erziehe

Die neue Atmungs-Orthopädie Original Schroth-Meißen

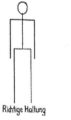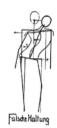

Richtige Haltung   Falsche Haltung

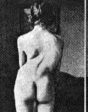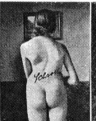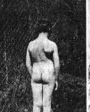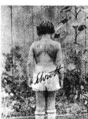

Correct posture   **Incorrect posture**
Schematic diagram illustrating proper body posture in a 'normal' person. Most curvatures of the spine are as shown in the next diagram: the upper torso is tilted over to the right and the ribs are twisted to the right and backwards.

Here we see a typical case: left hip raised, torso overhanging to the right, and rib hump twisted to the right and backwards. The new system of rotational breathing achieves a left shift in the torso that has sunk down on the right side. The above photo shows the outcome of 3 months' work to achieve a left shift.

Left-sided scoliosis also exists but is rarer (about 1 in 9 cases).
The new system of rotational breathing naturally moved this torso to the right. Outcome after 3 months.

Rule no. 1: Where the hump is on the right side, the torso overhangs to the right – it needs to be moved to the left.

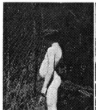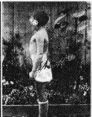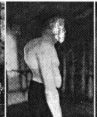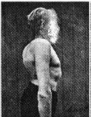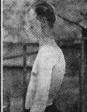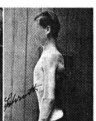

Third-degree scoliosis. 10-year-old patient. After 3 months' rotational breathing. "We cried with joy over Lisa's success."

Third-degree scoliosis, with extremely severe stiffening. Condition present for 20 years.

After 4 months' rotational breathing, original Schroth system, Meissen.

28-year-old patient, with simultaneous neuropathy.

After 2 months' rotational breathing.

Rule no. 2: The scoliotic skeleton is displaced like a line broken in several places. Mental postural control is absent. The rib hump is too far back. The new system of rotational breathing shifts it forwards.

Fig. 6 c (translated captions)

seine unmeßbare Verantwortlichkeit. Er muß den Leidenden aus der scheinbaren Unfreiheit, in die er sich seelisch geflüchtet hat, herausführen, ihm zeigen, daß dieser Selbstbetrug, „der sich lieber die Willensfreiheit abspricht und zum Gegenstand eines toten Naturgesetzes macht, als daß er die Verantwortung für seine Handlungsweise voll auf sich nimmt, ihn nicht von der Nötigung entbindet, immer wieder die Rückwirkungen seines eigenen falschen Denkens auf sich zu nehmen."

Erst dann, wenn es dem Erzieher gelungen ist, dem Leidenden klarzumachen, daß er sich den Folgen seines Verhaltens nicht entziehen kann, „daß er auch die Folgen von der Flucht vor den Folgen tragen muß", kann die eigentliche lokale Hilfe, die H e i l g y m n a s t i k, Früchte tragen.

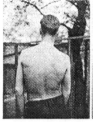 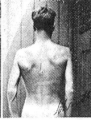 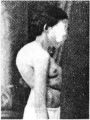 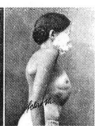 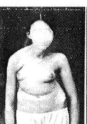 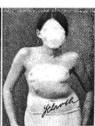

28 years old. Second-degree scoliosis.	After 2 months rotational breathing, Original Schroth System.	23 years old. Patient has been treated continuously since the age of 7.	After 5 months' rotational breathing.	The same girl seen from the front.	After 5 months' rotational breathing, Original Schroth System, Meissen. Her parents: "We were speechless."

Rule no. 3: If the body has improved, then the exercise principles of the new rotational breathing, Original Schroth System from Meissen, must be correct.

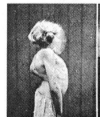 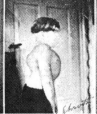 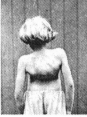 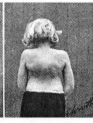 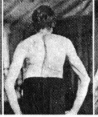 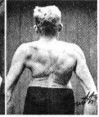

Extreme form of spinal tuberculosis, clinically healed.	After 3 months' rotational breathing. "Cried for joy."	The same child seen from behind. Doctor's verdict: "Just be glad she can walk."	After 3 months' rotational breathing. Mother's verdict: "I hadn't expected so much after you had given me no hope."	30 years old. Ossified scoliosis, present for 20 years.	After 4 months' rotational breathing, Original Schroth System, Meissen.

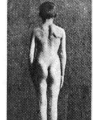 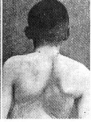 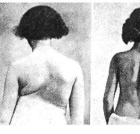 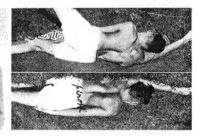

This is how this 12-year-old boy came for treatment to Prof. X. There he was prescribed a plaster cast, brace, 'seaside', and exercises.

After 4 years' treatment using all the resources of the best-equipped institution, this was how he looked.

This young girl had an identical experience abroad. Five years ago she had only first-degree scoliosis.
Prof. X. writes: "Before her orthopaedic gymnastics [a system that preceded Schroth], she had no scoliosis."

According to his original list of exercises, the 12-year-boy had to perform the exercise shown above.
Bottom photo: He is working on the same exercise according to Schroth.

**Rule no. 4: The function of the body yields its form. Working on the body can also be dangerous.
Under what circumstances?**

Fig. 6 d (translated captions)

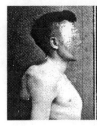 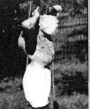 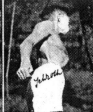 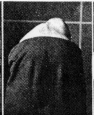 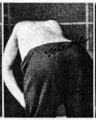 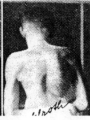

This is how the boy looked (side view) after the 4 years of treatment.

This is how he had to exercise, according to his original exercise list: right side backwards and side-bend to the right.

In contrast, the new system of rotational breathing enabled the rib hump to be 'breathed' forwards.

His former exercise list had also required him to do forward bends.

However, the new system of rotational breathing enabled the rib hump to be reduced in size through breathing.

After 3 months' rotational breathing he looked like this.

Parents' comment: "It is remarkable that Schroth was able to bring about a considerable improvement even though, as a severe case, his body must have been more difficult to treat; and this was not achieved before when his condition was mild."

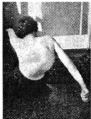 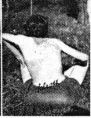 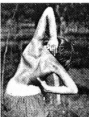 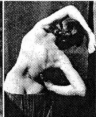 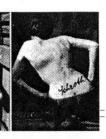

He also had to perform this exercise according to his former list: sitting straddled (legs apart), left arm to right foot, right arm behind.

However, the new system of rotational breathing actually 'breathes' the rib hump forwards and the left side backwards (= opposite effect).

According to his old list, he also had to perform this 'straightening' exercise.

Two more straightening exercises advocated by two other experts according to the same principle, published in a textbook for doctors, care nurses, welfare departments etc. This book explains why it was in such common use. 500 orthopaedic gymnastics instructors were trained in this way by a single institution.

The new system of rotational breathing also has the opposite effect here because it has to eliminate the 'waist triangle' on the right side and the high hip on the left.

Rule no. 5: Like the culmination of the exercise, so too is the body shape that is to be achieved by this exercise. "Positive criticism eliminates the bad by putting something better in its place."

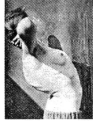 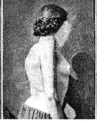 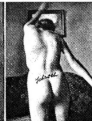 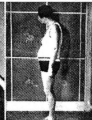 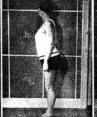 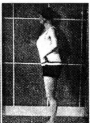

The boy in the previous frames also had to do the same exercise as this girl (backward bend).

This is how the young girl looks when she does nothing. Please look closely at the size of the rib hump and the lumbar region.

By contrast with the photo 'above', the new system of rotational breathing prescribes this exercise in the same case.

'Normal' body shape: posture displaced and ruined. Lack of skeletal training.

The body centre is still incorrectly positioned.

The principles of the new system of rotational breathing also apply in 'normal' bodies.

The result of 20 years of research.
(First tried out successfully on Katharina Schroth's own body with its abnormal curvature).

PART A
Theoretical basis of
the Schroth method

I. Division of the trunk (including shoulders and neck) into three segments (Figs. 7, 10)

Practical observation of persons with postural disorders showed that it was useful to divide the trunk into three segments, from caudal to cranial:

a) lumbar spine with pelvis
b) thoracic spine with rib cage
c) cervical spine with shoulder girdle (and head)

In a healthy person, these three segments can be represented by rectangles.

a) The caudal rectangle is formed by the pelvis, lumbar spine, hypogastric region including umbilicus, up to the lower ribs.
b) The next rectangle is formed by the chest and epigastric region. The lower border is the waist (12th rib) and the upper border the axilla (about the 3rd rib).
c) The third rectangle is bordered caudally by the upper border of the middle segment. The upper or cranial border is in the region of the acromion. The cervical lordosis lies outside of this upper segment. However, as the cervical spine belongs functionally to this third segment, it can be imagined as running cranially to the beginning of the occiput.

The three segments are stacked vertically on top of each other. The body is balanced.

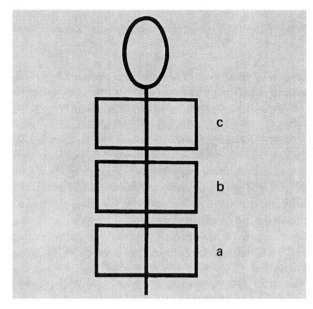

Fig. 7: Frontal view.

Viewed laterally, however, they are trapezoidal as a result of the physiological curves of the spine.
The caudal segment (trapezium a) has its lower border in an imaginary line passing through the two anterior superior iliac crest, extending dorsally to L5. With the pelvis in an erect position, this line runs horizontally. The upper border passes through the lower ribs and ends at T12.
The middle segment (trapezium b) includes the chest and epigastric region. The lower border is the upper border of trapezium a). The upper border runs along an imaginary line at the level of the armpits, the level of the cranial sternum between the clavicles and over one third of the shoulder blades dorsally up to T6. The upper segment (trapezium c) is bordered caudally by the cranial line of the middle segment. The upper border is formed by the shoulder level. Since the cervical spine is part of it functionally, one imagines trapezium c) elongated cranially to the occiput and mandible. This part is therefore called the shoulder-neck segment. These three segments are balanced over the centre of gravity.

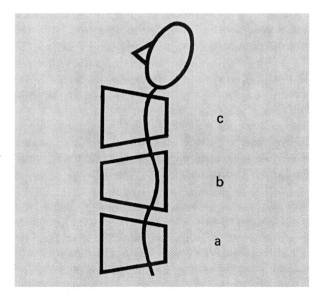

Fig. 8: Lateral view.

11

II. Symmetrical postural deviation in the sagittal plane

Symmetrical postural deviation in the sagittal plane, or kyphosis, results in the formation of three sagittal 'wedges'.

So far we have been describing the healthy locomotor system. In case of postural defects and even more in minor or major spinal deformities, these structural changes are more pronounced. For example, juvenile or adolescent kyphosis (Scheuermann's disease) or kyphoscoliosis. In these conditions, the physiological spinal curves show pathological changes in the sagittal plane. The spinal column appears compressed and shortened, giving rise to pathological vertebral deformations (Figs. 9 and 15-19)

In the case of malposture, these three segments are shifted against each other (sagittal plane), resulting in a line with two breaks (lateral view); beginning at the feet, running to the pelvis, from there to the back and continuing up to the head (Figs. 9, 14,15).

Due to the shifts of the three segments caused by the collapse of posture, the three segments appear as 'wedges' on top of one another – the short side of the trapezium becoming shorter and the long side of the trapezium increasing in height – and these really do have the appearance of wedges (Fig. 13). The more pronounced the deformity, the more extreme the wedging and the collapse of the back.

Lateral view (Figs. 15–17)

Wedge 1: The lumbopelvic wedge has its vertex in the lumbar lordosis. The wide side (abdominal wall) is formed by stretched abdominal muscles and the anterior iliac crest, sloping in the ventrocaudal direction forming the caudal border. The cranial border is an imaginary line beginning at the lumbar lordosis, passing the lower ribs and leading to the xyphoid process.

Wedge 2: The chest-rib wedge has its vertex below the nipple. The wide side is formed by the thoracic kyphosis. The caudal border corresponds to the cranial border of the lumbopelvic wedge. The upper border is an imaginary line running from the narrow anterior area below the nipple, passing the armpits up to the lower third of the shoulder blade.

Wedge 3: the shoulder-neck wedge: Since the shoulders are drawn forward, the anterior acromial processes form the wide side, while the exact position of the vertex is difficult to define. It lies in the region of the upper two ribs covered by the shoulder blades. The caudal border corresponds to the cranial border of the chest-rib wedge. The cranial border is formed by the

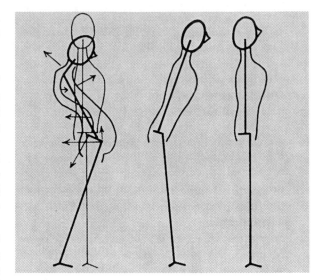

Fig. 9: Pathological body shape: wrong - overcorrection - correct

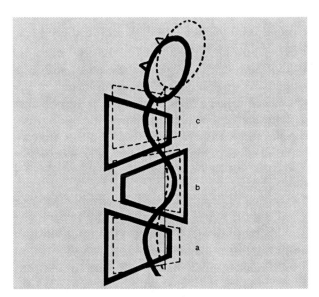

Fig. 10: Lateral view: pathological and normal shape.
c: neck-shoulder wedge
b: thorax-rib wedge
a: lumbar-pelvic wedge

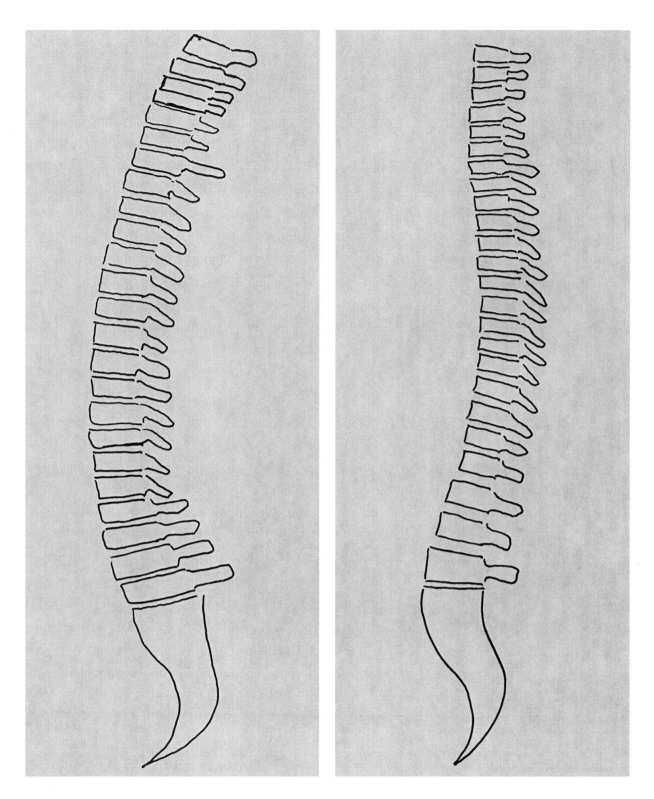

Fig. 11: Lateral view of a hollow back (thoracic lordosis). In hollow back, the physiological oscillations of the vertebrae are reversed. See page 188 and Figs. 533 and 583.

Fig. 12: Lateral view of flatback. In flatback, the physiological oscillations of the vertebrae are reduced. See page 173.

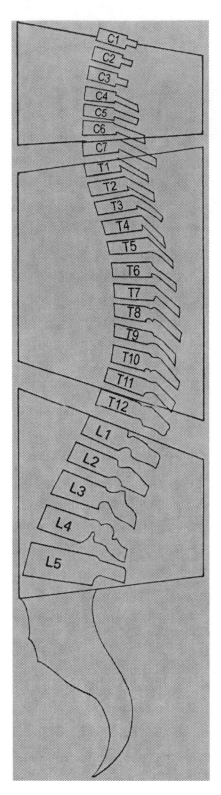

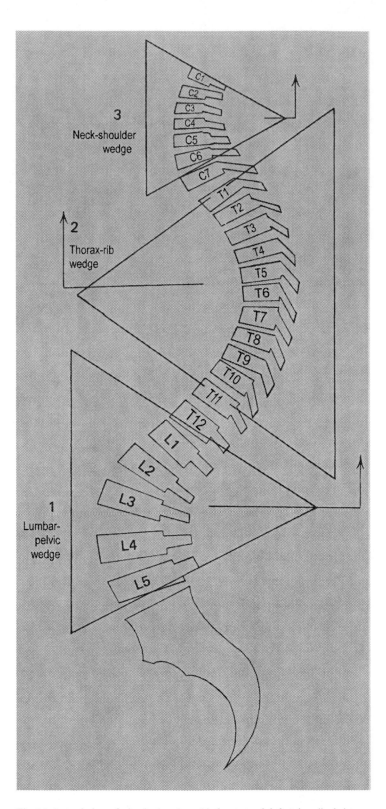

Fig. 13: Lateral view of a normal spine. Kapandji describes the lumbar lordosis of a dynamic type to be about 90°; the spine shown in Fig. 14 belongs to a static type, which is more often found in children (spine without a scoliotic component).

Fig. 14: Lateral view of a kyphotic spine with the postural defect described above. The right angles marked show the directions of the correction. See Figs. 9 and 472.

14

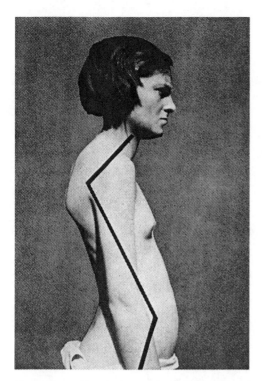

Fig. 15: Double 'broken' axis showing postural collapse.

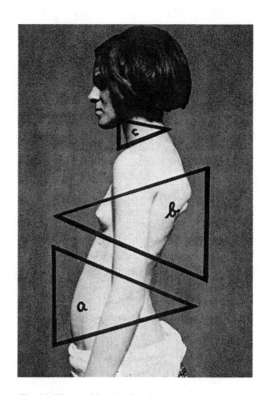

Fig. 16: The resulting 'wedges'.

shoulder level. Since the cervical spine forms a functional part of this wedge, the vertex is in the cervical lordosis and the wide side is formed by the hyperextended anterior neck portion. These two wedges may also overlap and in some cases can be seen as one large wedge theoretically.

The above applies to symmetrical postural disorders in the sagittal plane.

In the scoliotic body, the trunk also shows wedge-like deformities in the sagittal plane.

This is only true for the lateral view of the 'rib hump side'. This is because of the torsion of the trunk segments against each other.

For idiopathic scoliosis at least, it has been assumed that the lumbar spine has decreased lordosis while the thoracic spine tends to present a lordotic postural deformity (Dickson, Tomaschewski: see the sections on flatback).

Of course, there are structural changes of this type that cannot be corrected actively, such as cases with a partly fixed deformity (Meister, Heine). In the presence of deformity, different parts of the body segments adapt their appearance to the spine, and functional three-curve scoliosis can exist even in the presence of only minor lumbar and cervical countercurvatures. Treatment is adapted to the individual situation.

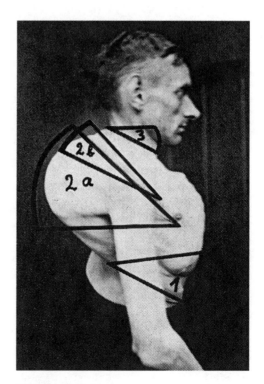

Fig. 17: Lateral view.

15

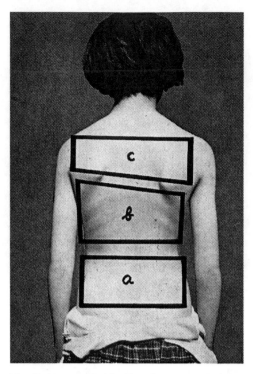

Fig. 18: 11-year-old girl with malposture and incipient left convex scoliosis.

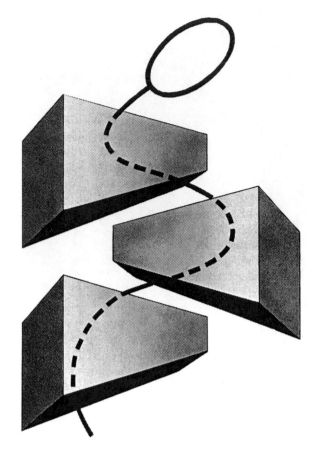

Fig. 20

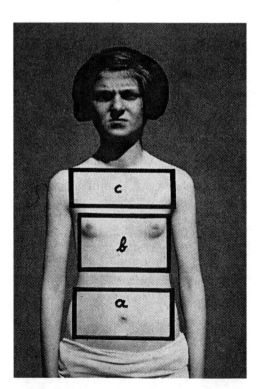

Fig. 19: The three blocks are still almost rectangularly superposed.

The 2nd, chest-rib wedge can be subdivided into two parts in cases of major scoliosis and kyphoscoliosis (Fig. 17). The vertex of wedge 2a is below the nipple and the wide side is bordered by the posterior rib hump; the vertex of wedge 2b is located in the region of the subaxillary rib portions. The corresponding wide side is formed by the kyphotic curve which begins at the shoulder. It shows the most cranially located thoracic hump. These two wedges can merge into one another.

Wedge 4, the wedge of the anterior rib hump, is on the dorsal concave side (Fig. 21). The vertex lies in the posterior concavity and the wide side is formed by the anteriorly-orientated ribs of the dorsal concavity. The caudal border is an imaginary line which begins at the concave posterior ribs and leads along the lowest ribs towards the umbilicus. The cranial border runs from the posterior concavity to a point below the nipple. This creates the scoliotic balance of the body and brings all body segments that deviate anteriorly or posteriorly above the centre of gravity. They balance each other out.

In the following, the terms 'concave' and 'convex' side always refer to the thoracic spinal curvature.

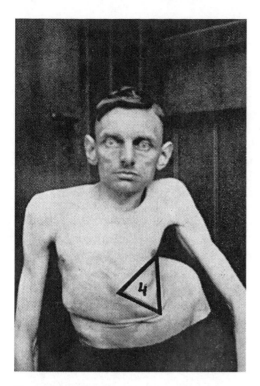

Fig. 21: Frontal view.

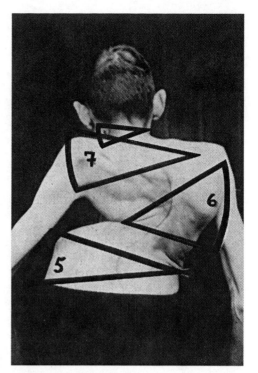

Fig. 22: Posterior view.

III. Postural deviation in the frontal plane

In scoliosis and kyphoscoliosis, the deviation in the frontal plane leads via a trapezoid to the formation of three lateral wedges (Figs. 20–23). While scoliosis is characterized more by lateral form deviations, in kyphoscoliosis, the sagittal and frontal deviations are present together. Looking at a scoliotic body from the back, we can see that the three trunk segments (pelvic girdle, rib cage, shoulder girdle) are not aligned as rectangles as they are in a healthy body. They have shifted against each other. These lateral deviations and the changed pressure and traction first twist the originally rectangular segments into trapezoids and then wedge-like segments (Fig. 23).

Dorsal view:
Wedge 5: lateral lumbar-pelvic wedge (Figs. 20, 22 and 23)
The vertex of the wedge is below the lateral rib hump 11th and 12th rib). The wide side is formed by the prominent lumbar convex-sided hip and, very often, also by the upper lumbar hump. Its caudal border is formed by the iliac crest sloping downwards on the side of the dorsal concavity due to the lateral shift. The cranial border can be seen as a line extending from the vertex of

the wedge leading to the ilia of the dorsal concave side, i.e., the highest point of the lumbar hump of this side.

Wedge 6: lateral chest-rib wedge (Figs. 22 and 23)
The vertex of the wedge is at the lowest point of the dorsal concave side. The wide side is formed by the lateral rib hump. The caudal border is also the cranial border of the 5th wedge, while the cranial border leads from the vertex of the wedge obliquely across the upper thoracic vertebrae to the middle of the shoulder blade on the convex side.

Wedge 7: lateral shoulder-neck wedge (Figs. 22 and 23)
a) Most often the vertex is located above the thoracic hump (covered by the shoulder blade). The wide side is formed by the shoulder on the side of the dorsal concavity. Its caudal border runs parallel with the cranial border of wedge 6. The cranial border is formed by the shoulder levels on both sides.

b) Functionally, the cervical spine forms part of this. The vertex is therefore in the shortened cervical muscles of the dorsal convex side and the wide side

17

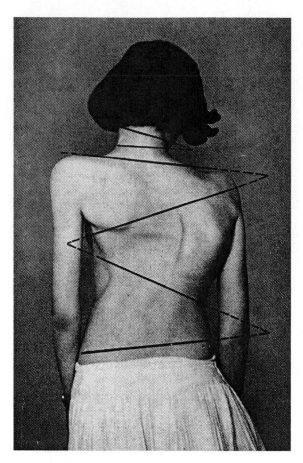

Fig. 23: 1. pelvic girdle 2. Rib cage 3. Shoulder girdle

formed by the overstretched opposite side. Sometimes, only one of these wedges is present, often both. They can merge and are then named the shoulder-neck wedge.

The three wedge vertices correspond to the three depressions of the rib cage. These postural abnormalities correspond to the three lordotic retractions.
a) Hip with floating ribs (11th and 12th ribs) below the rib hump;
b) Dorsal concavity;
c) Shoulder above the rib hump with narrow side of the neck.

The three wide sides correspond to the three thoracic elevations which represent the kyphotic bulges:
a) Hip of dorsal concavity with lumbar hump (for example left);
b) Rib hump of the opposite side (right);
c) Shoulder of the dorsal concavity (left). This very often seems to be a separate rib hump.

All wedge vertices are rotated forwards, all wide sides backwards within the lateral shifting, except wedge 4. The laterally shifted trunk segments are grouped around the centre of gravity and keep each other in balance. This is, however, a scoliotic and not a normal balance, that serves to keep the body upright, nevertheless.

IV. The three torsions of the trunk in three-curve scoliosis

Scoliosis is nearly always a three-dimensional pathological development. In addition to the three pathologically changed spinal curvatures and the three deviations in the frontal plane, there is a threefold torsion of the trunk segments against each other around the longitudinal axis. Since the spinal column adapts to the body, the various segments also show torsion of the vertebrae. The spinous processes point to the concave side within the curvature.

In a healthy person, the pelvic girdle, rib cage, shoulder girdle and head are in one frontal plane (Fig. 24). In the case of three-curve scoliosis, the pelvic girdle and shoulder girdle are rotated in the same direction, and the rib cage in the opposite direction. This creates the posterior rib hump on the right and the frontal rib hump on the left side (Figs. 23 and 25). In detail, therefore, the following is elements are present:

1. Shifting in the sagittal plane, resulting in exacerbation of lumbar lordosis, chest kyphosis, and cervical lordosis. This results in the above-mentioned wedges (Fig. 15). These wedges should be viewed from the convex side. They develop because of the rotation of the three trunk segments and have less impact on the spinal column on the entire trunk areas.
2. Shifting in the frontal plane causing the wedges to deviate laterally (Fig. 23).
3. Shifting in the transverse plane resulting in ventral rotation of the vertices of the wedges and dorsal rotation of the wide sides.
4. Sooner or later the shoulder girdle on the concave side will come closer to the pelvic girdle on the concave side (Fig. 22), as the ribs on the concave side move ventrally. They cannot support the shoulder girdle. Due to the distortions and shifting in the planes mentioned, shortening of the upper body is inevitable.

Analysis of the exact defects present in each patient is a complex process. This is the first step. Exercise treatment is then tailored to the particular condition at hand,

concentrating on the most important aim: to elongate the body. A certain deflexion of the frontal plane occurs at the same time. The stabilization of the correction then takes place in the form of isometric tension during the exhalation phase (see PART B).

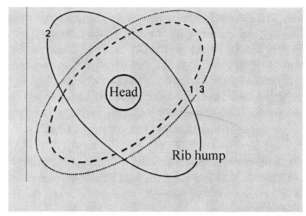

Fig. 25:
1 = pelvic girdle - 2 = rib cage - 3 = shoulder girdle

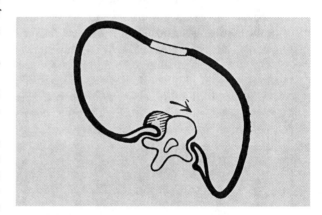

Fig. 26: Schematic horizontal section through the chest of a scoliotic person. It shows rotation and torsion of the vertebral body, a dorsal rib hump on the convex side, a frontal rib hump on the concave side, deformation of the rib cage and a shifted sternum.

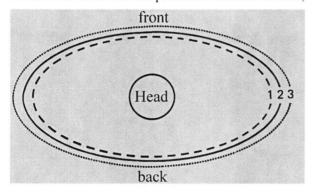

Fig. 24: From above:1 pelvic girdle; 2 rib cage; 3 shoulder girdle

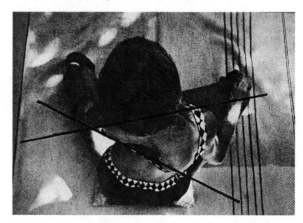

Fig. 27: Cranial view of the distorted trunk segments of a 17-year-old girl with right thoracic scoliosis.

V. Breathing as a formative factor in treatment

The movements associated with breathing are of major importance in the treatment of scoliosis. Breathing is also a mechanical problem, and thus we shall investigate the forces which become active during breathing movement.

On one hand, they are active forces working through the muscles in the locomotor system. On the other hand they are passive forces – partly the lungs – working through the elasticity of the soft tissue. Passive forces are always trying to reverse forced changes in the natural shape of the trunk. This is especially the case in exercises for scoliosis. The approach therefore has to be selective, activating the weak muscles, especially the weak muscle fibres of the diaphragm, until they are strong enough to counterbalance the strong muscles.

General physiological concepts distinguish between costosternal and abdominal breathing. It must first of all be stated that neither type of breathing is found exclusively on its own.

Scoliosis cannot be treated with only thoracic or abdominal breathing. The scoliotic shape of the rib cage and the chest needs three-dimensional treatment to widen the concave parts of the trunk and to flatten out the protruding parts. This is the concept of the Schroth breathing method: the diaphragm has to be active in each part of breathing movement. It has to be guided mentally to achieve a certain degree of deep or 'full' breathing. This is a learning process which leads to automatic movements by using visualization. Deep breathing is only

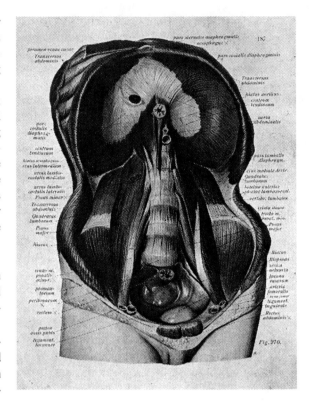

Fig. 28: Muscles of the posterior abdominal wall and the diaphragm as seen from the abdominal cavity.

possible with an upright body, with the pelvis straight and in an orthopaedically corrected position. To understand the many different mechanical problems, patients

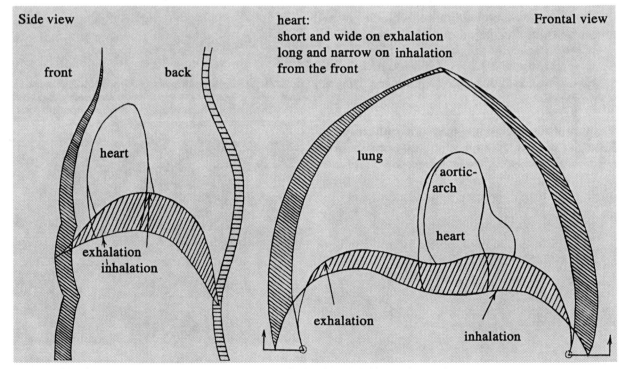

Fig. 29: Schematic presentation of diaphragmatic movement. Left: view from the left; right: frontal view.

20

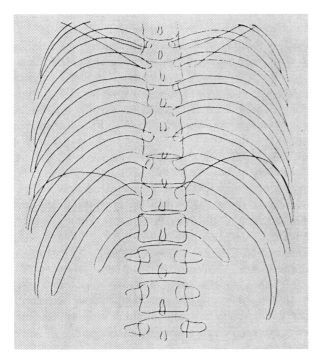

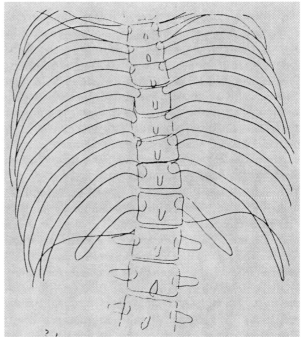

Fig. 30: Distance between the ribs on deep exhalation on the left and right side.
12th–11th 2.5 cm.
11th–10th 2.5 cm.
10th–9th 2.0 cm.
Position of diaphragm, left T10; right T9; erect spinal column.

Fig. 31: Deep inhalation on the right side. Distance of ribs on the left side, Same as Fig 30. Distance of ribs on the right side:
12th–11th 4.0 cm. - 11th–10th 3.5 cm. - 10th–9th 2.5 cm.
Position of diaphragm, left L1; right T12.
Spinal column pulled to the right while position of clavicles remains nearly unchanged.

have to be trained in a very precise and selective manner. Costal or rib breathing is possible, since the ribs are connected with the spine and move around an oblique axis. The rotational axes of each rib pair form an angle which opens dorsally. This angle differs however, depending on the height of the segment. In the exhalation position, the ribs point obliquely downwards. Lifting the ribs means also enlarging the sagittal diameter of the rib cage. The oblique position of the rotational axes also enlarges the horizontal diameter of the thorax in its lower part during inhalation. Improvement of the shape of the thorax is therefore always accompanied by an improvement in function, and vice versa.

This can be demonstrated by measurements and the pelvimeter. It is necessary to differentiate between *'external' breathing movement'* (i.e. of the rib cage) and *'internal'* breathing movement (i.e. lifting and lowering of the diaphragm). This approach can also be applied in other postural and breathing disturbances. Contraction of the diaphragm during inhalation flattens the cranially convex dome, thus increasing the volume of the pleural cavity. The lungs follow the movement of the diaphragm as well as that of the ribs – filling the complementary spaces. The flattening of the dome of the diaphragm is only possible by a simultaneous pressure and displacement of the intestines. When the pelvis is in a forward-downward position, the abdominal walls retreat forward during inhalation because the abdominal muscles yield to the pressure. This creates the impression that breathing with the diaphragm equals abdomi-

nal breathing. When the pelvis is brought into an upright position during exercise, the abdominal wall is relieved because the intestines move back into the pelvis. At the same time the lumbar lordosis decreases, which means that the spinal column receives an extension impulse. The latter may be enhanced voluntarily even more. Breathing using the diaphragm brings the abdominal wall lightly forward; at the same time, the lateral thorax expands down unto the lumbar region. This breathing movement is of critical importance for improvement of the scoliotic form. Very often, to breathe in this way is not possible because of thoracic rotation and counter-rotations, but it must be recaptured (Fig. 29). *During exhalation*, the diaphragm relaxes and moves back to the starting position. The shape of the thorax can also be influenced by specific exhaling movements, if the anterior iliac crest is raised, thus reducing the lumbar lordosis. It is very important for patients to maintain this *upright position* during exhalation. Afterwards they need to learn to maintain this better posture for 3, 5 and later 10 breaths. After the shaping results have been imprinted on the mind, all the muscles of the trunk are tensed as much as possible, by performing a so-called **'muscle mantle'** exercise. This is of prime importance to instill the feeling of 'posture'. Due to the attachment points of the diaphragm (origin in the ribs, sternum, lower ribs, and 1st to 4th lumbar vertebrae - see Schmidt and Kohlrausch 1981), the diaphragm also has to change position as well as the rib cage (see section A.VI, The Scoliotic Breathing Pattern).

The following has been observed with regard to the involvement of the *spinal column* during *breathing movement*: As long as a scoliosis is not fixed by ankylosis, it is possible to influence the spinal column positively. Erecting the pelvis leads to a reduction of the lumbar lordosis and the erector spinae muscles are activated. In addition, the patient is asked to visualize a straightened spine. This alone brings about a straightening. The more pronounced the spinal curvature, the more the trunk may be elongated during corrective inhalation. This has been demonstrated by measurements.

The combination of mechanical forces and mental cooperation is an essential requirement for the Schroth method and is decisive in success.

Figs. 30 and 31 show the effect of intentional unilateral breathing in a normal 52-year-old woman. Fig. 30: spine vertical. Fig. 31: maximum inhalation with unilaterally guided diaphragm on the right. It is clearly visible that the spine is being pulled to the right. Her shoulders are horizontal. The intercostal spaces have been widened distinctively (right side) and the diaphragm lowered about 8 cm.

It is, of course, possible to move the ribs without using breathing. Everybody can check it: inhaling, or exhaling, hold the air halfway (do not apply pressure). Now the ribs may be spread or contracted. This can be done several times; it is a purely muscular function. It has to be admitted, though, that spreading of the ribs is 100% better if the diaphragm is lowered intentionally during inhalation. The effect of the contraction of the ribs can be increased if the exhalation and elevation of the dome of the diaphragm are performed at the same time.

To improve shape, the muscles have to be activated, which brings back muscular as well as a static balance. This will result automatically in a better, i.e., more useful inflation of the lungs, because the hitherto unused parts of the lungs are activated as well.

Katharina Schroth observed the movement of the ribs 'at right angles' to lateral and cranial during inhalation and exhalation in her own body. It was not theory which made her believe that ribs move sideways and upwards during lowering of the diaphragm.

In a healthy body, ribs not only move to the sides (laterally) but also dorsally, ventrally and cranially during inhalation. Everybody can verify this by placing their hands on the attachment positions of the diaphragm (rib arches, free ribs, upper lumbar spine) and feeling what happens to the body. The scoliotic patient may not be able to do this immediately, and has to be trained to use the breathing movements with simultaneous correction of the exterior shape. A different body posture is therefore needed, including the relieving and widening of the concavities. In this situation, the question of what fills the hollow body segments is not important: whether it is the displacement of the intestines, or air, or the result of normal muscle activity. What matters is the fact that the visible recesses are flattened out.

Guiding the breath to the region of the lower ribs can easily be imagined since the diaphragm reaches down to this area, but this 'right-angled breathing' (RAB) does require a great deal of concentration, in order to lower the dome of the diaphragm, so everything can have a corrective effect. Prof. Vogel, Dresden, commented on this 'formative force of breathing' in 1937. See Appendix.

At this point, it is appropriate to mention a specific phenomenon that Katharina Schroth noticed at the beginning of her professional career: if a scoliotic patient only breathes deeper than usual (symmetrically and not in a certain direction), more air penetrates into the already stretched pulmonary half of the rib hump side. This worsens the scoliosis deformities, since breathing this way does not incorporate the orthopaedic moment of straightening and derotation. Breathing movements have to be modified for the treatment of scoliosis. Breathing has to be targeted, and it has to straighten, derotate, and influence the thoracic segments positively from the very beginning.

It is not difficult to conclude that three-dimensional breathing stimulates the inactive pulmonary alveoli. The positive result patients feel is that they become less susceptible to colds and that their physical performance increases, while their pulse stays in the normal range.

Even paradoxal breathing, during which the ribs contract in the inhalation phase, can be normalized.

Investigations into breathing excursions with the scoliometer (see Part D.II: Statistical evaluation of treatment results) show that RAB can bring about derotation. If we are successful in changing the scoliotic breathing pattern, each breath acts as a corrective exercise at the same time. By contracting the trunk musculature in the region of the protruding convex trunk segments, the breathing excursion is restricted in these areas and makes possible an increase of breathing excursion in the concave, recessed trunk segments. Patients can be trained only in RAB, but actually it forms the basis of the entire Schroth method.

VI. The scoliotic breathing pattern

In the resting position and, most of the time, when breathing deeply, the scoliotic patient has an asymmetric breathing pattern due to the scoliotic deformity (Fig. 32).

According to Schmitt (1985), the healthy patient shows an axially-oriented push of the ribs when contracting the intercostal musculature, thus stabilizing the spine at the same time by symmetrical breathing.

In case of asymmetric breathing or scoliosis, this push acts unilaterally on the spine and increases the rotation of the vertebrae because the shearing force of the corresponding ribs on the concave side is directed predominantly at the body of the vertebrae, and on the convex side via the costotransversal joint to the spinous processes.

The diaphragm is also impaired because its points of attachment (ribs) are displaced. It has to work within the 'scoliotic distortion'.

Thus, in the case of torsion of the thoracic vertebrae, symmetrical breathing increases the deformity. Each breath contributes to and exacerbates the scoliotic malposture and deformation. Already widened areas of the rib cage are influenced, and the lung is ventilated in already well aired parts.

The scoliotic has to learn to correct the breathing pattern. Consciously directed breathing into the concave parts of the rib cage mobilizes restricted ribs. Less ventilated parts of the lungs are filled with air and achievement of the correct posture is also facilitated. Contracting the convex areas prevents them from expanding further and directs breathing to the relaxed musculature of the concave areas. Scoliometer measurements (Weiss 1989) show that it is possible to alter the way a scoliotic breathes to achieve a more beneficial pattern (see chapter on changes in scoliometer values).

RAB cannot be integrated into the corrective techniques of the Schroth exercises unless the trunk is elongated as much as possible and the concavities are relieved of pressure. This means that the patient has to be able to straighten up first, come out of passive ligament-holding – within the existing range of spinal mobility – to achieve the desired effect.

We recorded the breathing movement values of several patients with the Heibrock-Seift Method (Figs. 33 and 34). Starting point was the beginning of a 5-week course of in-patient treatment. At the point of deepest inhalation and exhalation with a with a tape measure:
a) subaxillary
b) across the chest
c) around the waist (at the level of the floating ribs)
d) across the stomach below the umbilicus
Breathing movement was recorded in centimetres. Plots were made on graph paper.

Anja, 15 years, showed a major improvement in breathing under the axilla and around the waist (Fig. 34).

Karin, 20 years, showed a negative value of 1 cm. The intersecting lines across the waist show that her waist narrowed during inhalation. After 5 weeks, we recorded a positive value of 4 cm at this point. This increase can be attributed to daily breathing training including the diaphragm (Fig. 33).

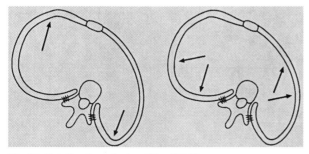

Fig. 32: Rotational angular breathing (RAB)
The scoliotic breathing pattern on the left. Transverse section of a scoliotically deformed thorax (Weiss). The scoliotic breathing pattern increases the torsion (modified according to Henke). The arrows indicate the direction of breath in idiopathic scoliosis.
Right: The corrective breathing pattern according to Schroth. The arrows indicate the direction of RAB.

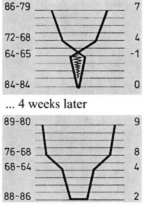
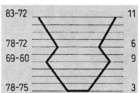

Karin, 20 years, start

86-79		7
72-68		4
64-65		-1
84-84		0

... 4 weeks later

89-80		9
76-68		8
68-64		4
88-86		2

Fig. 33

Anja, 15 years, start

81-74		7
73-69		4
64-62		2
79-78		1

... 5 weeks later

83-72		11
78-72		6
69-60		9
78-75		3

Fig. 34

VII. Increase in cardiopulmonary capacity during three dimensional treatment

Most scoliotic patients are affected by pulmonary and cardiac deficiency. We observed that patients show a reduction in or elimination of lip cyanosis during in-patient treatment. We also registered an increased vital capacity – which even doubled in many patients (with baselines around 350 cc). Patients often state that they feel better in general.

In 1974, the Institute of Sports Medicine at the University of Westphalia, Germany examined cardiopulmonary capacity in two groups of patients at our clinic, with the following results:

"At the beginning of the in-patient treatment, we did not note any pathological cardiopulmonary deficiency in the group (except in 2 patients). The spiroergometric values at the end of the 4-week treatment had increased markedly in each patient, although to different degrees. Most striking was the positive influence on the circulatory system. The pulse rate decreased with increasing effort, generally by 10–15 beats/min. The wattage of the effort threshold was able to be increased continuously. A highly significant improvement in PWC 170 was another result. The individual values for the physical work capacity (PWC at a rate of 170/min) in adolescent scoliotics showed a highly significant increase in the t-test.

This also applied to the endurance capacity below a pulse frequency of 130/min in the same patients. Another effect of training is the faster recovery in terms of pulse. All these factors are evidence that the circulation system is being used more efficiently. As far as cardio-circulatory capacity is concerned, the vital capacity cannot be seen as a measure of this, but it may be seen as a measure of restrictive functional impairment".

According to more recent studies (Weiss, 1989) a highly significant increase in vital capacity and rib mobility can be expected, even in adult patients.

Medical investigations in Bad Sobernheim confirmed that an intensive 4-week course of Schroth treatment can increase the organic capacity considerably. This indicates that the treatment is not only of value in terms of its orthopaedic effects, but also with respect to internal medicine.

Significant increases in cardiopulmonary capacity can be attained by endurance training or physical conditioning, but no significant increases in vital capacity (Bjure et al 1969, Götze 1976).

VIII. Effect of sun and air

Hippocrates pointed out: "Water, air, sun, conscientious nutrition, occasional fasting, the ability to relax and a joyful temper form the vital impulses which create health."

This is something we must always bear in mind. We exercise outside whenever possible. The famous physician for alternative medicine, Dr. H. Bottenberg (see Literature), illustrated wonderfully the connection between

Tabel 1: Average amount of air in one exhalation

Adolescents			Adults		
Boys	Age	Girls	Men	Height	Women
ccm		ccm	ccm	cm	ccm
1400	9	1400	2350	150	2200
1650	10	1500	2600	155	2400
1800	11	1600	2900	160	2600
1900	12	1750	3200	165	2800
2050	13	1900	3500	170	3000
2300	14	2100	3800	175	3200
2400	15	2200	4100	180	3400
Average values for sportsmen					
Competitive athletes		3950	Boxer		4800
Footballers		4200	Swimmers		4900
Athletes		4750	Rowers		5450

sun, air and health. He remarked: "The fresh air which we inhale and which touches our skin gently is the most elementary vital need for our organism. Many people need clean, living air more than nutrition. Next to natural nutrition, air, light and sun are the best physiological means to stimulate and increase the body's defences."
As early as 1795, Hufeland pointed out that a deficiency of light and sun may provoke scrofula and rickets. It is very important for scoliotics to bear this in mind.
Fresh air recharges the body and brings back lost muscle tone – therefore leads to health. It is recommended to sleep with an open window. It should always be borne in mind that we spend a third of our lives (8 hours sleep) in our bedroom. Leo Kofler illustrated the necessity for clean air with the following experiment: a sparrow locked under a glass bell was able to survive alone for 3 hours. Then the oxygen was used up.

The sparrow may have lived for 10 more minutes. Another sparrow was added – it died immediately after inhaling the stale air, whereas the first one stayed alive. Shortly before 3 hours had passed, it was set free. One may conclude that stale air from others is poisonous for us.
Clean, fresh living air has another physiological effect: it has the fragrance of nature. It stimulates all living beings to breathe deeply. Fritz Kahn describes vividly the most subtle regulating healing effects which influence a healing process.
Permanent outdoor treatment should have priority because it is a type of air-bath which represents the mildest and most uncomplicated biological form of treatment. A nude body can enjoy the air-bath thoroughly.
This is the reason why we have outdoor areas in addition to our exercise halls at the Katharina Schroth Clinic.

IX. Evaluation of spinal length loss in scoliosis in relation to vital capacity

To evaluate vital capacity in adults, we base our measurements on body length. Table 1 shows the standard values.
This most important point of reference to determine the theoretical value of lung content is different in scoliotic patients. The reasons are lateral shifting of the spine accompanied by rotation or torsion and corresponding changes in the rib cage. They cause a loss of height and restrict the pulmonary space.

Table 2: Rough values for the relationship between the angle of scoliosis and the shortening of the upper body

20 degrees	1 cm	90 degrees	8 cm
25 degrees	1 cm	95 degrees	8.5 cm
30 degrees	1.5 cm	100 degrees	9 cm
35 degrees	1.5 cm	105 degrees	9.5 cm
40 degrees	2 cm	110 degrees	10 cm
45 degrees	2.5 cm	115 degrees	11 cm
50 degrees	3 cm	120 degrees	12 cm
55 degrees	3.5 cm	125 degrees	12.5 cm
60 degrees	4 cm	130 degrees	13 cm
65 degrees	4.5 cm	135 degrees	14 cm
70 degrees	5 cm	140 degrees	15 cm
75 degrees	5.5 cm	145 degrees	16 cm
80 degrees	6.5 cm	150 degrees	17 cm
85 degrees	7 cm		

The diaphragm supports this defect functionally (see section A.VI regarding the scoliotic breathing pattern). In order to gain a theoretical value for the vital capacity that the patient should have in the upright position, we carried out spinal measurements by X-ray. Rotation, torsion and rib deformities were not taken into account. The course of the curvature was compassed at about the middle of the vertebrae and the vertical distance between caudal and cranial point of the curve was measured. The tape measure was then stretched to evaluate the difference. The difference represented the loss of height.

These measurements were done separately on the thoracic and lumbar spinal curves, since a single spinal curvature of about 100° Cobb shows a stronger contraction than two 50° Cobb curvatures. We then looked for a relationship between the angular values and the loss of body length.

The values in Table 2 refer only to the thoracic curvature (i.e. shortening and restriction of the rib cage). They are probable values. They should be added to the existing body length to evaluate the vital capacity. The theoretical body length is calculated by adding together the values for the thoracic and lumbar curvature. It is obvious that the standard values in Table 1 can hardly be reached in cases of major scoliosis. Less severe cases of scoliosis often exceed the standard values, especially when the patient is active physically.

PART B
Evidence-based theory

I. Influencing the scoliotic wedges with the aim of restoring rectangular blocks

1. Planes and axes of the body

Fig. 35 outlines the three planes (three directions, three dimensions) which define the space within which the body can move – as well as the axes around which the body can rotate.

1. The sagittal plane (sagitta = arrow) passes from posterior to anterior through the body and divides it into two halves.
2. The frontal plane (front = forehead) passes through the body from one side to the other.
3. The transverse or horizontal plane passes horizontally through the body.
4. The sagittal axis runs through the body from posterior to anterior. The body rotates around this axis in the frontal plane (for example right upwards or left downwards)
5. The frontal axis runs through the body from one side to the other. The body rotates around this axis in the sagittal plane (for example front upwards, back downwards)
6. The longitudinal axis runs from cranial to caudal. The body rotates around this axis in the transverse plane (for example right backwards, left forwards)

In the case of malposture and scoliosis, it is important to be aware of the changes in postural appearance caused by the shifting of individual body segments in the above mentioned planes and rotating around the corresponding axes. The three-dimensional changes that ensue are especially evident in scoliosis. It is therefore necessary to correct these changes in a three-dimensional manner. We describe this in the following chapters.

The most important element in postural correction is the upward direction, i.e. elongation cranially. This elonga-

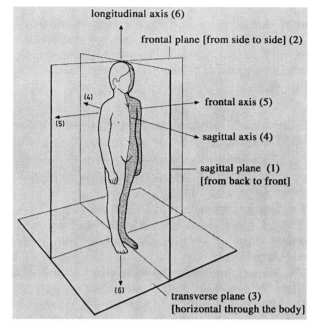

Fig. 35

tion leads to an opening of the concavities. Space is also defined by length x height x width. Each deviation in shape to the side, back or front results automatically in a shortening of the trunk and therefore an increase in the angle of the deformity. Since the lifting forces of the intervertebral discs are being wrongly directed, the scoliosis increases according to the deviation of each of the body segments from the midline. It is therefore of utmost importance to actively elongate the trunk and the spine. Our method provides this by starting each exercise with small serpentine movements of the spine upwards and sideways like slow wriggling.

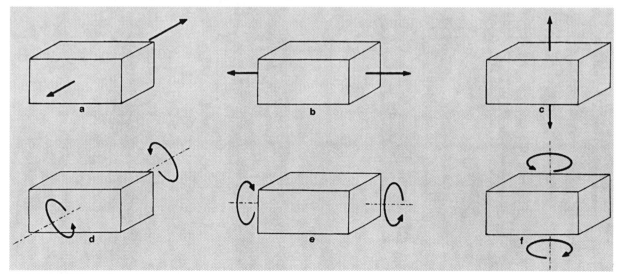

Fig. 36: Possibilities of repositioning and turning the pelvis:
Fig. 36 a, b, c: the three main axes, sagittal, transverse, longitudinal;
Fig. 36 d, e, f: movement around these axes.

2. Conceptual division of three-curve scoliosis into three blocks

In scoliosis, the rectangular blocks that are normally superimposed vertically, shift and rotate against each other. In three-curve scoliosis, the shoulder and pelvic girdle blocks shift in the frontal plane to one side and the rib cage block to the other side. At the same time, the laterally shifted blocks rotate dorsally, as shown in Fig. 37.

3. Principle of pelvic corrections in three-curve scoliosis (Fig. 36)

The first two pelvic corrections are made in the sagittal plane. The pelvis, pointing forward, is drawn back above the heels (a).

The frontal pelvic rim is then raised (e).

The third pelvic correction is a lateral movement in the frontal plane. Patients are instructed to draw in the prominent hip (b).

The fourth pelvic correction moves in the transverse plane. The convex-side hip is brought backwards (f).

The fifth pelvic correction is, like the third, a movement in the frontal plane. Patients are instructed to lower the hip below the convexity (d). Pelvic corrections for 4-curve scoliosis appear in section C.VII.

4. Correction of deviations in the sagittal plane: postural improvement, first and second pelvic correction

The axis of the legs, which runs obliquely forwards to the forefoot due to shifting of the weight has to point obliquely backwards for the purposes of correction, and the tilted pelvis has to be brought upright. The body-weight is brought onto the heels = **first pelvic correction**. This moves the pelvis backwards.

The frontal pelvic rim is raised = **second pelvic correction**. This brings the upper trunk forward, leading to a reflex that activates lumbar and dorsal erectors. At the same time, the rib hump is flattened visually (Fig. 39).

5. Corrections of deviations in the frontal plane: third pelvic correction and shoulder countertraction (Figs. 40–46)

The pelvis, having shifted laterally, has to be moved back across the midline in the opposite direction, creating an overcorrection: **third pelvic correction**. It is not enough to find only the vertical line, since we have to attempt to facilitate a new postural image. We aim at overcorrection to achieve this. This is not an overcorrection of the spine, but of the body statics. The inactive muscles have to be activated and stimulated and strengthened. When first performing this correction, there is the danger of increasing the cervical curvature (shoulder on the concave side is pulled too far laterally). **Shoulder countertraction** therefore has to be applied. The shoulder on the convex side is moved diagonally sideways and upwards, aiming also to lift the cervical curve while the trunk moves in the opposite direction. The shoulder blade should never be pressed towards the spine, but pulled away from it. The shoulder blade turns around its sagittal axis, the lower angle pointing towards the spine, and the upper outer angle laterally. At this point, the shoulder girdle is held in position, and the rib cage is derotated in a three-dimensional way: forwards, upwards, and then internally (see section B.I.8, 'Rotational angular breathing', below).

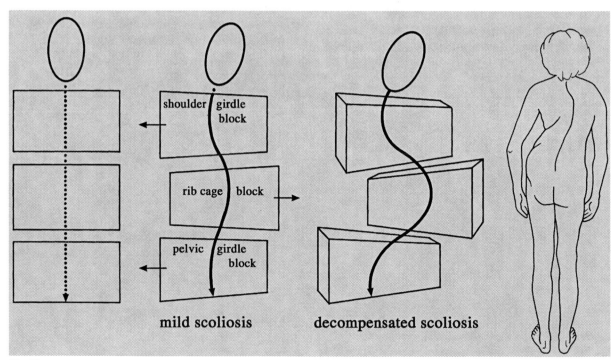

shoulder girdle block

rib cage block

pelvic girdle block

mild scoliosis   decompensated scoliosis

Fig. 37

30

Fig. 38 (right): 12.5-year-old girl with idiopathic scoliosis. As one can see on this a-p X-ray in the standing position, she also has a rotated pelvis: the wing of the left ilium seems wider than the right. This explains why the wing of the left ilium has turned backwards and the other, which appears narrower, has rotated forwards.

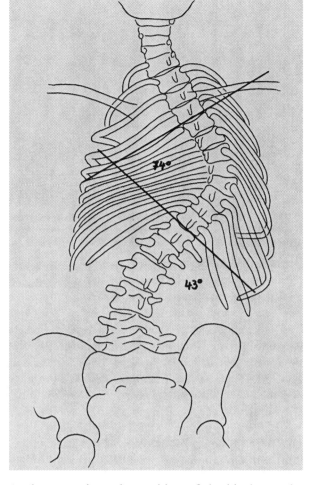

Exception

While exercising upright between two poles or in a lying position, both arms are at the same height, provided the shoulders are horizontal. If the shoulders are not at the same height, the hand of the side on which the shoulder countertraction is being applied grasps higher.

If the shoulder on the concave side is lower and the curvature starts in the upper thoracic spine, the shoulder countertraction is applied on the opposite side. The arm on the concave side is pushed outwards and upwards, and the lumbar countercurvature is contracted forward inwards (Fig. 46). It is also possible to pull the same shoulder upwards and sideways, and to move the hip below the convexity diagonally backwards and downwards ('Oblique torsion', Figs. 187 and 204-205).

Very important: avoid purely lateral pressure. Due to rotation of the convex-side middle trunk segment, the lateral ribs and muscles also rotate backwards. The parts found laterally are actually ribs and muscles of the front. They must be neither pushed nor contracted, because they would push or rotate the rib hump even further dorsally, and this would exacerbate the rotation of vertebrae. The goal is to rotate them into the correct position and widen the spaces between the ribs. Only then can the muscles of the protruding rib hump be contracted (intercostal muscles and M. latissimus dorsi). The diagonal lateral movement is created by the upper part of the M. serratus anterior (pars horizontalis) and the middle part (pars divergens). Once this technique is mastered, the laterally protruding rib hump decreases, and in some cases disappears completely.

At the same time, the position of the hip has to be corrected (outwards, backwards and downwards). (Figs.187, 205)

Note: in the case of four-curve scoliosis, do not lean towards the concave side, since this would move the hip below the convexity even further laterally.

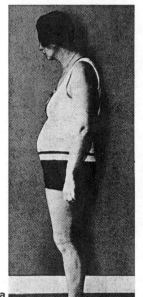 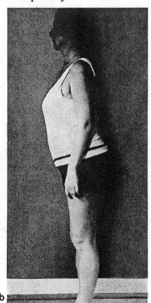 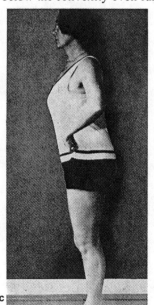 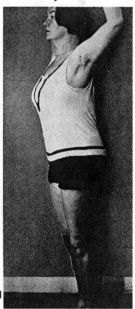

Fig. 39 a, b, c, d Postural correction: a) The pelvis is too far forward. b) Incorrect pelvic posture causes a lumbar lordosis. .
c) Correct posture. Pelvis erect, corrected lordosis. d) The pelvis has to be kept in corrected position during exercises.

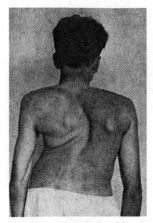

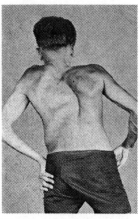

Fig. 40: Scoliotic body with pelvic malposture. The bodyweight rests on the right leg.

Fig. 41: Same patient exercising the third pelvic correction. See explanation in text.

6. Derotation of the trunk as part of the fourth pelvic correction and derotation of the shoulder girdle in three-curve scoliosis

First, the patient must master the technique of derotation of the pelvic girdle. From this fixed point, leverage can then be used to correct the upper trunk segment (rib cage). Once this has been mastered and the rib cage is derotated, this forms a solid basis for derotation of the shoulder girdle.

The **three kyphotic elevations** of the trunk:
trunk segment 1 is the hip and lumbar hump below the dorsal concavity;
trunk segment 2 is the dorsal rib hump;
trunk segment 3 is the shoulder girdle of the dorsal concave side;
They have to be moved forward.

The **three lordotic parts** of the trunk:
trunk segment 1 is the hip below the rib hump including the lumbar part and floating ribs on this side;
trunk segment 2 is the concavity;
trunk segment 3 is the shoulder above the rib hump.
They must be rotated backwards.

Fourth pelvic correction: the gluteal muscles should be firmly contracted.
a) Contraction of these muscles on the dorsal concave side brings the hip forward
b) Manual pressure on anterior thigh of the rib hump side brings this hip backwards (Fig. 47)

The derotated pelvis now forms a firm point against which the second trunk segment can rotate. This derotation also remains as a fixed point. Now the shoulder girdle has to rotate in the same direction as the pelvis: above the rib hump backwards; above the concave side forwards.

7. Horizontal positioning of the aleae (crista iliaca) of the ilium: the fifth pelvic correction

In most cases, the pelvis moves out of its corrected horizontal position during the third pelvic correction, which means that a fifth correction is necessary. The leg on the convex side appears to be shorter. This **fifth correction**, however, consists only of **lowering the heel** on the convex side, thus widening the space between the ribs and pelvic rim (Figs. 40, 41, 116-120). Besides achieving an improved clinical appearance, this correction causes the important deflexion of the lumbar spine into the upright position, a basic correction for the spinal segments located more cranially.

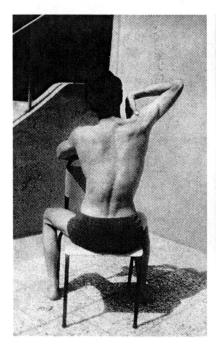

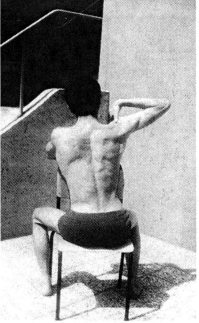

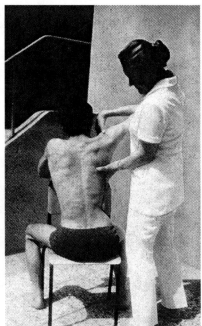

Fig. 42: Shoulder countertraction. Incorrect position of the head and shoulders

Fig. 43: Correct position of the shoulders and head.

Fig. 44: With manual assistance: rotation, lifting and pushing grip.

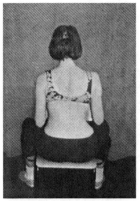
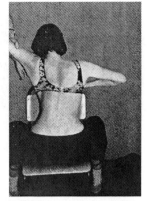

Fig. 45   Fig. 46

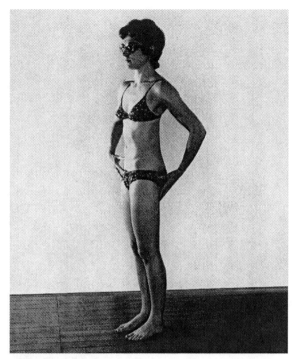

Fig. 47: Fourth pelvic correction

8. Targeted 'rotational-angular breathing' with counterrotation of derotated trunk segments (most important point in postural improvement for all patients!).

Rotational angular breathing (RAB)

After pelvic correction has been established, breathing movements of the rib cage are performed in a 'right angled' manner. This means that the breathing directions follow the sides of an imaginary right angle (the second side of this angle always runs cranially). The RAB starts at the 'vertices of the wedges' and is combined during inhalation with the mental image of lowering the diaphragm. RAB is accompanied by a countermovement of the body segments located above or below.
The procedure for kyphosis and scoliosis is as follows.

A) LUMBAR REGION BACKWARDS AND UPWARDS
   (WEDGE 1, FIG. 49)

With hands on the lumbar lordosis, the patient inhales and checks whether the region flattens while lifting the anterior pelvic rim. Flattening of the lordosis relieves pressure from the abdominal wall, since the intestinesthen rest mostly in the pelvis. This has to be reinforced by tightening the abdominal muscles during exhalation through the mouth (forming the letter 'f' or 's'). Imagining the following is useful: intestines backwards and along the spine upwards = right angle. The countermovement takes the form of downward movement of the posterior iliac crest, increased straightening up of the pelvis, and leaning forward of the upper trunk to open the vertex of the wedge in the lumbar region.

B) 'FLAT ANTERIOR CHEST' FORWARDS AND UPWARDS
   (WEDGE 2, FIG. 49, 52)

The patient's hands are now gently rested on the recessed anterior side. These ribs are then brought forward by breathing forwards and upwards into the area. At the same time, the diaphragm is lowered and sinks down to the intestines, and the rib hump flattens. The patient can

feel this very easily. The countermovement is pushing the shoulder and hip backwards.

C) CERVICAL LORDOSIS BACKWARDS AND UPWARDS
   (WEDGE 3, FIG. 49)

During inhalation, the neck moves gently backwards and upwards (oscillatory movements of the spine), giving the head a strong occipital push. This decreases the lordosis. Countermovement: upper trunk forwards, widening of the chest. The following breathing movements have to be performed additionally in the case of scoliosis:

D) FLOATING RIBS (11TH AND 12TH) BELOW THE RIB HUMP
   SIDEWAYS AND UPWARDS (WEDGE 5, FIGS. 50, 51)

In the case of severe scoliosis, these ribs point almost vertically downwards. The patient puts his/her fingers into the recessed area and pushes until the ribs are found. Then they are moved sideways and upwards and backwards and upwards by breathing and the diaphragm is lowered mentally (and physically). Countermovement: the lateral rib hump is pulled towards the centre.

E) THE SAME FLOATING RIBS BACKWARDS-UPWARDS (WEDGE 1)

The thumb pushes strongly from the back against the last ribs, which arch towards the thumb during inhalation. Now the concavity below the rib hump is filled with air, because the diaphragm lowers and forces these ribs outwards. Now the previously inactive ribs can give support again. Countermovements: pelvis downwards, trunk forwards, contraction of the posterior rib hump.

33

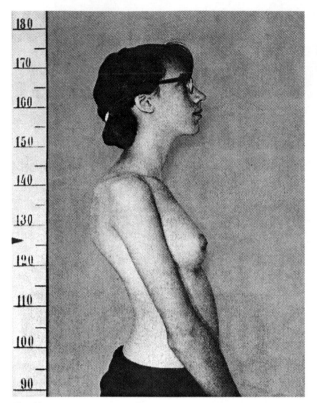

Fig. 48

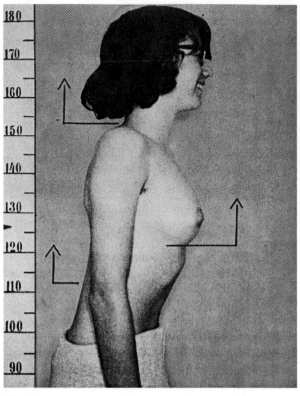

Fig. 49

F) NARROW ANTERIOR SIDE FORWARDS AND UPWARDS (WEDGE 2A, FIG. 52)

Similar to breathing movement b) unilateral at the convex side. It is important to visualize lowering the diaphragm at the same time to even the lumbar lordosis and create a support from which the narrow front can be pushed out. Counter-movement: counterhold of ipsilateral hip and shoulder.

G) NARROW ANTERIOR SIDE FORWARDS AND UPWARDS (WEDGE 2, FIGS. 52 AND 53)

If the trunk is very rotated, (sternum has shifted to the convex side), an additional inward movement is necessary until the sternum is across the midline (Fig. 53). It is equally important to lower the diaphragm. The inward movement is lateral and may be done only after

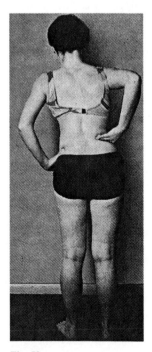

Fig. 50

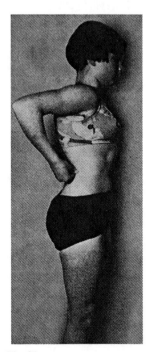

Fig. 51

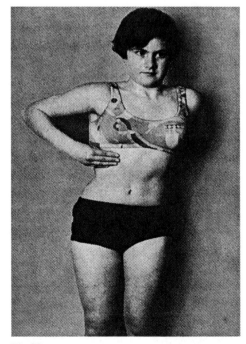

Fig. 52

34

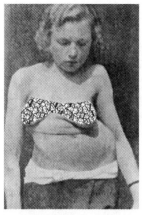

Fig. 53:
18-year-old girl at the beginning of treatment.

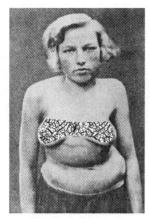

Fig. 54:
After 3 months of treatment.

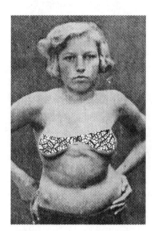

Fig. 55:
After 4½ months (notice her facial expression). The part of the rib cage which had deviated to the right, laterally and dorsally, has been moved forwards, upwards and inwards with RAB. The three blocks are now superposed vertically.

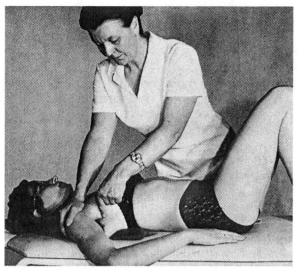

Fig. 56

derotation. If the sternum lies in the middle, the derotational breathing is omitted. Instead, only the lateral intercostal muscles are contracted during exhalation as for shoulder countertraction (Fig. 44). Countermovement: hip and shoulder of the convex side outwards. If the sternum has twisted to the concave side (Fig. 52), see section C.VIII.6, Correction of the shifted sternum.

H) SUBAXILLARY RIBS FORWARDS AND UPWARDS (WEDGE 2B, FIG. 56)

This area is especially narrow if the shoulder above the rib hump is rotated far forward. Widening and relief of pressure is only possible with proper alignment of the shoulder and scapula, with the latter in a vertical position. Here, too, we must make the connection downwards to the diaphragm. Countermovement: shoulder level (exterior angle of scapula) backwards, inferior angle forwards, to help push the rib hump forward.

I) CONCAVE SIDE LATERALLY AND UPWARDS (WEDGE 6, FIGS. 41 AND 58)

These very closely-spaced ribs are spread by inhaling sideways and upwards over the concave-side hip (checking movement with the fingers). Lowering the diaphragm, the ribs can be felt to move outwards one

after the other. This phase is important, since only after widening the inter-rib spaces can the ribs be moved backwards and raised. Countermovement: contraction of the concave-side lateral hip muscles (M. tensor fasciae latae, M. glutaeus medius and minimus) from sideways to inwards. The outer shoulder girdle on the same side should also be contracted. This is very difficult to achieve, but shoulder countertraction on the convex side contributes to it.

K) CONCAVE SIDE BACKWARDS AND UPWARDS (WEDGES 4 AND 6, FIG. 58)

The ribs on the concave side cannot be rotated immediately because they then hinder each other. Moving them backwards can only be achieved after they have been lifted laterally. Afterwards there is an upward movement which causes the concave area to arch backwards. This also evens out the thoracic lordosis. Voluntarily contracting the diaphragm leads to a faster and more complete corrective movement. Countermovements are concave-side gluteal contraction to move the hip forward (fourth pelvic correction), and forward rotation of the concave-side shoulder.

It is important to combine all countermovements with depression of the diaphragm and an occipital push. With these countermovements, the kyphotic and lordotic trunk segments are brought back into one plane. The trunk is visually balanced.

L) RAB WITH TRUNK HANGING FORWARD (FIGS. 244, 250 AND 490-494)

Asymmetry of the back is most visible in this position. However, it submits to good correction since the spine is at maximum elongation. Four kilos of head weight draw it out, and the concave side is freed of the shoulder-girdle pressure. Diaphragmatic breathing can flow unobstructed. Ribs on the concave side are rotated laterally,

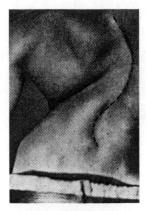

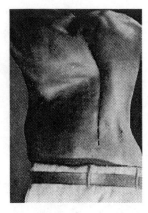

Fig. 57: The concave side (left) is badly depressed most of the time. The shoulder girdle on the same side rests heavily on the concave ribs, often even on the pelvic girdle.

Fig. 58: The concave side is widened with simultaneous pelvic correction and RAB. Now the ribs on the concave side can straighten the vertebral bodies

cranially and dorsally. Figs. 491–494 show ventral rotation of the convex side when the concavity is pushed out dorsally by breathing. This action reverses thoracic spinal lordosis. The patient should breathe in this way for as long as possible and try to perfect the result with each breath. As mentioned earlier, one characteristic of major scoliosis is a lordotic spine in the area of the strongest curvature. This means that it is not useful to concentrate exclusively on the rib hump while exercising. Derotational movement of the vertebrae is often more important. As we see in Fig. 494, the rotational breathing movement is more successful with added tactile stimulation.

9) Postural correction of the neck and head

The head should be held in a position that extends the median scoliotic curve. The larger this curve, the more the head is held towards the side of the convexity, thus enlarging the cervical curve (Fig. 23, 59). The head must thus lean towards the concave side during exercise. The following rule can be applied in almost all cases: incline the head towards the concave side and turn the chin towards the convex side (Fig. 61). The smaller the main curvature, the straighter the head may be held. In any case, even with kyphosis, it also has to be inclined back if there is cervical hyperlordosis (see Part C). For cervical kyphosis, the head should only be held upright without extension of the cervical spine, i.e., no occipital push.

10) Isometric tension for stabilization following postural correction

Flattening out the raised areas using relaxing movements can only be successful if isometric tension is applied to the newly-obtained 'normal' shape as an integral part of each exercise.

Exercise: On inhalation, the best possible correction of the posture is adopted, whatever exercise is being performed. On subsequent exhalation, all muscles of the trunk are tensed as much as possible (without movement), and the patient should count to four mentally, steadily increasing the tension. The tension is held during the next inhalation, and should be increased even more during the subsequent inhalation, until – according to individual capacity – reaching a count of twelve. The muscles should then be allowed to relax a little, without the influence of breathing, until the latter has returned to normal. The tension should be applied from the lower to the upper body, starting from the front of the thighs, via the groin up to the ribs, and from there sideways and backwards. The exercise is then repeated. After three or four of these "Twelve-Count-Tensing" exercises, the patient should relax for a while until breathing has returned to its resting rhythm and the muscles have recovered. This takes place

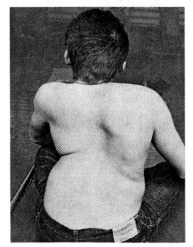

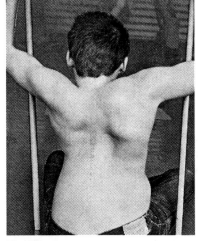

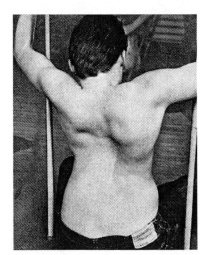

Fig. 59:
Before exercising. The hair covers the neck.

Fig. 60:
By pressing the hands against the poles, the upper body is lifted from the pelvis and the lateral parts of the trunk are elongated. After this, RAB is applied.

Fig. 61:
We then correct the positioning of the head: it is inclined to the concave side, while the chin is pointed towards the convex side. These corrections are stabilized by firmly pushing the poles against the ground.

in corrected position lying supine. In doing so the patient should 'think' the concave back sections wider and apply them to the floor. The effect of this imagining is highly visible and occurs to an astonishing degree.

Every exercise can be combined with these "Twelve-Count-Tensings" and, depending upon the patient's strength, can be increased up to 16–20 repetitions. It is an excellent way of shortening over-stretched muscles and restoring a better posture. It can only be successful, however, if it is performed with the best possible (corrected) starting position. Any strong tensing of the muscles results in the formation of new muscle fibres. Care must therefore be taken to ensure that not only the rib hump side is contracted, because this would only make it look bigger. After derotation therefore, it is necessary to tense both sides during the exhalation phase – the concave side after lengthening,

and the convex side after shortening. While these Twelve-Count-Tensings can be performed at the end of any exercise, patients should not imagine that because they have just exerted themselves so much, they can sit or stand as they please in their leisure time (meals, watching television, etc.). Those who think this way will surely soon fall back into their previous malposture. This means that they are performing an incorrect exercise that unfortunately reverses the correct results they just achieved. The outcome is as if they had never exercised. Patients must make a great effort to ensure that their previous posture is a thing of the past. When all is said and done, their own bodies should tell them, so that they never again consciously think of re-adopting their old habits. If they get tired, it is much better to simply lie down and rest. Patients need to increase their proprioception of the new posture.

II. Appropriate starting positions and orthopaedic aids for trunk derotation exercises (three-curve scoliosis)

Four cushions are needed: postcard-size, filled with rice or grain, weighing about 200 grams, preferably wedge-shaped (Fig. 574). They should be firm but also flexible to adapt to body shape. They are used to derotate specific trunk segments. The cushions not only serve passive correction, but also as a mnemonic device for everyday activities. "What do I have to bring forward? What has to go backwards?"

1. Flat supine position without pillow under the head

Bent legs. One cushion under the concave-side hip; one cushion under the shoulder blade on the same side (Fig. 62); one cushion sideways under the rib hump (Fig. 63), but not underneath or across the spine. The pressure should be applied where the rib hump begins to deviate caudally to the back and to the side. If there is a thick lumbar hump under the dorsal concave side, an additional cushion should be put under it (Fig. 64). Particularly in four-curve cases, it must lie crossways so that the concave ribs are not pressed forwards. The upper trunk is inclined obliquely towards the concave side. If patients sleep on their back, the position described above is good, otherwise attach foam cushions to the pyjama top. To avoid lateral

deviation of the rib hump (i.e. lumbar hump), a wedge-shaped cushion may be put underneath it (Fig. 575).

2. Prone position

Generally, the pelvis is elevated by a large cushion, a roll or a little footstool. Take care that it is not too far up under the thighs, which could promote lumbar hyperlordosis. An additional cushion under the hip on the convex side, a thick cushion under the shoulder joint or elbow on the convex side; one to three cushions under the frontal rib hump (concave side), the size of these cushions depending on the size of footstool or roll. The forehead should rest

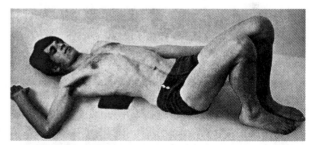

Fig. 63

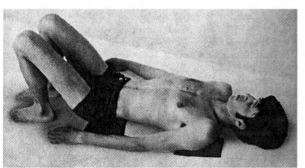

Fig. 62

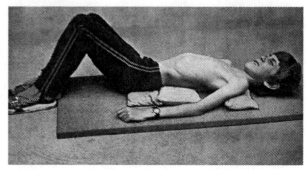

Fig. 64

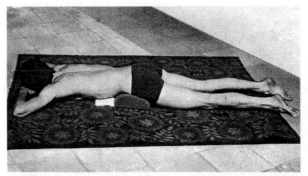

Fig. 65

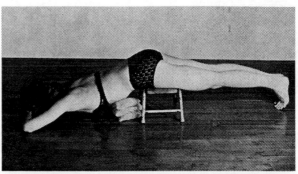

Fig. 66

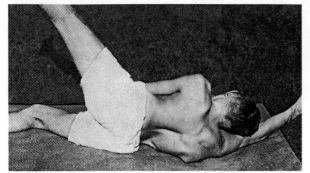

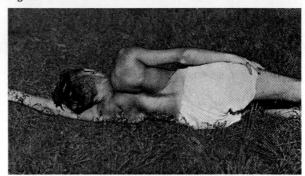

Fig. 67: Unsuitable position. The convexities are increased. The thoracic convexity moves backwards.

Fig. 68: Suitable position on the concave side. The spine is stretched

on the hands; the chin is directed towards the sternum and the convex side (Figs. 65 and 66). If the pelvis is aligned, i.e. there is no prominent hip, the legs should lie straight. If the hip on the thoracal concave side is prominent, the legs should be about 10° to the concave side, thus opening the 'weak spot' underneath the dorsal convexity. This stretches and activates muscles in this area and enables the hip to move towards the convex side. Pay attention to the concave side – it must stay wide and open. Do not perform lateral flexion. Patients with a lumbosacral counter-curvature straddle the leg on this side (section C.VII).

3. Lateral position

Never lie on the side of the rib hump, even when sleeping! Spinal torsion and the rib hump will be exacerbated by lateral pressure. Even books or pillows placed under the lateral rib hump will further compress the narrow ribs and intercostal spaces on this side. This may produce a fold in the ribs and a 'pointed rib hump'.
The patient should ideally rest on the dorsal concave side, with that arm underneath the head, stretched up

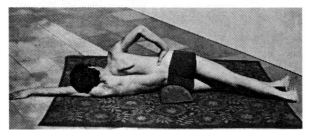

Fig. 69:
The cushion underneath the hip leads to overcorrection and is not necessary in every case, since the floor pushes the pelvis inwards.

or outward. The head lies on the upper arm or a pillow. If the hip on this side is prominent, place a cushion under it. If the hips are straight, lay the cushion somewhat higher to the side under the lumbar convexity, but not under the concave ribs. These must lie free so that at that rib rotation may be promoted there by means of corrective breathing. The weight of the rib hump now works correctively. RAB is now possible (Fig. 68–70).

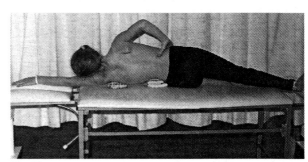

Fig. 70:
In the case of pronounced lateral shifting of the shoulder girdle, put a corrective cushion underneath it. In the case of a large lumbar hump and rotational vertebral slippage, the lumbar hump is derotated manually forwards and then cushions are put underneath – as many as needed to bring the lumbar spine into a median position.
Note for sleeping: Patients with a lumbosacral curvature (see sections C.VII and C.VIII) usually have a high lumbar hump. When lying on the side this should be supported, even when sleeping, by a 20-cm-long, thin, sand-filled cushion, otherwise it wells outwards. If this happens, lying on the side is not only an unfavourable position, but is dangerous, since the lumbar curve bends outwards and twists further. A sand-filled cushion does not usually slip so easily, and remains in the same position when the patient turns onto his back. Once the patient has imprinted the Schroth philosophy on his mind, he develops a 'hygienic conscience' that makes him wake up if he turns onto the 'wrong' side when sleeping. In this way, sleeping at night also becomes a corrective exercise.

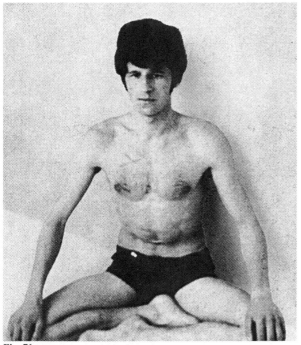

Fig. 71

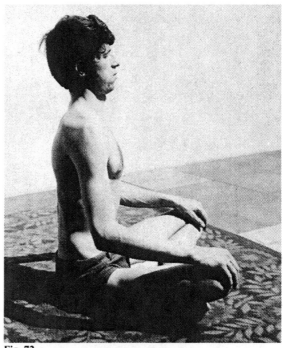

Fig. 72

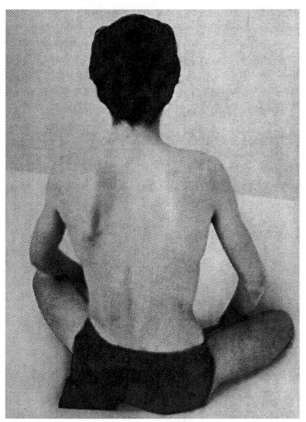

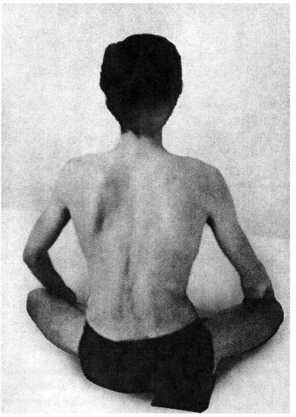

Fig. 73:
Corrective cushions in accordance with the 5th pelvic correction for three-curve scoliosis; applied only if the hip below the rib hump has to be lowered or if the lumbar convexity is inflexible and cannot be influenced. The statics must not be shifted towards the right. If a fourth curve is present, this cushion is omitted because it would increase the lumbosacral curvature.

Fig. 74:
A cushion is placed underneath the thoracic convex side only if there is unilateral gluteal atrophy (caused by polio and such disorders). A horizontal pelvis is the goal. In the case shown, the cushion has to be omitted because it increases the lumbar curvature. A cushion may be necessary in the case of a correction of four-curve scoliosis when the leg on the side of the lumbar convexity is splayed. This will move the pelvis into a horizontal position.

39

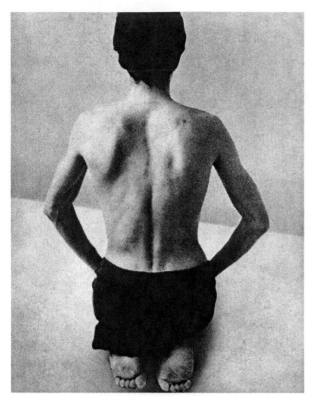

Fig. 75:

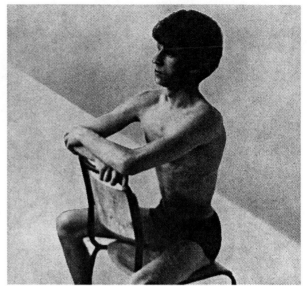

Fig. 77

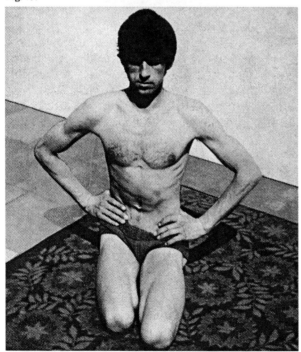

Fig. 76:
In the case of three-curve scoliosis, the lower leg is pushed a little backwards at the side of the convexity to derotate this hip.

4. Sitting position (Fig. 71)

Always sit on the ischial tuberosities, either on a chair – without leaning back – or cross-legged on the floor. The lower leg on the concave side is placed across the lower on the convex side. If the lumbar curvature cannot be influenced by exercise, we must put a cushion under the hip on this side (Fig. 73). The bodyweight then rests on

this side. The hip on the convex side is now lowered until it has contact with the ground; it is also brought backwards to derotate the pelvis. Sometimes the patient feels it would be easier to place a cushion under the opposite side to create better balance. This would narrow the vertex of the wedge even more and the lower wedge would be enlarged (Fig. 74). Additionally, this would support the scoliotic pelvis and make derotation impossible.

The table at which one sits should be adjusted to body size to support the corrected upright posture during meals. We have tables of different heights at our clinic (Fig. 571).

5. Sitting on the heels (Figs. 75 and 76)

If a cushion is used, it should be on the heel of the lumbar convexity. Do not use in cases of four-curve scoliosis.

6. TV position (Fig. 77)

Straddled on a chair, femurs horizontal, feet pointing slightly outwards; forearms resting on the back of

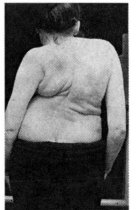

Fig. 78

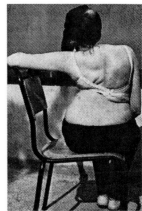

Fig. 79

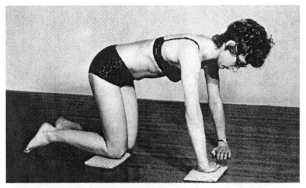

Fig. 80:
No cushion under the knee in the case of four-curve scoliosis.

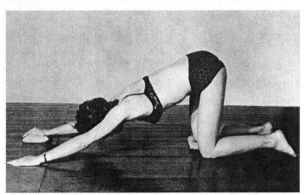

Fig. 81:
No cushion under the knee in the case of four-curve scoliosis..

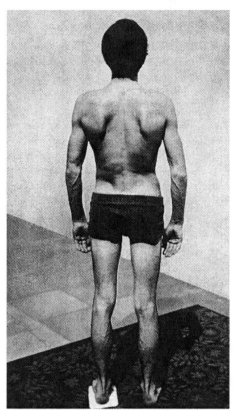

Fig. 83:
No cushion under the foot in the case of four-curve scoliosis.

the chair; pelvis back as far as possible; if necessary, a cushion under the hip of the lumbar convexity. This position prevents the trunk from 'sinking in', and the patient can pay close attention to other things. This is a very suitable position for studying, listening, etc.

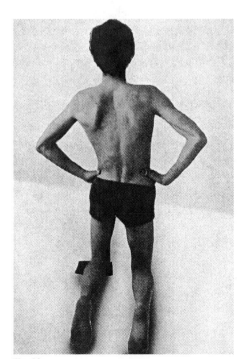

Fig. 82:
No cushion under the knee in the case of four-curve scoliosis.

7. Corrective sitting position when the concavity is extreme (Figs. 78 and 79)

Concave side towards the back of the chair; the hip on the convex side as much as possible to the side, down and back. Arm on the concave side rests on the back of the chair to support this side and to widen it. The hip on the concave side carries the weight.

8. On all fours (Fig. 80)

The knees are held apart as wide as the hips, with the thighs in a vertical position; the arms are extended vertically under the shoulders, with the fingers pointing inwards. A cushion is placed under the knee of the convex side; a second cushion under the hand of the same side accomplishes passive derotation of the shoulder girdle and pelvic girdle. Internal rotation of arms is used to create a better starting position for exercises, which include shoulder countertraction. When performing only breathing exercises (no change in body position along axes), the arms and fingers point straight ahead.

9. Low-sliding position (Fig. 81)

As above; however, arms extended forwards and clavicles pointing towards floor. Cushion under wrist and knee on convex side.

10. Kneeling position (Fig. 82)

If a cushion is needed (will not usually be the case), it should be under the knee of the lumbar convexity (see "sitting cross-legged").

11. Standing (Fig. 83)

If one leg is shorter, the whole foot and not just the heel must be elevated (danger of pes equinus – dropfoot).
The following distinction should be made: trunk in upright position – cushion under one foot moves the hip cranially and means the pelvis is no longer horizontal. Trunk leaning forwards (Fig. 84), the cushion pushes the hip dorsally and derotates the pelvis. Always think carefully: what is achieved by using a cushion? In the case of three-curve scoliosis, a cushion must be placed under the foot on the convex side to bring the hip backwards while exercising with the trunk inclined forwards. The hand grasps the next higher bar, for example, to derotate the same-side shoulder girdle. When in doubt, omit cushions (section B.I.1, Planes and Axes).

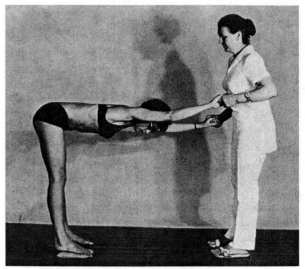

Fig. 84: Omit the cushion in the case of a four-curve scoliosis.

III. The scoliotically changed locomotor system

Explications of muscular movement are always based on measurements taken from non-scoliotic persons. This means that it is sometimes difficult to explain the movements of the muscle and ligament apparatus in scoliosis. The scoliotic patient has a number of contractions of the soft parts and changes in bones with unilateral ankylosis, and the entire system reacts differently.

A multitude of muscles are involved in a scoliotic curvature. Thus, correction of a scoliotic curve cannot be limited to correction of one muscle only. If we only concentrated on individual muscles, important parts of the corrective process would be ignored. Additionally, many synergistic and antagonistic effects lead to a balanced corrective system. In the following, we shed light on the activity of some muscles.

a) Pathological elements

Scoliosis is characterised by a more or less pronounced change in the balance of forces, starting already in the feet, legs and hips, with inequality of muscles in terms of length and size. The greater the deviations from the midline, the longer the affected muscles become and the more volume is lost. They become flaccid and finally inactive. They lose their supportive function. Shape changes are only possible because the muscles permit them to happen. They become longer or shorter depending on the direction in which the trunk is moved and rotated. In other words, deviations of the trunk to the side or backwards can only develop if the corresponding supportive muscles give way and become elongated. Figure 113 shows that muscle inequality already starts in the lumbar segment and continues through as far as the cervical spine.

Therefore, treatment must primarily improve posture so that the body can regain its original perpendicular axis. This can only happen by developing and training the corresponding muscle groups responsible for upright posture. To restore the balance of the body muscles, those that have grown longer must be shortened and those that have become shorter must be lengthened. In

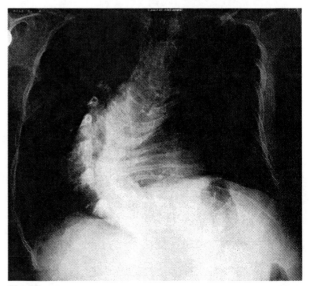

Fig. 85

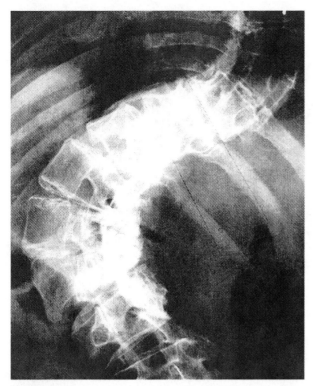

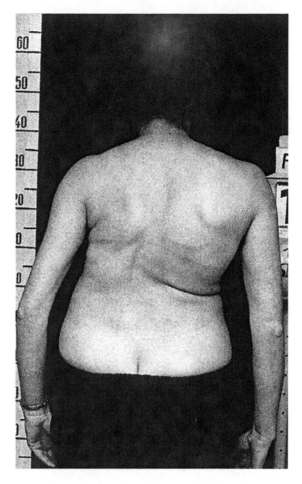

Fig. 86:
Congenital scoliosis presenting diffuse changes in vertebral bodies that cannot be altered by our method. We could, however, certainly achieve improvements in breathing and posture.

Firg. 87 (right): Same patient as in Fig. 86.

order for these to be able to hold the spinal column and ribcage in their normal perpendicular position again, they need to be strengthened – and on *both* sides. It is absolutely essential that the inactive shortened muscles have to perform strength work in the lengthened state.

In his thesis to become a university lecturer, Brussatis described the difference between electrical activity in the muscles on the convex and concave sides (Brussatis 1962). He found that the activity in the muscles on the convex side was greater. This can be explained by muscle mechanics. According to Schmidt/Thews (1976), there is a connection between pretension and contraction of a muscle. Investigations done with isolated frog muscles demonstrate that a muscle can only reach its maximal tension after a certain degree of pre-stretching. The latter corresponds roughly with its resting position.

Increased stretching decreases the contractive capacity as much as further contraction would.

Applying this to scoliotic malposture, the only conclusion that can be drawn is that the strongly contracted muscles on the concave side of the curvature are as insufficient as the over-stretched ones on the convex side. Strong myoelectric activity of the muscles on the convex side results from the fact that they alone have to bear the load of the parts of the body that lie cranially. They hypertrophy but do not increase in strength, as we used to believe. They are in a much too severely prestretched state. They cannot bear the stress alone and,

instead of strengthening, weaken continuously until bony disposition has been reached to stop the progression of the scoliosis.

The electromyographically 'silent' muscles in the concavity shorten and show decreasing function as the curvature increases. Pre-tension decreases here, and we can also assume that this results in an increase in insufficiency.

The corrective starting positions of the Schroth method ensure that near-physiological pre-tension is reached, in both the concavity and the convexity. This enables muscles to contract almost to the maximum extent.

Scoliosis is always preceded by an incongruity between maximum weight tolerance and actual workload of musculoskeletal system. Once the different parts of the skeleton are no longer properly aligned, they gradually enforce the 'scoliotic balance' of the body, so-called 'static decompensation'. This, however, is only possible because the defective ligamentous structures (overall connective tissue weakness) allow this to happen. The physiological function of the vertebral and costovertebral joints, and often also the sternocostal junctions, are disturbed. Vertebral slippage combined with rotation and even subluxation may result. This opens up the way to extensive deformities.

The scoliotically changed locomotor system is held in place by sets of muscles, some of which are overloaded

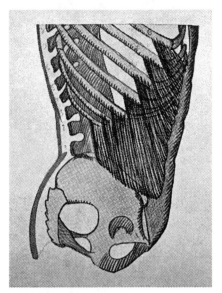

Fig. 88

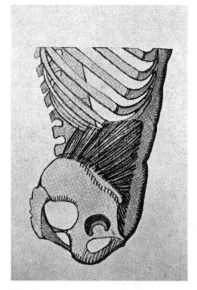

Fig. 89

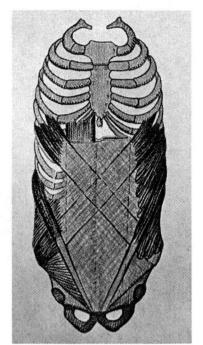

Fig. 90 (right)

and stretched and others which are contracted and atrophied. This allows multiple torsion of the spine to occur to an incredible degree. The greater the pathological effects of pressure and traction, the greater the effect on the bones. Initially, intervertebral discs become wedge-shaped, and later they suffer pressure atrophy, with bony ankylosis in the most severe cases.

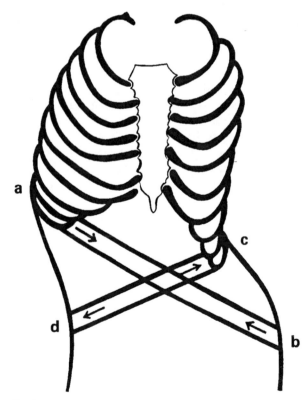

Fig. 91:
Schematic representation of the length difference of the abdominal musculature. The arrows show the direction of exercises.

b) Individual muscles involved in scoliotic malposture

1. ABDOMINAL MUSCLES (FIGS. 88–91)

The pelvic girdle and ribcage (and shoulder girdle) are counter-rotated in scoliosis. All abdominal muscles are therefore involved. Our working hypothesis: in right-convex scoliosis, fibres of the M. obliquus abdominis externus on the right (Fig. 91, a) and those of the M. obliquus abdominis internus on the left (b), which run diagonally parallel in one line, are over-stretched. Consequently, the rib hump can move laterally and dorsally. On the other side, the hip on the concave side shifts outwards and backwards (b).

The opposite muscles, c–d, are shorter and bring the frontal rib arch (so-called anterior rib hump) and the hip below the dorsal rib hump forwards and inwards.

The exercise treatment has to restore muscular balance by shortening the elongated diagonal a–b and elongating the shortened diagonal c–d. This principle applies to all exercises. Short diagonals seem longer than previously overstretched diagonals on the other side. The remaining abdominal muscles which had also moved obliquely, normalize at the same time. The result is normalization of the entire trunk.

First exercise to stretch line c–d (Fig. 92)
Supine position with corrective cushions. With one hand, the patient pushes the hip below the convexity outwards (laterally), backwards (dorsally) and downwards (caudally). The other hand brings the anterior rib hump outwards (laterally), upwards (cranially) and then backwards (dorsally). This is done gently and with accompanying corrective breathing. The patient should

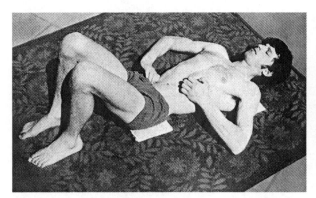

Fig. 92

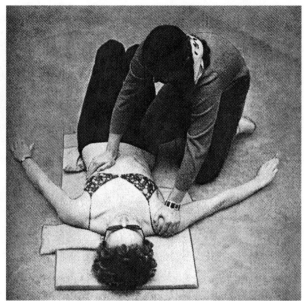

Fig. 93 (right)

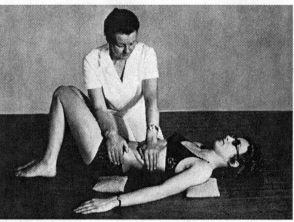

feel oblique traction inside (if necessary, the fingers can be hooked underneath the frontal rib arch to help). During exhalation, the patient relaxes and then repeats the exercises with a new breath. To intensify the exercise, corrected position may be held during the following breath.

Second exercise to stretch line c–d (Fig. 93)
Supine position with corrective cushions. The therapist kneels on the convex side and holds the hip back, using the knee (or a sand-filled cushion). One hand moves the frontal rib arch laterally and cranially and, additionally, dorsally and cranially (derotating and lifting with manual aid). The patient supports this with RAB which spreads and widens hollow areas of the back. Now the dorsal ribs find room to move and align.
Lumbar spine and corrected hip stay on the floor.

Third exercise to untwist b–c (Fig. 94)
Supine position with corrective cushions. The therapist kneels on the convex side, pulling the hip on the concave side forwards and inwards. The other hand pushes the frontal rib hump outward and upward (laterally and cranially) and backwards and upwards (dorsally and cranially) creating two 'right angles'. The patient inhales during rotation and tries to maintain the position during exhalation for as long as possible. In the case of a lumbar hump above the hip on the concave side, it also has to be pulled forwards and inwards.

Fourth exercise to shorten line a–b (Figs. 95, 98 and 101)
Supine position with corrective cushions. At first, the patient may support manually on his own. He places one hand on the laterally deviated rib hump, moving it forward, upward and inward. The other hand moves the prominent hip on the concave side forward and inward. This movement is assisted manually only at the beginning, afterward the hands 'glide' in the right directions, and then visualization alone produces the desired results.

Fig. 94

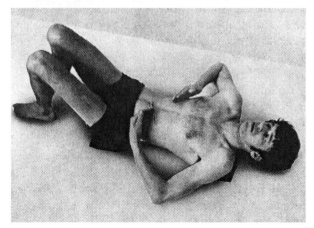

Fig. 95

Fifth exercise for derotation a–d (Fig. 102)
Supine position with corrective cushions. The therapist kneels at the patient's concave side and pushes the convex-sided hip to the outside, backward and downward. The patient assists with this movement. The other hand of the therapist moves the rib hump forward, upward and inward. The patient senses these corrective movements and tries to reproduce these sensations later on

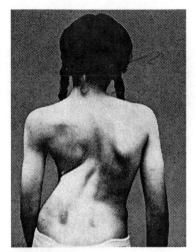

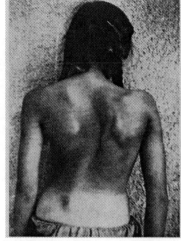

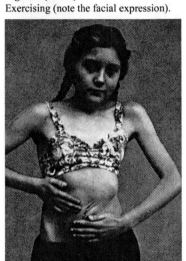

Fig. 96: Start

Fig. 97: After 8 weeks.

Fig. 98: Exercising.
Fig. 101 (below):
Exercising (note the facial expression).

Fig. 99 (below): Start

Fig. 100 (below): After 8 weeks.

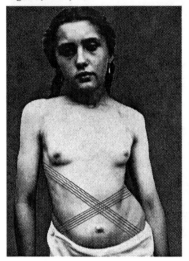

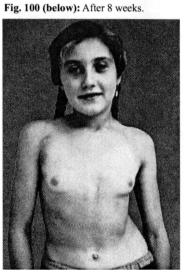

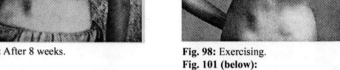

while practising.

2. M. QUADRATUS LUMBORUM AND THE DEEPER HOLDING MUSCULATURE (FIG. 103, 104)

Together with erector trunci, this muscle has the function of keeping the lumbar spine in medial position. It is attached to the 12th rib as well as the transverse pro-

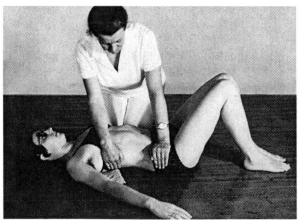

Fig. 102

cesses of the lumbar vertebrae. In scoliosis, this muscle works unilaterally, pulling transverse processes of lumbar spine to one side (see section B.III.3, Erector trunci). Result: shifting of the lumbar spine and torsion, thus creating lumbar scoliosis. (See section C.VII.4, Accessory rotation.)

In case of inactivity, this muscle no longer pulls on the transverse processes (Fig. 104). It occurs on the convex side, where vertebrae glide over to the opposite side and create a compensating lumbar curvature.

The upper body which has deviated to the convex side has to be kept in balance by M. quadratus lumborum and erector trunci. These muscles are then forced into increased (supportive) activity. Due to continuous pathological muscle tension and overall weakness of connective tissue, vertebral articulations deviate from the vertical axis in scoliosis. At times they even subluxate and create torsion of the lumbar spine, including a rotation of spinous processes towards the lumbar concavity. The transverse processes rotate – with the hip – forward on the convex side. The lumbar musculature shortens while a muscular hump forms on the opposite side (it is possible to palpate the transverse processes – Fig. 104).

46

"A laterally deviating spine is only possible in connection with torsion. The spinal column does not have a central point of rotation but an eccentric one, similar to that of an ellipse. A vertebral body, without posterior arch and spinous process, has its centre in the middle. However, because of the posterior vertebral arch, spinous process and zygapophyseal joints with additional axes of rotation, a corresponding rotational centre is created, located at the posterior margin of the actual vertebral body. This centre of rotation does not lead to real rotation but to torsion. This can easily be demonstrated: Fix two steel rulers of equal length next to each other (about 1 or 2 cm apart and parallel) and try to bend them. Each ruler will show torsion, similar to the effect of scoliosis." (K. F. Schlegel, Prof. of Orthopaedics, Essen.)

Before starting the next exercise, the 'muscle cylinder', the patient should observe his lumbar spine carefully. Practising getting down into starting position as well as getting up has to be performed carefully. It is important to be aware of the leg that leads to getting up or down. Inattention at this point may lead to reversing the exercise results. No problem arises when one gets up or down with both legs at the same time.

Most often the patient will use the 'comfortable' leg: the leg on the concave side, to go down, and the convex-sided leg to get up. This will increase the lumbar convexity. (Figs. 105, 106).

It is most important to practise between two mirrors. From standing position to kneeling:

1. Kneeling: leg of convex side starts the movement.
2. Simultaneously leaning trunk to concave side and extending leg on convex side.
3. Ending: first pull leg towards body and bring trunk into upright position.
4. Standing up: foot (leg) on the concave side starts the movement.

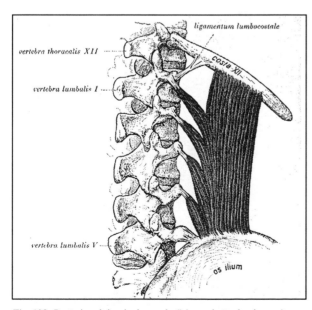

Fig. 103: Posterior abdominal muscle (M. quadratus lumborum).

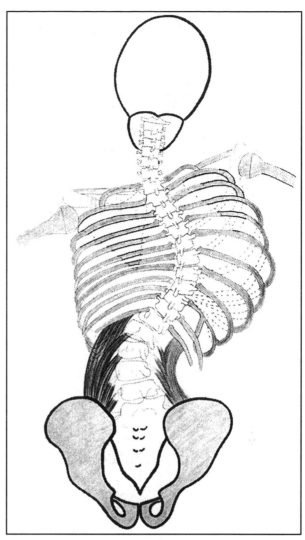

Fig. 104 (Drawing by Lehnert-Schroth)

Goal of exercise treatment is the activation of musculature below the convexity by forcing it to 'work' into a corrective position.

Exercise to increase the tonus of M. quadratus lumborum and of deeper holding musculature in three-curve scoliosis (muscle cylinder) (Figs. 107 and 108)

Kneeling or standing position; hands on hips; pelvis upright; trunk leaning over to concave side (do not bend over!). Leg on the convex side is stretched out, rotated outwards and placed laterally. The leg and upper body form one straight line. The hip on the concave side is contracted to the midline (the 3rd pelvic correction) and rotated forwards (4th pelvic correction); extended leg pushes hip caudally at the same time (5th pelvic correction). These pelvic corrections force the M. quadratus lumborum to work. The following is happening:

1. The previously atrophic part of the lumbar musculature begins to work again and to develop powerfully.
2. The lumbar spine moves back to the midline again because the concavity is released from pressure.
3. The transverse processes of the lumbar vertebrae, from

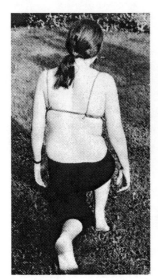

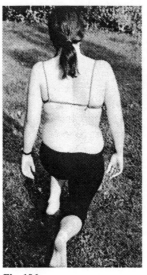

Fig. 105:
Left leg kneeling (incorrect).

Fig. 106:
Right leg kneeling (correct).

which the M. quadratus lumborum originates, rotate sideways – in some cases even a little backwards.

4. This musculature and all other muscles which have atrophied due to scoliotic torsion are now forced to support the weight of the upper trunk. They are activated and increase in *length and strength*.

The upper body, which is positioned diagonally, should now perform very tiny up-and-down movements so as to stimulate the inactive lumbar muscles specifically. It is always better to perform tiny movements than large, impressive-looking ones that are incorrect.

A glance in the mirror will immediately indicate that the 'shoulder countermove' (Fig. 107) is now required in addition.

However, what has been described above is just the starting position. Next come the rotational angular breathing movements with the deliberate lowering of the diaphragm in each case.

Each strengthening exercise should be followed by a break to allow recovery.

Patients with four-curve scoliosis exercise these inactive waist muscles differently (section C. VII, Exercises to correct the lumbosacral curvature and scoliotic pelvis), while still making the inactive waist muscles work.

This exercise rapidly produces a good muscular balance of the entire musculature below the thoracic convexity. In this corrected starting position, the different orthopaedic RAB techniques may be applied, beginning at the vertices of the wedges. Simultaneously, the trunk segments above and below are counter-held and shoulder countertraction is applied (Figs. 44, 107, and 108).

Exception: (Fig. 109). If the main curvature is very low, extending into the lumbar region, there is no atrophic musculature below the rib hump. Therefore these muscles do not have to be activated. They are supported by a pole which the patient pushes with the hand of the concave side into the floor. Thus the concavity is opened and space is created for corrective breathing.

3. ERECTOR TRUNCI (M. LONGISSIMUS DORSI; M. ILIOCOSTALIS), THE BACK EXTENSORS (FIG. 111 AND 112)

These are two overlapping longitudinal muscles, located on both sides of the spine. The M. iliocostalis is divided into lumbar, thoracic and cervical segments. The M. longissimus dorsi is divided into M. longissimus dorsi, M. longissimus cevices, and M. longissimus capitis.

Contracting the erector trunci bilaterally results in an elongation of the spine which pushes the ribs forwards (elongation of the thoracic spine). Unilateral contraction of the M. iliocostalis can also produce lateral flexion of the rib cage. In the case of scoliosis, these two muscles are also out of balance. Their activity and length differ on the two sides. In the case of thoracic scoliosis with a convexity on the right (Fig. 113), the left lumbar extensors have to hold the upper body, which is shifted over to the right. Due to overstretching, this muscle can no longer fulfill its function and allows the lumbar curvature to increase and the ribs to shift more and more ventrally.

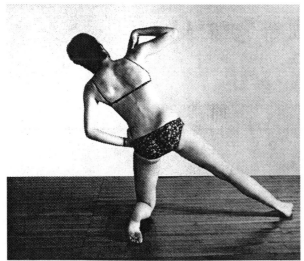

Fig. 107

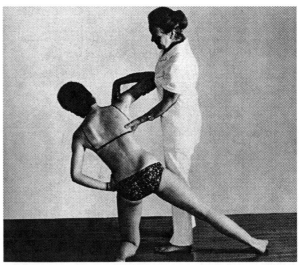

Fig. 108

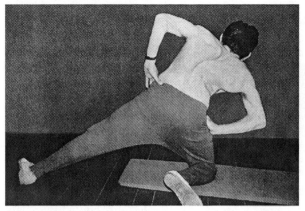

Fig. 109

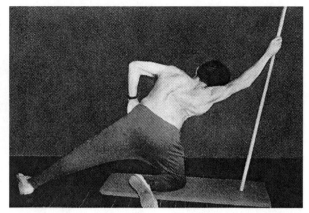

Fig. 110

The 'rib valley' may also appear due to insufficiency of the lumbar part of the M. erector trunci. Insertions of this muscle – the ribs on the concave side – can now shift ventrally.

The insufficient thoracic part on the right side cannot compensate in the long run (weight of the head, neck and shoulder girdle hanging over to the left), and gives

way to the ribs on the convex side to move backwards. The situation is similar in the cervical region. Compensatory bending of the cervical spine to the right overstretches the left cervical part of this muscle. Weakened by pathological overstretching, this muscle will also not be able to uphold the weight of the head in the long run and it will not be able to counteract curvature of the cer-

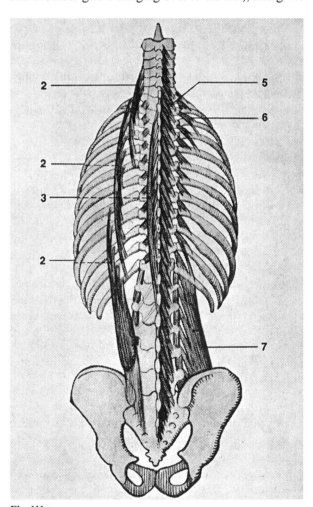

Fig. 111:
2 = m. iliocostalis
3 = m. spinalis
5 = m. rotators
6 = m. levator costae
7 = m- quadratus lumborum

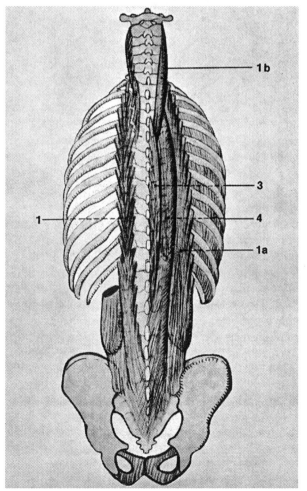

Fig. 112:
1a = m. longissimus dorsi
1b = m. longissimus cervicis
3 = m. spinalis
4 = m. multifidus

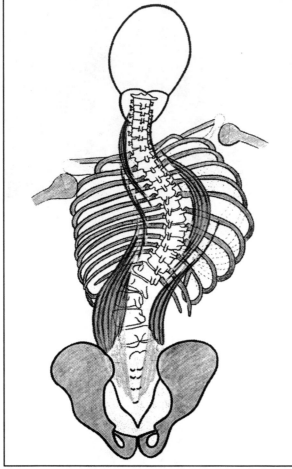

Fig. 113
The torsion relationships of the scoliotic spine, with resultant strengthening of the muscles on the convex side. These left lumbar spinal erector muscles are overly strong, thus the right thoracic group becomes stronger as well, and finally the left cervical group, resulting in a typical three-curve scoliosis posture. (Drawing: Lehnert-Schroth).

vical spine. The goal of our exercises has to be reversal of the scoliotic balance of the body. We start with correction of the lumbar and pelvic region, and strengthen the intrinsic part of M. erector trunci because of its ability to derotate the lumbar spine. This activates the left part of M. erector trunci because it is now in an almost normal pre-stretched position. This allows corrective static changes to the posture.

The right-sided thoracic part of this muscle can, with the help of RAB, move the ribs on the convex side ventrally and thus the concave-sided ribs dorsally. Be careful not to enhance flatback, and always exercise into extension and elongation to make derotation possible.

Shortened parts of this muscle on the left side are stretched by spreading the ribs and then using RAB to make space for the ventrally sunken ribs and to enable the thoracic lordosis to move dorsally.

Exercise treatment has the goal of creating muscular balance in all segments. We start with the lumbar region, then the cranial segments follow automatically.

As mentioned above, exercise always starts with active elongation, which leads automatically to deflexion

and creates room for derotation of the pelvis, ribcage and shoulder girdle. All corrective measures are then stabilized by a final 'muscle mantle', a firm contraction of all thoracic muscles. In the end, all muscles are strengthened, those on the concave side and those on the convex.

Continuous repetition facilitates corrected posture. The observation point may be the septum of the M. latissimus. It shows activation during the stabilization phase on both sides, and demonstrates that the overstretched and shortened lateral musculature is activated to achieve its physiological length. The left-sided lumbar part of the erector trunci holds the laterally shifted trunk and has a static holding function.

The same muscle is shortened on the right side.

Looking at the intrinsic lumbar parts of the M. erector spinae (Figs. 113, 127 and 128), we see that it is overstretched in the right-sided lumbar region and shortened on the left because of its dorsoventral direction from pelvic crest to the transverse processes. One may continue to theorise: it might be that the intrinsic musculature does not show either shortening or overstretching because of the many ligaments. This seems logical because of its dorsoventral direction. The fact is: the right sided lumbar part is shortened and needs to be elongated or stretched. The right-sided thoracic part of the erector trunci holds the shoulder girdle, which shifts over to the concave side. This is especially the case when weight is carried on one side.

The same muscle on the right side is shortened.

The left-sided cervical part of the erector trunci holds the head, which hangs over to the right. This muscle also has a static function in this overstretched position. On the right, these muscles have shortened. Reversal of these faulty static relationships must begin in the lower segment by creating opposite relationships. We strengthen and activate the static function of the right-side lumbar part of the erector trunci.

During the exercise, this muscle should activate more on one side than on the other. This means a correction across the midline, or overcorrection. The patient has to develop a strong 'muscle mantle'.

Exercise treatment reproduces muscular balance in all segments, starting at the lumbar region. Other segments follow automatically.

Exercise influencing all segments correctively: "Rotational sitting" (Fig. 115)

Omit in the case of four-curve scoliosis. Sit on a chair. Leg on the thoracal convex side is extended backwards and rotated so the instep of the foot touches the floor. This heel pushes backwards and downwards. The other leg in front, knee bent, forming a right angle. Upper body leaning (not bending!) forwards forming one line with the extended leg. Bodyweight rests on the hip of the concave side. A cushion in front of the hip on the convex side (these are all 5 pelvic corrections!).

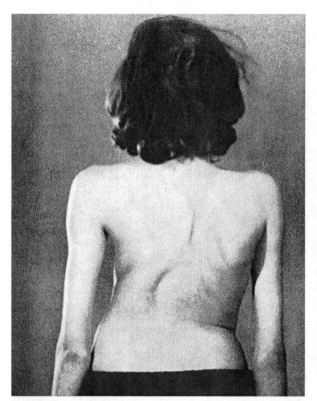

Fig. 114
14-year-old girl with right-sided dorsal kyphoscoliosis and a markedly twisted compensatory lumbar curve. Lumbar surface ratio 1:2.

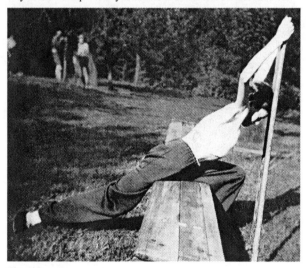

Fig. 115
The same patient performing rotational sitting. This exercise is not used for four-curve scoliosis.

The upper body leans obliquely to the concave side without narrowing it (this strengthens inactive musculature below the thoracic convexity). The head pulls into the same direction (a compensation for cervical scoliosis); the chin is turned to the convex side (activating unilateral weak neck musculature - intensified by weight carrying activity). Gives derotation impulse to the cervical spine. Fig. 114 shows clearly how far the lumbar spine has shifted from the midline. Fig. 116 shows 1) the lumbar spine approaching the midline and 2) activation of the lumbar segment of the erector trunci. Fig. 117 shows

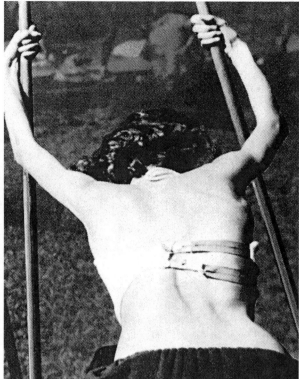

Fig. 116
The same patient doing the same exercise viewed from behind. Lumbar surface ratio: 2/5:3/5.

severe scoliosis in a 24-year-old female patient with very restricted movement and VC. Her left side is completely atrophied anteriorly, laterally and posteriorly. The very pronounced rib hump depresses the lumbar musculature on the right as well as the false ribs, and creates a deep furrow.

The sitting position described above is only a starting position for RAB, which always begins in the concave areas (vertices of wedges) and is combined with conscious depression of the diaphragm:

1. Convex side: floating ribs sideways and upward, and backward and upward (laterally and cranially, dorsally and cranially).
2. Concave side: sideways and upward and backward and upward.
3. Convex side, ventral: forward and upward (ventrally and cranially).
4. Subaxillary ribs on the convex side: forward and upward with counterhold of aligned shoulder girdle in a horizontal direction – obliquely outward, upward and backward (the shoulder countertraction, Fig. 44). Shoulder girdle is rotated *en bloc* against the rib cage.

Attention: shoulder girdle
During these exercises the trunk has to lean towards the concave side at all times and to be widened or 'opened'. There is the danger of pulling with the shoulder on the concave side. This is *not necessary* and in most cases even wrong. Forced lifting of the shoulder girdle will

51

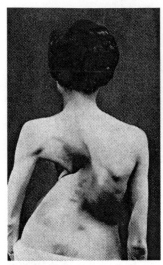

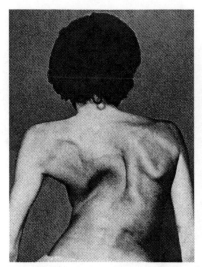

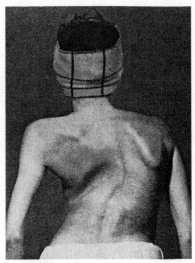

Fig. 117: Very severe scoliosis; 24-year-old patient.

Fig. 118: Same patient after three courses of treatment (3 months each).

Fig. 119: The same patient after 4 in-patient courses of treatment.

create a cervical curve automatically. The concavity is widened by breathing into it and keeping the width by isometric tension: During rotational sitting, for example, the arm of the concave side pushes against the back of the seat or a table after correction of all three trunk segments. The shoulder is not lifted, but has to be brought forwards actively. RAB moves the concave ribs apart and backwards and upwards this lifts the shoulder This way they form a holding and supporting posterior wall (Figs. 58 and 120).

4. M. ILIOPSOAS (FIG. 125 AND 126)

The muscle consists of the M. psoas major, M. psoas minor and the M. iliacus. We believe that these muscles are mainly responsible for derotating the lumbar vertebrae during our exercises. Kapandji gives a vivid description of this muscle and its effect in healthy people:
"As M. iliopsoas, it is the strongest flexor in any position. The M. psoas major's longitudinal fibres have a great lifting capacity. This muscle is positioned ventrally to the M. quadratus lumborum. It has two origins: a deep portion at the transverse processes of the lumbar vertebrae, a superficial one at the vertebral body of T12 and the lumbar vertebrae; aimed at the upper and lower edges of two neighbouring bodies of vertebrae, as well as the corresponding disc, which serves as the area of origin. The muscle pulls obliquely downward and laterally into the pelvis. It nestles against the inside of the hip bone. The ligament of the muscle fastens to the tip of the trochanter minor (inside of the thigh). When the hip joint is fixed (the fixed point at the thigh), this muscle has a great impact on the lumbar spine. It effects lateral movement to the side of the contraction and at the same time rotation to the opposite side. Since the muscle originates at the apex of the lumbar lordosis, it also creates ventral flexion in relation to the pelvis. It creates hyperlordosis in the lumbar spine".

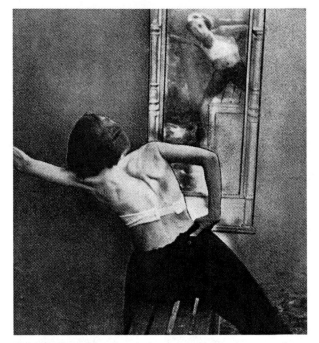

Fig. 120: The above patient during exercise using mirror control.

What good is all this theory? Everything is different in a scoliotic body. There are synergistic and antagonistic effects in the abdominal musculature and autonomous back musculature. Thus it is impossible to describe the effect of only one muscle during our exercises. There is a derotational momentum due to the muscle attachment at the frontal region of the vertebral body. In the following isometric exercises, this muscle does tremendous work while being elongated (as in the 'muscle cylinder' exercise). This may neutralize the hyperlordotic effect in the lumbar convexity. The train of thought described here cannot completely explain the corrective effect. There is no better teacher than observed facts. (Figs. 548 – 565)

52

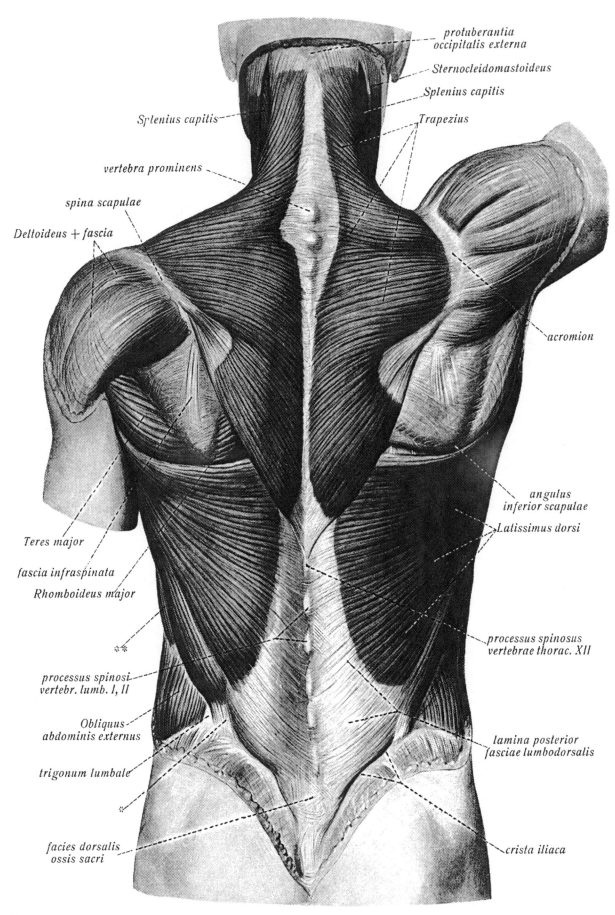

protuberantia
occipitalis externa

Sternocleidomastoideus

Splenius capitis

Splenius capitis

Trapezius

vertebra prominens

spina scapulae

Deltoideus + fascia

acromion

angulus
inferior scapulae

Latissimus dorsi

Teres major

fascia infraspinata

Rhomboideus major

processus spinosus
vertebrae thorac. XII

processus spinosi
vertebr. lumb. I, II

Obliquus
abdominis externus

lamina posterior
fasciae lumbodorsalis

trigonum lumbale

facies dorsalis
ossis sacri

crista iliaca

Fig. 121

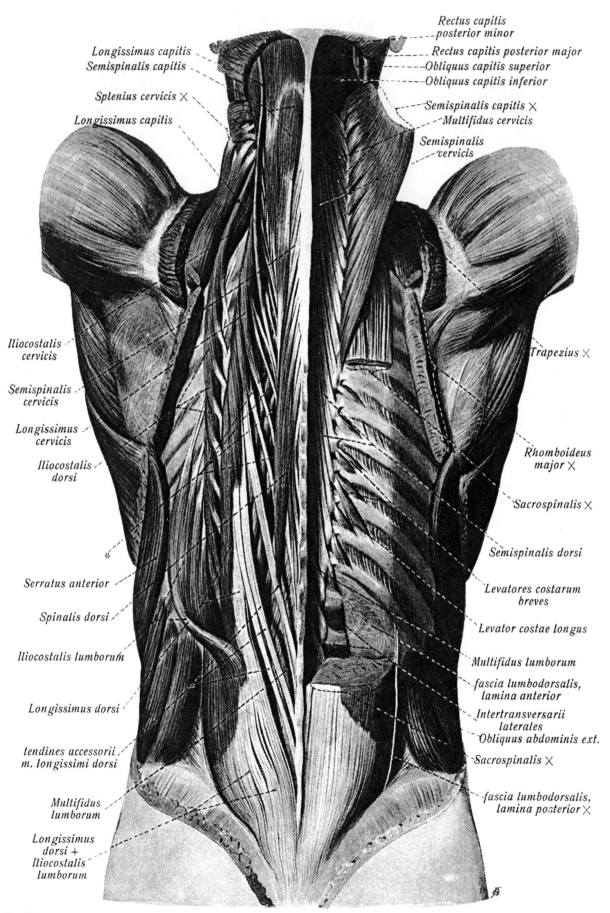

Longissimus capitis
Semispinalis capitis

Splenius cervicis ✕

Longissimus capitis

Rectus capitis
posterior minor
Rectus capitis posterior major
Obliquus capitis superior
Obliquus capitis inferior
Semispinalis capitis ✕
Multifidus cervicis
Semispinalis
cervicis

Iliocostalis
cervicis

Semispinalis
cervicis

Longissimus
cervicis

Iliocostalis
dorsi

✳

Serratus anterior

Spinalis dorsi

Iliocostalis lumborum

Longissimus dorsi

tendines accessorii
m. longissimi dorsi

Multifidus
lumborum

Longissimus
dorsi +
Iliocostalis
lumborum

Trapezius ✕

Rhomboideus
major ✕

Sacrospinalis ✕

Semispinalis dorsi

Levatores costarum
breves

Levator costae longus

Multifidus lumborum

fascia lumbodorsalis,
lamina anterior

Intertransversarii
laterales
Obliquus abdominis ext.

Sacrospinalis ✕

fascia lumbodorsalis,
lamina posterior ✕

Fig. 122

54

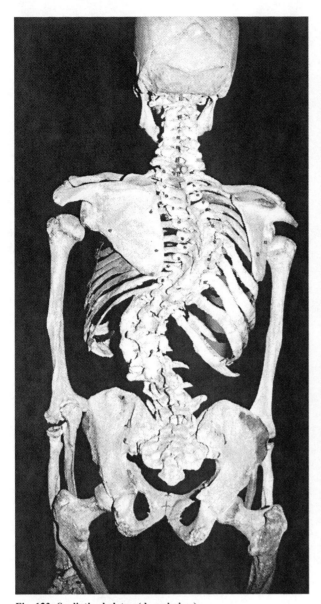

Fig. 123: Scoliotic skeleton (dorsal view)
Nerves for the autonomous muscles come directly from the spinal cord and innervate directly: M. iliocostalis, M. longissimus, M. spinalis, Mm. rotatores, Mm. intertransversarii, and M. erector spinae. Comparing the above figures, one can visualise how these innermost muscles must have been pulled and twisted in the scoliotic body, and the nerves are irritated. Gymnastic exercises that derotate the thorax against the pelvic and shoulder girdles may well free these stretched or pinched nerves and relieve the patient's pain.

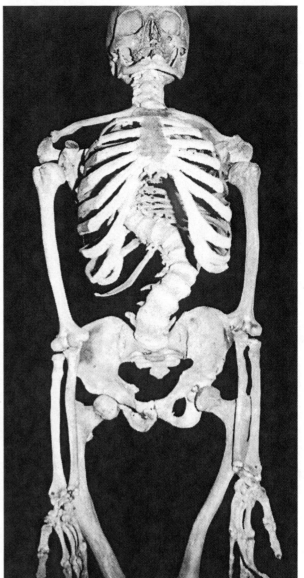

Fig. 124: Scoliotic skeleton (frontal view)

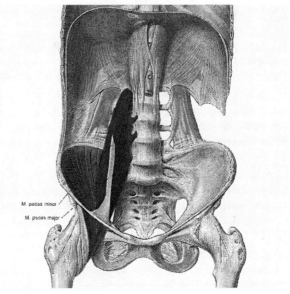

Fig. 125: Frontal view

5. INTRINSIC MUSCULATURE (FIGS. 127 AND 128)

Macintosh and Bogduk (1987) found that the M. longissimus dorsi and M. iliocostalis (erector spinae) have an intrinsic lumbar part. The intrinsic lumbar musculature of M. erector spinae originates on the dorsal parts of the iliac crests and the dorsal upper spina, attaching to transverse processes of the lumbar vertebrae. In lumbar scoliosis, the spinous processes rotate toward the interior side of the arch (concavity). The transverse processes move ventrally on the concave side, thus increasing the distance from posterior iliac spine to the transverse pro-

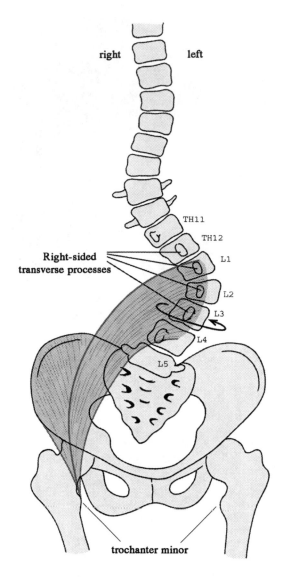

right   left

TH11
TH12
L1
L2
L3
L4
L5

Right-sided
transverse processes

trochanter minor

Fig. 126: frontal view (drawing S. Adler)

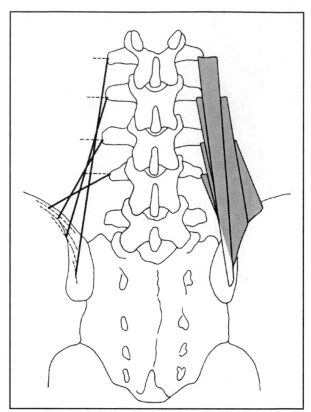

Fig. 127: Intrinsic lumbar parts of the M. erector spinae. Schematic representation of the lumbar fasciae of the M. iliocostalis lumborum. The broken lines mark the extension of the areas of attachment.

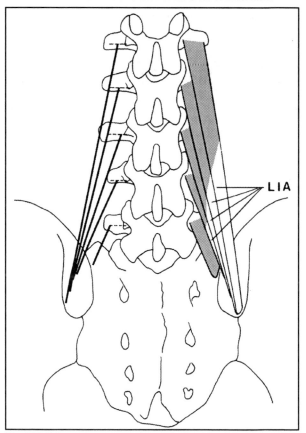

LIA

Fig. 128: Schematic representation of the fascicle of the M. longissimus thoracis pars lumborum. Fascicles 1–4 have long caudal tendons which form the lumbar aponeurosis. The broken lines show the cranial attachment.

cess of the lumbar vertebra. This means stretching of this muscle group on the concave side and shortening on the convex side.

We may draw the following conclusions for Schroth corrections from these biomechanical facts. It has been shown that lateral stabilization (as in lateral flexion, for example) is created significantly more by lateral parts of the autonomous back musculature than by medial parts (M. multifidus and rotatores). Looking at the muscle cylinder exercise, we observe this when leaning over toward the concave side. Activity of intrinsic lumbar musculature of the M. erector spinae increases more than that of M. multifidus at the same height on the convex side. Thus this muscle will untwist lumbar transverse processes which have been twisted ventrally on the convex side and, in addition, straighten the lumbar curvature. We find no such an oblique direction of the M. erector spinae in the thoracic region, but rather a more parallel alignment to the axis organ. Increased activity on the thoracic convex side is visible here as well.

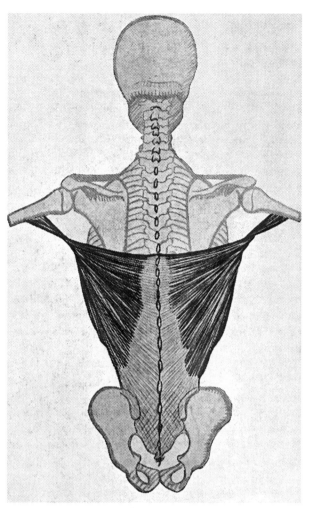

Fig. 129

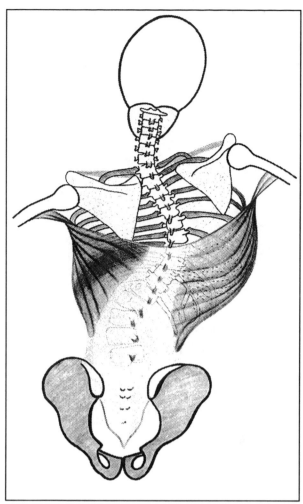

Fig. 130

According to biomechanical facts, we find here a tendency to lateral straightening of the curvature and a straightening of the thoracic convexity, above which the M. erector spinae is stretched. However, if torsion is too pronounced, the opposite effect may take place, if the thoracic convex-sided M. erector spinae pushes across the arch vertex on the thoracic concave side. In this case, preliminary corrections have to be made so that the origin and insertion points of the autonomous musculature are brought closer so that the above effect does not occur.

6. M. LATISSIMUS DORSI (FIGS. 129 AND 130)

This muscle originates from the spinous processes of T6–12, extends laterally and cranially, and has its point of attachment on the tuberculum minoris of the upper arm. It has a flat insertion at the lower inferior angle of the scapula by which the latter is held to the ribs. Through inactivity of musculature, the lower angle of the scapula does not receive pressure and can deviate backwards. A wing-shaped prominent scapula results (scapula alata).

In scoliosis (Fig. 130), this muscle is active only unilaterally or is shortened. On the side of the dorsal con-

cavity, it may press the lower angle of the scapula against the ribs in a way that it forces them to deviate forwards. Then, the upper border of the scapula becomes prominent posteriorly beyond the normal position. On the convex side, this muscle is overstretched and allows the ribs to sag backwards (Fig. 131). The lower angle of the scapula is lifted backwards and upwards, and the entire scapula turns in its upper part forwards. As the outer part of shoulder level has been brought forward, the rib hump increases in a way that its cranial part often lies horizontally (Figs. 17, 23). Due to the three torsions of the trunk, the septa of the M. latissimus dorsi are no longer lateral, but have deviated in the middle and lower trunk segments. The M. latissimus dorsi is short on the concave side and long on the convex side (Fig. 468).

Exercise treatment has to elongate the muscle on the concave side first, then activate it forcefully. On the convex side, it has to be forced to contract together with the M. serratus lateralis. This is only possible after correcting the three torsions of the trunk.

Exercise: Small cranial oscillatory movements upwards between two poles (Figs. 60, 61)
Sitting on the ischial tuberosities. Corrective cushions. Upper body leaning forward and sideways towards the

57

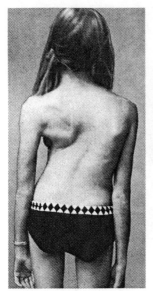
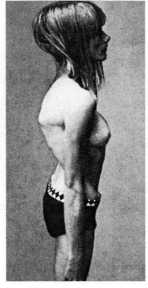

Fig. 131   Fig. 132

concave side. The patient's spine is straightened by continuous small wriggling movements, since a derotation of individual rotated trunk segments is only possible after straightening the trunk. Maintaining the corrected position of shoulder girdle, the poles are pushed into the ground. The oscillatory movements upwards (straightening of the back) have to be slow and allow intense concentration on the concave areas of the trunk. Only after this can RAB exercises begin. During exhalation this result is stabilized by isometric tension and a muscle mantle. The position is then correct for the next inhalation. The second side of the 'right angle' always runs

cranially to give the spinal column maximum length and elongation. Additionally, an occipital neck elongation musculature increases the straightening effect.

Having reached best possible height, the poles are pushed against the floor during exhalation. The pelvis might lift a bit from the floor. The corrected hip below the convexity should push forcefully towards the floor as well. Once the margin of the M. latissimus dorsi activates on both sides, the concave side is sufficiently stretched and the laterally overhanging convexity is tensed and contracted.

7. MM. SCALENI (FIG. 133)

The function of these muscles is to elevate the 1st and 2nd ribs onto which they insert. In kyphosis of the upper thoracic spine, they are partly inactive. Consequently, the first two ribs have lowered anteriorly, narrowing the apices of the lungs. The back deviates dorsally and cranially. The head sinks forward. The same is present in scoliosis, but is often worse on one side.

Exercise treatment has to train the Mm. scaleni to bring the upper chest forward and widen the apices of lungs again. Succeeding in this brings the protruding parts of the upper back forwards and flattens the kyphosis (Figs. 280-287).

Isometric head and neck elongation exercise

Omit in case of cervical kyphosis or flatback (Fig. 295). Supine position. Corrective cushions. The hollow parts of the back are brought in contact with the floor from caudal to cranial. This is done by performing small, oscillatory movements with the spine in combination with RAB. An additional occipital push elongates the cervical spine even further. During exhalation, the patient pushes the head and elbows against the floor. This contracts the upper back, and the shoulder girdle lifts slightly from the floor. At the same time, minimal contractions of the dorsal intercostal musculature ("pulling it together") are performed. A short resting period follows, then the exercise is repeated.

Additional Exercise: Figs 288-290

Same starting position as before, except the head is turned alternately to left and right. The patient soon notices which rotation is more difficult. That side is then exercised more often. In the case of scoliosis, the head has to be bent in continuation of the main curvature to the concave side, with the chin pointing to convex side. – There are exceptions.

This is an essential exercise and has to be practised in the supine position, sitting up, standing, and with or without wall resistance. The section on exercises shows more neck exercises aimed at individual muscles. Dur-

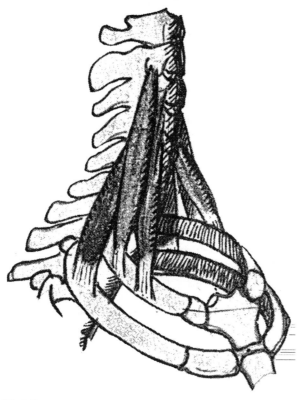

Fig. 133

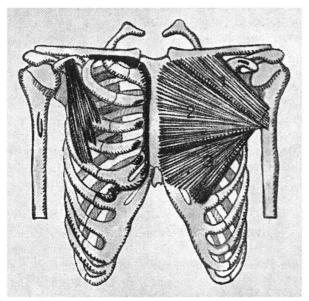

Fig. 134

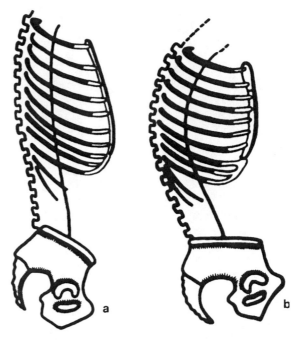

Fig. 135: Schematic representation of the skeleton: sitting on the ischial tuberosities.

Fig. 136: Sitting on the coccyx.

ing all exercises, the information given here should be taken into consideration. It is very important, since the position of the head is an essential element in good or bad posture. It makes the rib hump appear either larger or smaller. Uninterrupted transition of the thoracic spine to the cervical spine up to the occiput is of special importance.

8. PECTORAL MUSCLES (FIGS. 134, 589, 590)

The pectoral muscles pull shoulders forward, particularly in scoliosis, when antagonists (M. trapezius; Mm. rhomboidei) have lost their tone. The more the latter are weakened, the more the shoulder girdle is brought forward and the apices of lungs are inhibited.

Exercise treatment has to counteract this process. Only after the pectoral muscles have been lengthened sufficiently are the upper back muscles in a position to contract, because they are no longer restricted from the front (see Part C).

Exercise: The starting position is the low-sliding position (Fig. 81) Corrective cushions. Kneeling, thighs at right angles, trunk and arms in one line, stretched forwards, hands on the floor. In lumbar hyperlordosis, the pelvis is pulled back a little towards the feet (caudally). In order to stretch all pectoral muscle fibres, the extended arms glide gradually more and more sideways, reaching a diagonal position. The position of the arms which produces the strongest stretching effect is maintained. The patient performs small oscillatory movements to elongate the spine.

In scoliosis, the trunk leans towards the concave side. The hip below the thoracic convexity pulls caudally. Circles are performed with the narrow front (especially by subaxillary ribs). Omit this exercise in case of flatback.

9. COCCYX AND ISCHIAL TUBEROSITIES (FIG. 135 – 143)

It is not unimportant how someone with scoliosis or malposture sits, because the visual impression they make depends on this. The size of the rib hump may seem larger. Sitting on the coccyx might round the lumbar spine, but it also has an effect on the back. It is the same as bending over. The abdomen protrudes forwards, the chest sinks ventrally, and breathing is inhibited. Sitting on the ischial tuberosities causes a more upright position, leading to elongation of the spine and flattening of the convexities.

Sitting on the coccyx indicates fatigue of the body and lack of support. Asking the patient to sit straight up will result in straightening for a short period only, and it will be very tense. Sitting on the ischial tuberosities, on the contrary, is done without strain, as it is a natural position. Figs. 142 and 143 show sitting on the coccyx and ischial tuberosities in scoliosis, viewed from the back:

a) in the presence of a dorsally overhanging rib hump, the spinal curvatures and torsions are increased

b) the spine in a more upright position with curvatures straightened.

These are reasons why the patient should be careful about sitting posture at table, in school, at work, or during leisure time. Since we sit for long periods, it is obvious that the sitting position is important for the back. Each minute of wrong sitting or crouching may be compared with

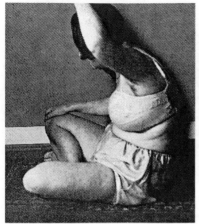

Fig. 137: 40-year-old woman. Sitting on the coccyx produces a kyphotic lumbar spine and kyphosis in the thoracic region.

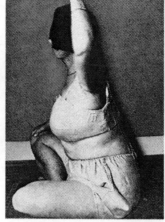

Fig. 138: Sitting on the ischial tuberosities produces straightening of the entire spine.

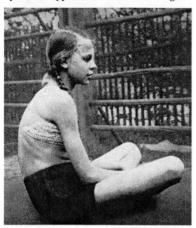

Fig. 139:

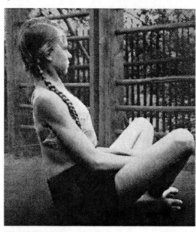

Fig. 140: Wrong: too tensed.

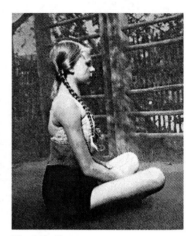

Fig. 141: Correct.

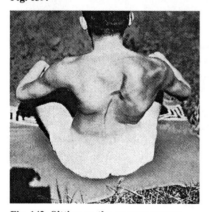

Fig. 142: Sitting on the coccyx: wrong.

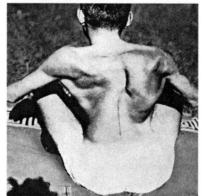

Fig. 143: Sitting on the ischial tuberosities: Correct.

an inadequate exercise. Poor posture of many years cannot be changed if one falls back into a 'relief' position. It facilitates wrong movement and old postural patterns. These patterns have to be changed immediately. It is quite easy because there are 'lifting' forces within intervertebral discs which help straightening up. Once the patient has a clear picture of this, the wrong posture will be avoided at all times. Striving for an upright position will lead to better health and strength.

The patient has to live with scoliosis. It is important to overcome this handicap now and strive for an upright posture which will eventually influence the spinal column, and this is of most importance while sitting.

60

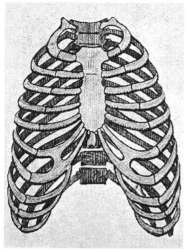

Fig. 144: Thorax during exhalation.

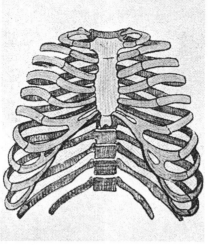

Fig. 145: Thorax during inhalation

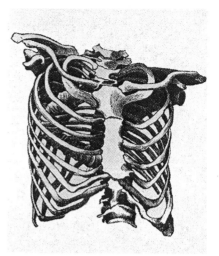

Fig. 146: Scoliotic thorax.

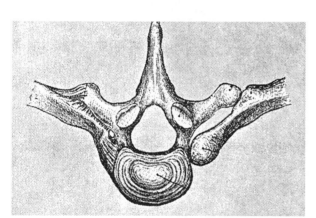

Fig. 147: Attachment of the ribs at a thoracic vertebra viewed from below. The left shows the ligaments.

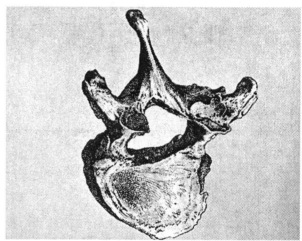

Fig. 148: Results of changed pressure and pulling in severe kyphoscoliosis with soft bone tissue.

10. FLOATING RIBS (FIGS. 150, 152, 477)

Ribs 11 and 12 end laterally in soft tissue musculature. They run almost horizontally. In severe scoliosis, these two ribs reach vertically into the abdomen because the soft tissue musculature does not offer support and is atrophic. The weight of the overhanging rib hump produces a deep fold. The lumbar spine is displaced and pushed over to the opposite side.

Exercise treatment has to return these two ribs to their designated place to enable them to fill the waist segment below the rib hump and to support.

Exercise: (Figs. 150 and 152) fingers push into the fold beneath rib hump until they feel ribs. They offer resistance, against which the patient breathes sideways and upwards while lowering the diaphragm. Fig. 152 demonstrates how spinal curvatures straighten. The head touches the pole above it. Variation: exercise with splayed leg and laterally leaning trunk (Fig. 152).

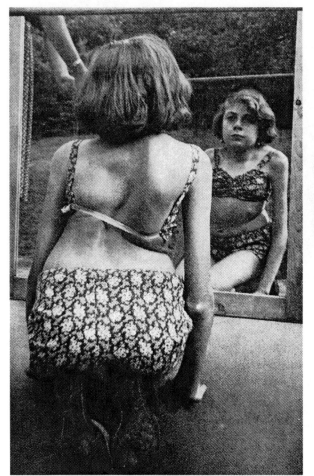

Fig. 149

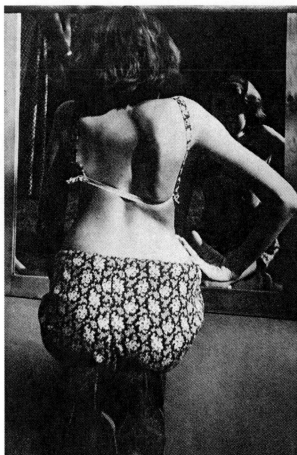

Fig. 150

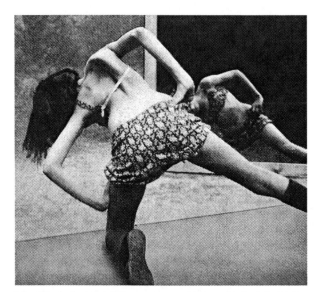

Fig. 151 Lateral inclination: unfavourable because the left side becomes narrow

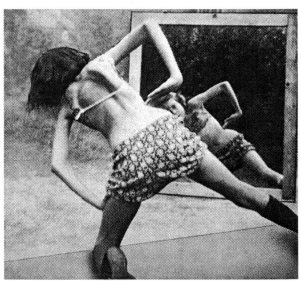

Fig. 152 Favourable because both sides are being elongated.

IV. Summary of the physical corrections using the Schroth method for three-curve scoliosis

The term 'three-curve' originates from the three shifted blocks of the trunk that each pull the spine to their side. The basis of correction is always a properly aligned pelvis and correction of the body statics in all three planes.

First pelvic correction

The entire pelvis is moved backwards, which constitutes a correction of statics in the sagittal plane.

Second pelvic correction

Lift anterior pelvic rim; pelvis horizontal. This achieves delordosation of lumbar spine and correction in the sagittal plane about the frontal axis.

Third pelvic correction

Pulling in the prominent hip on the concave side contracts the musculature in the area of the major trochanter. The result is lateral shifting of pelvis and correction of statics in the frontal plane. If there is no prominent hip, the third correction is omitted.

Fourth pelvic correction

Pelvis on convex side moved backwards, hip on concave side forwards. This corrects pelvic distortion and the twisted lumbar spine, and results in correction in the transverse plane around the longitudinal axis.

Fifth pelvic correction

Heel on the convex side is pushed against the ground. This lowers the pelvis on the convex side, deflexes the lumbar spine with accompanying derotation of lumbar spine, and results in correction around the sagittal axis. Standing, it is necessary to perform these pelvic corrections with the weight of the body on the leg of the concave side. If the weight is not shifted to one side, it is not possible to accomplish satisfactory correction of the scoliotic statics in the frontal plane.

Once the pelvic position has been corrected, attention is paid to active elongation of the spine. This is achieved by lateral deflexion of the thoracic curve towards the concave side. This is followed by active derotation of the thoracic spinal region, supported by contraction of the intercostal muscles on the convex side. RAB is then performed: forwards and upwards on the convex side, and backwards and upwards on the concave side.

Counterrotation to achieve correction has to be performed with the shoulder girdle: the convex-sided shoulder is moved backwards and the concave-sided one forwards (exactly like the pelvis). Additional shifting of the entire shoulder girdle to the convex side is also necessary (shoulder countertraction). The corrective effect is on the upper spinal curve and also on body statics in the frontal plane.

The culmination of the corrective procedure lies in an orderly alignment of the head, which in logical sequence is inclined towards the thoracic concave side to deflex the cervical spine, and the chin is turned to the thoracic convex side to derotate the cervical spine. Thus the thoracic spinal curvature is further extended.

The optimal preconditions for RAB are not present until all of these corrections have been made. The pelvic corrections therefore constitute the basis of the Schroth rotational breathing procedure.

Using directional breathing in this way, the floating ribs on the convex side are moved sideways and upwards and backwards and upwards (laterally and cranially and dorsally and cranially). This is accompanied by lowering the diaphragm. The procedure is the same on the concave side. Sunken ribs are moved by breathing.

Breathing in this way not only corrects the deformed thorax but also the spine. The individual vertebrae are physically pulled into an almost horizontal position medially and are rotated by dorsal tension of the ribs connected to the transverse processes. It is also an important correction of flatback. After achieving correction and the appropriate starting position, the entire corrected system is stabilized as follows:
a)   by isometric tension
b)   reflex holding of muscles
c)   isotonic tension.

The corrections are monitored continually by the patient and therapist using mirrors and by physical sensations. If necessary, the corrections should be repeated. In the prone, supine and lateral positions, correction is supported by corrective cushions. (Fig. 574)

We use:

A) IN THE PRONE POSITION

The starting position is with the legs straight backwards or 5–10° towards the concave side, which stretches the concavity below the rib hump.

A footstool under the pelvis (not under the thighs) shifts the pelvis back, making the first pelvic correction in the sagittal plane.

A corrective cushion under the hip on the convex side results in the fourth pelvic correction, detorsion of the lumbar spine, and thus a correction in the transverse plane.

A corrective cushion under frontal rib hump on the concave side to derotate the middle segment of the trunk and spine achieves a correction in the transverse plane.

A corrective cushion under the convex-side elbow achieves derotation of the shoulder girdle and upper spinal curvature, which is simultaneously a correction in the transverse plane.

B) IN THE SUPINE POSITION

The starting position is always with the legs pulled towards the body, achieving a delordosation of the lumbar spine and support for the second pelvic correction (in the sagittal plane).

A corrective cushion under the hip of the concave side (dorsally) achieves the fourth pelvic correction (transverse plane).

Place a wedge-shaped cushion under the dorsal convexity (lower angle of the scapula) to derotate the thoracic segment including the spine, creating correction in the transverse plane and support for correction in the sagittal plane. Passive stretching of ventral chest parts. Omit in case of flatback.

Place a corrective cushion under the scapula on the concave side to derotate the shoulder girdle and to support correction in the sagittal and transverse planes in case of a shoulder hump. It has a corrective influence on rotation of the upper spinal curve.

Place a wedge-shaped cushion, if necessary, under the lumbar hump to reverse lumbar convexity by derotation in the transverse plane and deflexion in the frontal plane.

C) IN THE LATERAL POSITION

Starting position: as a rule, always lying on the concave side for correction of body statics in the frontal plane and for deflexion of all spinal curves.

Place a corrective cushion laterally against the hip for the third pelvic correction. A corrective cushion placed against the shoulder girdle deflexes the upper spinal curve and corrects lateral shifting of the shoulder girdle.

The upper body is inclined forwards to make the first pelvic correction.

The corrective cushions derotate and deflex primarily the individual trunk segments. Secondly, they also affect the corresponding spinal deformities, similar to the principle of using a brace. Manufacturers have taken up this idea and have incorporated spacers into their braces.

Here again, it is necessary to point out that the patient has to be aware of the scoliotic patterns of the trunk described to be able to perform the necessary measures willingly and adequately. This demands high standards of the therapist. The advice to practise in front of and between mirrors should be taken seriously. The exercises aim to achieve a new corrected posture founded on quite a different structure from that which the patient is used to and which leads to a new feeling for joints and muscles and a different awareness of the body. Self motivation and complete concentration (compliance) are required.

V. Theoretical reflections on four-curve scoliosis with lumbosacral curvature and its correction

Different types of scoliosis exist: one-curve thoracic or lumbar scoliosis. Different double-curve forms of idiopathic scoliosis. Three-curve scoliosis is quite frequent. And it seems that different scoliotic deformities have developed over the past few decades. From the 1970s onwards, we started to see more cases of scoliosis with a separate lumbosacral curve. As far as we are concerned, a spinal curve in this position was a new manifestation in scoliosis, and therefore we called it the fourth curve. These patients also show a structural deformity of the lower vertebral bodies. L4 and L5 tilt laterally, sometimes more than 40°; the reasons for this are still unknown. In some patients, L5 shows unilaterally enlarged articular processes and bony intermediate parts that are responsible for this curvature. The affected intervertebral discs are wedge-shaped, and this further increases the curvature. The spine now tries to balance above the centre of gravity and forms additional curves: the lumbar, thoracic and cervical curves. The hip on the convex side is most often very prominent (Figs. 153 and 154) and shifts cranially and dorsally.

A very specific exercise for this form of scoliosis has proved to be effective. The emphasis of the exercise must not be too far to the concave side and should predominantly involve vertical, upward movement. Otherwise, the lumbosacral curve would be pulled in the same direction and the curvature would be increased. Leaning too much to the convex side would further increase the lumbar curvature. This may lead to the patient making very little use of the lateral lumbar musculature. Imagination, directed breathing, manual help, mirror control and the therapist are therefore very important.

There are major differences between four-curve scoliosis and three-curve scoliosis (the following examples refer to thoracic, right-sided scoliosis).

In a typical three-curve scoliosis, the upper trunk overhangs to the right. The weight of the body rests on the right leg. The pelvis moves to the left, increasing the impression of convexity. The statics of the body are incorrect.

In typical four-curve scoliosis, the lumbosacral curvature is pulled into the direction of the sacrum and coccyx, since the trunk has shifted in the lumbar spine and pelvis segments laterally (to the right). The bodyweight rests on the left leg and the trunk leans to the left. This forces the right hip to shift laterally to the right. Usually the lumbar convexity is very large and the angle of the thoracic curvature is smaller.

In three-curve and four-curve scoliosis, the trunk segments deviate laterally and are also rotated dorsally, which is also the case in this caudal segment.

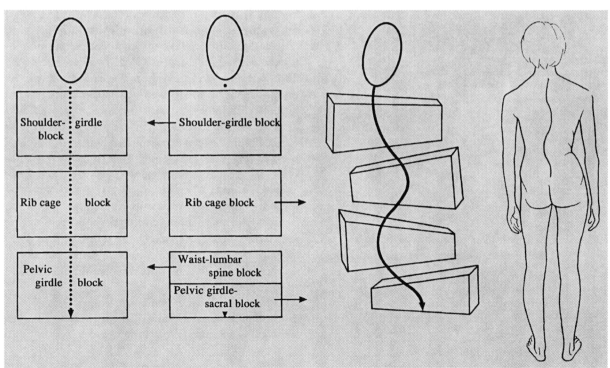

Fig. 153: The four-curve scoliosis.
Imaginary division of the trunk into three 'blocks' that shift and turn against each other in scoliosis. In the case of four-curve scoliosis with an additional curvature in the lumbar spine, the pelvic block is divided into a lumbar and pelvic section. The thoracic sections have shifted laterally and dorsally. The lateral shifted trunk areas are simultaneously turned backwards, as seen in this diagram.

65

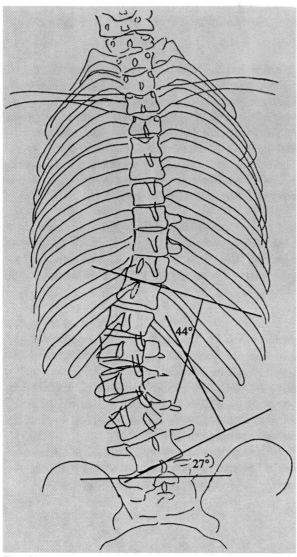

Fig. 154:
X-ray of entire spine. The pelvic shift and twisting is obvious: The right wing of the ilium seems larger than the left. This indicates that the right one has turned dorsally (Fig. 38).

2 ····	Lumbar section	4 ------	Shoulder girdle
1 ——	Pelvic girdle	3 –·–	Rib cage

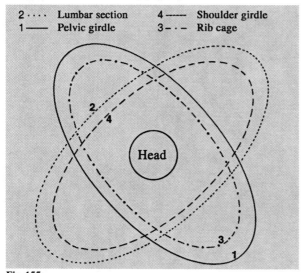

Fig. 155:
View from above: the pelvis (1) and rib cage (3) have turned in the same direction. The lumbar section (2) and shoulder girdle (4) have also turned, but in opposite directions.

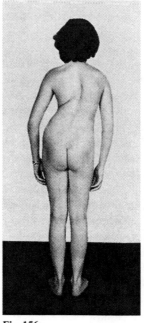

Fig. 156:
11-year-old girl with idiopathic three-curve scoliosis (cervical left, thoracic right, lumbar left). The bodyweight rests on the right leg. The lumbar curvature leads vertically into the sacrum. This form is often called 'one-curve' scoliosis.

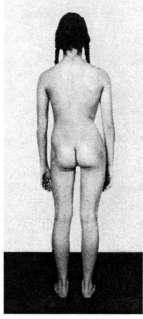

Fig. 157:
15-year-old girl with static-related four-curve scoliosis (complicated because of a shortened left leg as a result of a hip luxation): cervical left, thoracic right, lumbar left, lumbosacral right. The body rests on the left leg.

The following examples of exercises show the subtle but effective powers of the Schroth method in activating positive changes in the patient's statics. They can be practised in different starting positions, but always aim to derotate body segments shifted laterally or ventrally. They aim to align the body in the vertical above the body's centre of gravity – which means redistribution of the body's statics.

The bodyweight must be on both legs in general (sitting or standing). Placing the weight on the leg of the thoracic concave side – as required for three-curve scoliosis – would force the hip below the thoracic convexity further outwards. There is no specific rule for this – the most important part of all exercises is alignment of the lumbar spine and the prominent hip inwards. The first and second pelvic corrections are naturally also practised. In the case of a large lumbar hump, the frontal pelvic rim may only be raised to the middle position, of course.

An up-to-date X-ray should be studied repeatedly to guide thoughts and aid visualising corrective possibilities and the direction of the exercises.

Additional symptoms found in four-curve scoliosis (Figs. 161 and 162)
We checked 115 patients with a lumbosacral counter-curvature in our clinic for the following clinical signs:

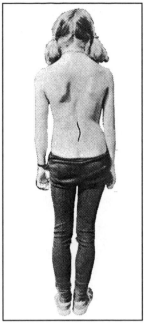

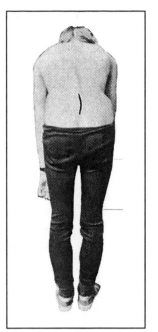

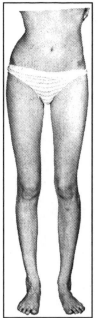

Fig. 158:
As the pelvis is shifted towards the right side, the caudal spine also moves in this direction.

Fig. 159:
Anteflexion allows diagnosis of a sacral countercurvature (see spinous processes).

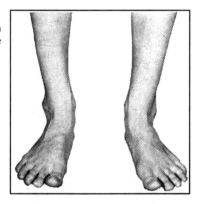

Fig. 160:
The protruding hip is the most obvious sign on clinical observation.

Table 3: Protruding hip

Total	thoracic convex	no findings
115 Pat.	109	6
percent	94.7	5.2

right scoliosis	right prominent	no findings
101 Pat.	96	5
percent	95.05	4.95

left scoliosis	left prominent	no findings
14 Pat.	13	1
percent	92.86	7.14

1. Pes valgus (increased on the side of the thoracic concavity)
2. Possible internal rotation of the leg (more marked on the thoracic concave side)
3. Pelvic prominence on the thoracic convex side
4. Increased weight on the leg on the thoracic concave side
5. Unequal level of spinae (possible pelvic distortion)
6. Evaluation of walking pattern

87.8% had a thoracic convexity on the right, 12.2% on the left.

Direct signs of a lumbosacral countercurvature
(Fig. 157, 159)
The most striking characteristic of the clinical picture is pelvic prominence on the thoracic convex side. 96 patients showed this sign; 5 patients showed no lateral deviation. 13 of the patients with a thoracic convexity on the left showed a prominent hip on the left. 1 patient showed no deviation of the pelvis. Other pelvic malposition was less obvious.

Indirect signs of a lumbosacral countercurvature
(Figs. 160–163)
Pes valgus is found more often on the thoracic concave side (70.3%). 20.8% of patients had bilateral pes valgus. An apparent internal rotation of the leg on the concave side was present in 79.1% of patients. 5.2% showed

Fig. 161
Pes valgus, most often found on the side of the thoracic concavity.

Table 4: Pes valgus

Total	thoracic concave	thoracic convex	bilateral	no findings
115 Pat.	75	5	27	8
percent	65.21	4.34	23.47	6.95

right scoliosis	left	right	bilateral	no findings
101 Pat.	71	4	21	5
percent	70.29	3.96	20.80	4.95

left scoliosis	right	left	bilateral	no findings
14 Pat.	4	1	6	3
percent	28.57	7.14	42.86	21.43

Fig. 162 (left), Fig. 163 (right):
Inner rotation of the leg on the side of the thoracic concavity.

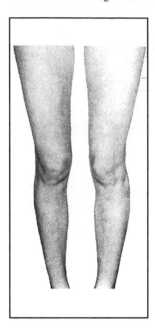
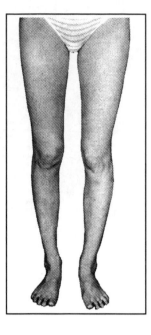

Total	thoracic concave	thoracic convex	bilateral	no findings
115 Pat.	91	6	2	16
percent	79.13	5.21	1.73	13.91

right scoliosis	left	right	bilateral	no findings
101 Pat.	83	4	1	13
percent	82.17	3.96	0.99	12.88

left scoliosis	right	left	bilateral	no findings
14 Pat.	8	2	1	3
percent	57.14	14.29	7.14	21.43

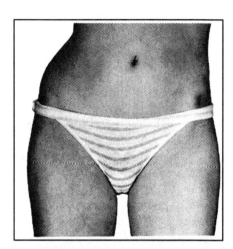

Fig. 164 a: The protruding hip is the most obvious sign on clinical observation.

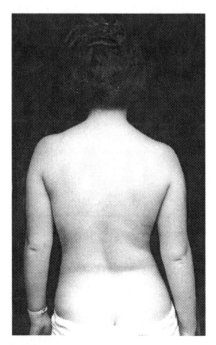

Fig. 164 b (left):
15-year-old girl, before treatment began.

Fig. 164 c (right):
The same patient after a treatment of
five weeks.

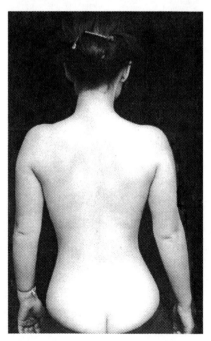

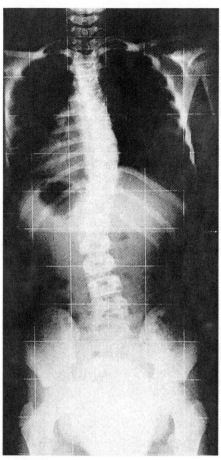

Fig. 166

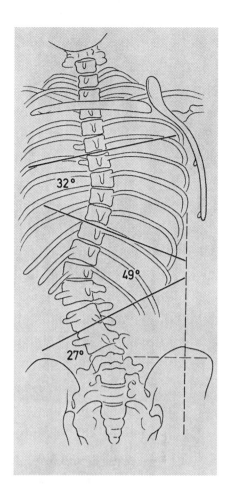

Fig. 165:
Shifting of the upper trunk to the thoracic concave side is clearly visible in the X-ray. A plumb line drawn from the outer ribs would pass outside the hip on the thoracic concave side, but would cut through the hip on the convex side.

increased internal rotation of the leg on the convex side. One patient had bilateral rotation. 13.9% had normal findings. We believe that interior rotation of the leg on the concave side is caused by a changed pelvic position. Due to forward rotation of the pelvis on the concave side, the acetabulum and thus the entire hip joint is turned forward. This is made worse by distortion of the crista of the ilium around the frontal-transverse axis.

Apparent pelvic distortion (Fig. 164)
Unequal level of the spinae, similar to the pelvic distortion described by Lewitt (1987), was found in over 80% of our patients with lumbosacral countercurvature. 77.2% showed an upper frontal spina which deviated caudally on the concave side, and the posterior upper spina had shifted cranially. 19.8% showed no evidence of this type of scoliotic pelvis; 2.9% showed distortion in the opposite direction. 10 of 14 patients with the convex side on the left also showed the typical scoliotic pelvis. 4 patients did not show corresponding findings. We observed increased bodyweight on the concave side in almost all patients (normal posture). This study was concerned only with visually apparent signs.

All these symptoms occur more often in patients with right than left thoracic convexity. Patients with left-side thoracic convexity had bilateral pes valgus twice as often as patients with right-sided convexity. We believe that indirect signs of the lumbosacral countercurvature, mainly pelvic distortion, are consequences of the typical scoliotic pelvis. For example: the acetabulum and the entire hip joint will rotate inwards as much as the thoracic concave sided pelvis turns ventrally and caudally. This causes the apparent interrotational position of the leg on the concave side.

As described above, the hip on the concave side points ventrally (compared to the opposite side). In relation to the opposite side, this causes an increase of tension in the ventral femoral muscles on the thoracic concave side. The wing of the ilium is forced to move caudally on the concave side, especially due to the M. rectus femoris. This could serve as explanatory model for the observed pelvic distortion. The Schroth method reverses this by exercises – pelvic corrections – and assumes pelvic distortions as described by Lewitt.
The patient is observed for direct and indirect signs of a lumbosacral countercurvature so it can be detected and corrected. This enables the physical therapist to select the appropriate corrective measures for each patient, provided they are acquainted with the program.

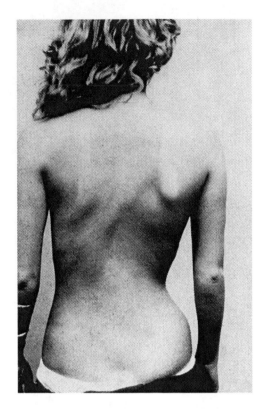

Fig. 167

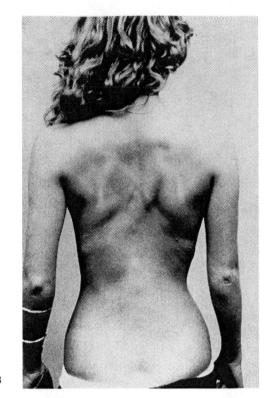

Fig. 168

Fig. 169

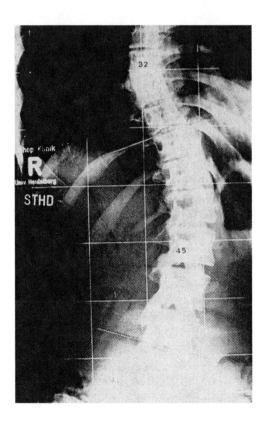

Fig. 170

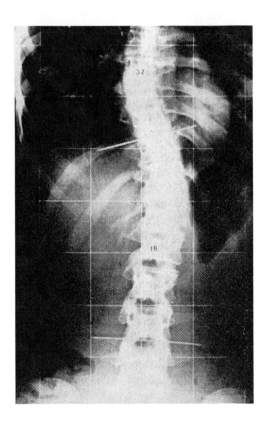

Figs. 167 – 170 were given to me by Prof. Niedhardt. He photographed and X-rayed this patient after a six week course of in-patient Schroth treatment.

Figs. 167 and 169 The normal upright position.

Figs. 168 and 170 The corrected posture. The lumbar curvature has been reduced from 45° to 18°. Corrective movements are possible within the range of the patient's pelvic mobility. They are not obtained at the cost of loosening of the pelvis or ligaments. The corrective exercise is finished off by tightening the entire musculature (muscle mantle).

70

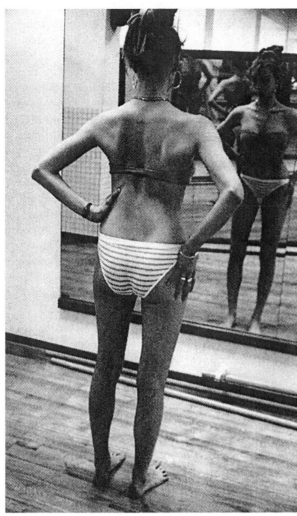 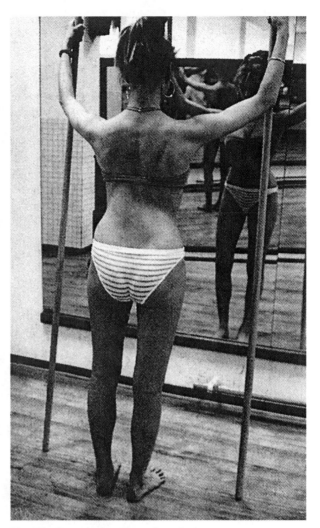

Fig. 171: Correction by manual self-help and mirror control.   **Fig. 172:** Correction by using poles and mirrors.

VI. Summary of the physical corrections using the Schroth method for four-curve scoliosis (with lumbosacral curvature and displacement of pelvis, Figs. 173–175)

The expression 'four-curve' was chosen because the four trunk blocks shift against each other and pull the spinal column to one side. The alignment of the pelvis and the defect in body statics differ strikingly from three-curve scoliosis, thus demand a different approach to treatment. Clinical observation shows a pelvis that has moved forward in the sagittal plane. The anterior pelvic rim has dropped. In the frontal plane, the hip below the rib hump has moved laterally (1) and cranially (2). The opposite hip has shifted caudally (3). In the transverse plane, the hip below the thoracic convexity has moved dorsally and the other hip ventrally. The result is counterrotation and distortion on the frontal-transverse axis.

An anatomical leg length difference is very rare. The pelvis has adopted a functionally oblique posture with countermovement or counterhold, pulling on the spinal column (7):

a) hip sharply turned towards the lumbar hump

b) lumbar hump less twisted towards rib hump

c) rib hump slightly turned towards the shoulder girdle

d) shoulder girdle minimally turned towards the head

To try to compensate for this functionally scoliotic pelvis using heel elevation may exacerbate the existing pelvic malposture, which would also increase the lumbosacral curvature. Testing the height of the pelvis with a pelvic level in the standing position shows that the height difference can be evened out by the Schroth pelvic corrections.

Fig. 174 shows lumbar and pelvic segments rotated and shifted in opposite directions. This causes the 'wedge-like trunk section' to move in opposite directions.

The clinical picture not only shows rotation in the transverse plane, there is also reciprocal rotation of both cristae of the ilium around the frontal-transverse axis, (4) and (5), with simultaneous lateral shifting as a result of misdirected statics in the frontal plane. The leg on the concave side shows interrotational positioning and pes valgus (6). The result is a compensatory lumbosacral spinal curve.

Our goal is to eliminate these multiple three-dimensional counterrotations and to turn the entire lumbar and pelvic region into a rectangular block. The following are the five pelvic corrections.

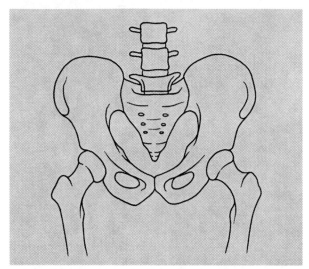

Fig. 173: Normal pelvis; frontal view.

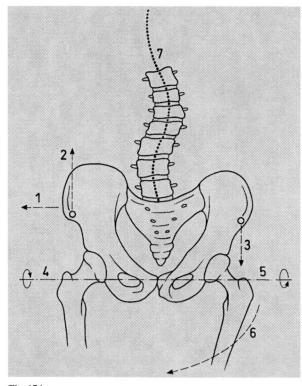

Fig. 174:
Malposition of legs, pelvis and spine due to a lumbosacral curvature.

First pelvic correction:
Standing position; feet parallel, spread to hip width; weight equally on both feet; entire pelvis shifted backwards. Makes a correction in the sagittal plane.

Second pelvic correction:
Rotational movement outwards and backwards with the femur on the concave side (1) resolves the counterrotation of the hip bones around the frontal-transverse axis (pelvic distortion). The hip on the concave side moves automatically upwards and backwards (2), the hip on the convex side moves forwards and downwards (3). The latter still protrudes laterally, therefore we make the third pelvic correction below.

Third pelvic correction:
Pulling in the protruding hip (4) is effected by contracting muscles in the area of greater trochanter (correction in the frontal plane). Lateral shifting only before resolving the counterrotation would not produce the desired correction because of the pelvic distortion. The second and third pelvic corrections have to be made at the same time. Now the lumbar block and the pelvic block form an entire wedge shaped block, especially if the hip on the convex side moves too far ventrally during correction of the scoliotic pelvis.
This block is now rotated in its entirety to pull on the area below the rib hump and to derotate the lumbar hump. The following correction supports this goal.

Fourth pelvic correction:
a) Shift lumbar-pelvic block backwards on the convex side (5), and forwards on the concave side. Correction occurs in the transverse plane. Mid-position in the frontal plane is the target position.
b) Lifting the upper frontal pelvic rim achieves delordosation of the lumbar spine, a correction in the sagittal plane (which can only be successful after derotation of the lumbar hump).

Fifth pelvic correction:
'Isometric heel pushing' of the leg on the convex side without lowering the hip.
In the starting position, the leg on the concave side is abducted and rotated outwards. This straightens the lumbar spine and resolves the pelvic counterrotation. The pelvis has to be moved in its entirety to the midline (see **Note** at the end of this section, p. 74).
Cranial correction is now necessary – including RAB – directly following the basic pelvic corrections. As the lumbar curve is usually the larger curve in four-curve scoliosis, it may be that only minimal curves are present cranially. In this case, the direction of the exercise is straight upwards.
In the presence of a large thoracic curvature, the direction of the exercise should be towards the concave side, but the starting point is above the lumbar hump. Inclining the head and turning it is only necessary if there is a cervical curve and a distorted cervical spine, otherwise the head is held straight.
We support corrective movements using corrective cushions as follows.

a) Prone position
Footstool under the pelvis (not the thighs!) is the first pelvic correction in the sagittal plane.
The leg on the thoracic concave side is abducted and rotated to the outside for the second pelvic correction. The hip of the convex side is tucked in for the third pelvic correction. A corrective cushion is placed under the hip on the convex side (ventrally) to equilibrate the pelvis in the frontal plane for the fourth pelvic correction.

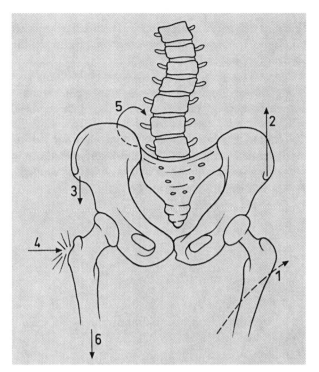

Fig. 175: Directions of corrective movements.

A corrective cushion is placed under the frontal rib arch on the concave side. If the lumbar hump is large and includes several segments in the thoracic region (thoracolumbar scoliosis), this cushion can be omitted.
A corrective cushion is placed under the shoulder girdle or the elbow on the convex side to derotate the shoulder girdle and upper spinal region.

b) Supine position
The leg on the convex side is pulled towards the body with the foot on the floor. The leg on the concave side is abducted and rotated outwards, the pelvis is in the horizontal position and the hip on the convex side is pulled inwards with gradual and firm tension.

A (wedge-shaped) corrective cushion is placed under the lumbar hump to derotate and deflex the thoracolumbar section. If the curves in the upper spine are minimal, corrective cushions are placed under both scapular angles. Otherwise according to the type of scoliosis. No cushions in case of flatback.

c) Lateral position:
The patient lies on the concave side. The leg on this side is bent at an angle of 90°. The leg on the convex side is kept straight, with the foot resting on a footstool at the height of the hip.
Two or three cushions are placed under the lumbar hump (lateral). Prior manual derotation – pulling the lumbar hump forward and upward – is absolutely necessary!

73

Enough corrective cushions should be used to bring the lumbar spine into the midline position (corrective cushion laterally under shoulder girdle).

When exercising in the seated position, on all fours, or in the low-sliding or similar positions, abduction and exterior rotational positioning of the leg on the concave side is necessary (see note below).

To counteract increased use of the knee and foot joints, the patient should first perform general physiotherapeutic elongating and stretching exercises as well as strengthening exercises for the hip leg and foot muscles.

Malposition (distortion) of the pelvis may lead to blocking of the iliosacral joints. This can be resolved by the above-mentioned pelvic corrections or by using Schroth leg and hip exercises.

Note: Abduction and external rotational position of the leg of the concave side must always involve the pelvis while contracting the area of the trochanter major of the convex side. Otherwise the sacral part of the lumbosacral curve is increased and pulls the coccyx with it. Pelvic correction is always three-dimensional.

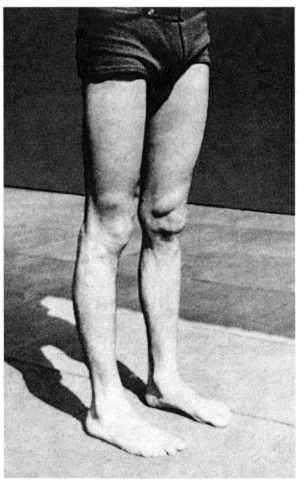

Fig. 176

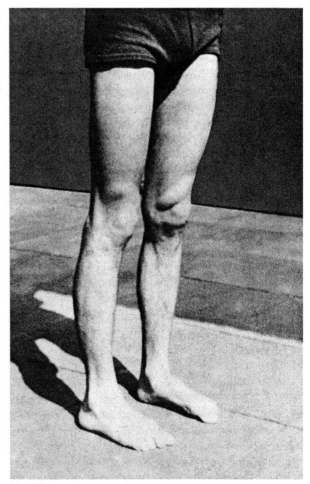

Fig. 177

Most scoliotics suffer from weakness of connective tissue, not only of the trunk but also of the legs. They should have a daily exercise program including foot exercises. One of the causes for scoliosis may be unilateral pes planus or pes valgus.

Even though in many cases the shape of feet cannot be influenced, the pain caused by fallen or low arches may be relieved (pes valgus, transversus, and planus). In daily life, we should take care that the feet are always parallel, because standing and walking with feet pointed outwards contributes to flattening of the longitudinal arches and promotes fatigue and pain.

Exercises in heel position should always be done with the toes open.

Exercises to strengthen the arches of the feet
(Figs. 176 and 177)

Standing position: feet apart, parallel and in line with the hips. The inner and outer edges of the feet are raised simultaneously to increase muscle tone as follows: While the toes push against the floor, the soles are contracted at short intervals. These contractions may be accompanied by long or short breaths.

Hallux valgus is of special significance. It is combined with a major change in the metatarsophalangeal articulation of the big toe which causes the latter to grow into an incorrect position.

Exercises to counteract complaints caused by Hallux valgus (Figs. 178 – 180)

Sitting position. 'Bring up' the heel. Lift the heel and bring it a little to the inside, then put it down again, keeping the toes spread on the floor all the time. This increases the arch. Practise this until the exercise is mastered.

In this corrected position, press the entire foot (all the toes and the heel) isometrically down on the floor. The muscles are tensed and this influences the longitudinal and transverse arches and the muscles of the lower leg. Reinforce this with small muscle contractions as if you were making a fist with the foot. Each contraction moves the instep higher and shortens the foot. The lateral muscles on the ball of the big toe contract. This exercise has impressive results; it normalizes and beautifies the foot – especially if hallux valgus has not yet developed (Fig. 179). The thumb presses the ball of the foot from the outside and the index finger pushes the big toe against this to move the toe into the correct position. Now all the muscles of the foot are contracted firmly and isometrically. The feet are then shaken to relax them. The feet now feel better with blood flow, and the sensation while walking is more sensitive.

The isometric contractions described above may be done from the feet upwards (observe in a mirror), up the lower leg, posterior, lateral, medial, M. quadriceps; M. tensor fasciae latae, M. biceps femoris; adductor musculature and lower abdomen. Priority should be given to the exhaling phase to avoid pressure in the larynx blocking reflux of the blood.

Training all leg and pelvic muscles in this way automatically creates a vertical leg axis, brings the pelvis into an upright position and has a positive influence on posture.

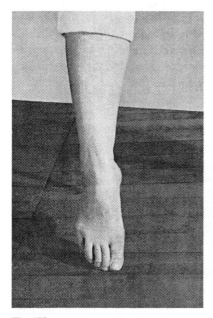

Fig. 178

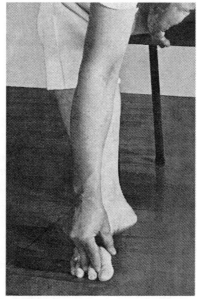

Fig. 179

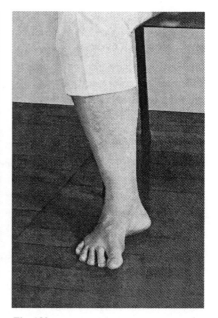

Fig. 180

VIII. Summary of theoretical considerations

There are always three factors to consider in scoliosis. The human body has **three physiological curvatures**: lumbar lordosis, thoracic kyphosis, and cervical lordosis (section B.II)

Accordingly, the segments of the trunk form **three "blocks"**: lumbar, the lumbar spine and pelvis; thoracic, the thoracic spine and rib cage; and cervical, the cervical spine and shoulder girdle (section A.I).

The **three sagittal displacements** of these blocks against each other are caused by malposture. The result are the **three 'wedges'**.

Due to lateral shifting of the three trunk segments, **three lateral wedges** exist (section A.III).

The **three wedge vertices turn forwards**, and the **three wide sides of wedges are turned backwards**, thus creating **three torsions of the trunk** around the vertical axis (section A.IV).

This creates the **three kyphotic elevations** and the **three lordotic retractions** (see section A.III).

For treatment of scoliosis it is important to activate the **three different parts of the erector trunci** which influence the three trunk segments separately (see section B.IV).

Corrective breathing movements are made in **three directions** (see section B.5).

Three basic requirements have to be fulfilled when exercising:

1. Achievement of the best possible elongation of the spine and sides.
2. Derotation of trunk with the help of breathing movements.
3. Isometric strengthening during elongation and derotation.

The basis for *targeting the weakest* point is created by adopting the *best possible starting positions* for the thoracic breathing movement.

If not treated, scoliosis tends to worsen. Our treatment aims to improve faulty posture and hinder progression of the deformity. We do this by influencing the defective scoliotic statics and reversing the 'inner picture' which the patient has of his or her posture. The opposite of the existing defective posture is the goal: the vertices of the wedges have to be widened and the wide sides have to be compressed to attain an upright position, which means that the concavities become convex and convexities become concave.

Using guided breathing movements, less ventilated parts of the lungs are activated, improving performance of the heart and circulation.

Whenever possible, exercises are performed outside to ventilate the lungs and enrich the blood with oxygen. **None of the exercises are performed without intentional and guided breathing movements. We are not performing 'general' breathing exercises.**

Transformation of the scoliotic 'normal' posture happens with the help of three factors:

1. Recognition of the malposture (mirror, photographs).
2. Imagining and being aware of the malposture.
3. Modulation of faulty movements, aiming for change and added stabilization.

Acceptance of the scoliotic posture as 'normal' over a long period creates an obstacle to treatment again and again. This is the reason why photos and mirrors are of such importance. At the beginning, patients do not feel straight and upright, but continuous exercise and activation of weak muscles changes their awareness. When exercising, it is also important to watch fellow patients and recognize their faulty posture. The Schroth method is not only a treatment, but a learning process for the patient to perform exercises in the correct manner, without the therapist's help. Figs. 117-120 show the effect of orthopaedic-breathing exercises in a patient with progressive scoliosis. The left lumbar side of this patient is overstrained because the weight of the trunk hangs over to the right. This has produced a very prominent lumbar curvature which has caused a countercurvature of the cervical spine. In comparison, the muscles below the rib hump are less developed.

It is our goal to straighten the whole body, starting at the heels, proceeding to the ankles and knees, to make it unnecessary for the lumbar hump to deviate so far (the lumbar curvature being the main one in this case). This is the reason for the foot exercises described above. They are of great importance.

A strong corrective exercise is tightening the middle section of the left lateral thigh muscle. The left hip is pulled in intentionally, which then results in an outward movement of the right hip (laterally). Previously, this right hip had moved forwards and medially. It is helpful to use the visualization of the lateral middle part of the left thigh pushing the right thigh outwards, and it must remain there. Now, the left pelvic muscles move the left side of the pelvis forwards (it had turned backwards before). At the same time, the lateral pelvic muscles on the right side contract and move this side of the pelvis backwards. These contractions are performed successively. Once each position is achieved it is maintained, to further develop and refine correction.

All these measures help to 'rearrange' the pelvis correctly (Fig. 58). To achieve a lasting result, this has to be followed by intense muscular contraction. It is interesting to watch the right M. erector trunci in the lumbar region at this point. It has been activated and stimulated to work again. Now, the reduction in the lumbar curvature enables the middle spinal curve to be straightened. The M. latissimus dorsi immediately starts to interact on the left and pulls the curve to the midline. The lumbar hump on the left side flattens. Having proceeded so far, the bodyweight is intentionally kept on the left leg. Fig. 58 shows the effect: the left side widens and opens up. We have witnessed a change from a subluxated hip (with pain at each step) into a symptom-free hip. After all these preparations, we have finally gained space to integrate the ribs on the concave side. This happens at two 'right angles': ribs sideways and upwards, and backwards and upwards, with the diaphragm moving downwards. The ribs turn the transverse processes of the vertebrae, since they are connected to them. This can be seen on an X-ray screen. An orthopaedic surgeon once remarked about this: "Your method is like mathematics – there will always be a result." Patients become aware of the different effects of an exercise with and without the use of the diaphragm. It is not possible to 'lift' the trunk out of the pelvic girdle without the support of the diaphragm. This is then followed by stabilization by tensing the muscles.

Each exercise represents an education in posture. Body awareness of 'right' and 'wrong' posture has to be learned in front of mirrors to enable patients to feel and sense their bodies without visual control (mirror).

First, the correct right posture is created by exercises. It should then automatically be adopted in daily life and activities. This has to go as far as the sleeping positions, since we spend one third of our life in bed. The best possible positions within the range of anatomical possibility have to be reached and incorporated in our lives. Once the weakened muscles have been strengthened and exercised, overloaded muscles are relieved and a muscular balance and harmony is reestablished.

Specific exercises should not be favoured. The programme should be versatile to avoid neglect of certain muscle groups. Feedback from a therapist should always be sought at certain intervals. Postural changes occur rapidly, sometimes – depending on the severity of the condition – within 4–6 weeks. Friends and family often comment spontaneously on this. Another effect is the more positive attitude towards oneself and life.

IX. Objectives of Schroth treatment

Children and adolescents

a) Correction of scoliotic malposture
b) Stabilization of the corrected posture by improvement of postural capacity
c) Maintenance of the corrections during daily activities by facilitating a corrected body awareness
d) Halting progression
e) Cosmetic correction of body silhouette
f) Improvement of breathing function
g) Improvement of cardiopulmonary capacity and reduction risk of illness
h) Improvement of the psychic attitude to scoliosis through group interaction in our clinic
i) Acquired knowledge results in more confidence and assurance in dealing with one's own scoliosis

Adults

a) Increase and conservation of cardiopulmonary capacity
b) Improvement of pulmonary activity by breathing training and active rib mobilization
c) Pain reduction or relief through active and passive physiotherapeutic measures
d) Development of a corrected posture
e) Halting progression
f) Cosmetic improvement
g) Improvement of psychic attitude towards one's disorder
Adults and adolescents must learn how to think in terms of the Schroth corrective principles and incorporate them into daily living.

X. Learning to observe in the Schroth manner

A critical observation of exercise and follow-up pictures (Figs.181 a-c).

Katharina Schroth attached great importance to looking at pictures. She wanted the patients to 'see' their photos the right way. She wanted them to 'learn' to see.

In the early years, most patients had very severe scoliosis, and many had a prominent hip on the thoracic concave side. It seemed that that a certain type of scoliosis had developed because of the 'Swedish bending exercises' practised at that time.

To make them more familiar with scoliosis and to enable them to exercise more confidently, Katharina Schroth had the patients photographed almost naked and they exercised in very little clothing. This proved to be very appropriate in motivating the therapist and patient to continue along the path begun.

Try to imagine the two halves of the trunk in three-curve scoliosis parted in the middle and vibrating against each other (Fig. 182).

Rib humps do not occur on their own. They only become obvious when the segments of the trunk above and below shift forwards in the opposite direction. Concavities also do not appear on their own. They become obvious when the trunk segments above and below shift backwards.

Fig. 181a shows the condition at the beginning of course of Schroth therapy (the three pictures were taken in Meissen where the Schroth method was developed). The patients realised what is, and imagined what should be. Fig. 181b shows an exercise.

Fig. 181c shows the treatment result after 3 months. What can we learn from these pictures?

Fig. 181a: (baseline)

The patient puts increasingly more weight on the right leg than on both. The trunk therefore becomes heavier on the right, and is held by the left hip so it does not lose its balance completely. This creates the 'scoliotic balance'. Since the head needs to be above the centre of gravity, it swings towards the midline, and the rib hump on the right side is formed. The right shoulder joint shifts forwards. This creates a seemingly larger rib hump when you look at it from the right. A perpendicular line from the right axilla will drop beside the right hip.

The left shoulder, i.e. the entire left shoulder girdle, has shifted backwards and blocks breathing in the left lung. This blockage increases as the left shoulder girdle moves more and more behind the left (concave) ribs towards the pelvic girdle and pushes the ribs forwards. The left prominent hip has moved upwards at the same time. A belt would show this obliquity in the waist. From the beginning, Katharina Schroth's objective was:

'Create the opposite of what the body shows at this point' to build new movement and postural images in the brain. One hopes that after exercising, the scoliotic body has adopted a vertical posture. The existing displacement and distortion of the trunk will be reversed. This must happen.

Fig. 181b:

An attempt to realise her maxim:

1. The weight is shifted from the right to the left leg,
2. The left hip is pulled in,
3. The trunk, which had moved past the right hip, is shifted in the opposite direction. An imaginary perpendicular line from the right axilla will now touch the right hip,
4. The lumbar spine, which swung in the cervical plane sharply towards the right, is now more vertical,
5. The depressed concavity is now open to be ventilated.

Those are 5 positive points that we can see she has

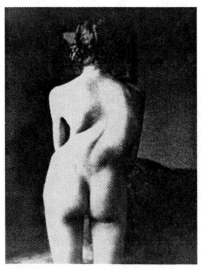 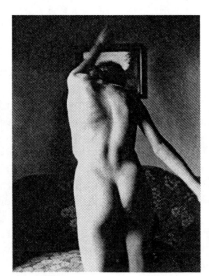 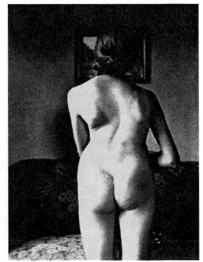

Fig. 181 a   Fig. 181 b   Fig. 181 c

achieved. At the same time, however, she has made nine mistakes:

1. It is right to pull in the left hip and move it downwards, but the right hip must not move upwards.
2. The hip must also not move forward: the gluteal fold is now oblique.
3. The right hip has narrowed the lumbar concavity on the right.
4. Turning this right hip forwards hinders activation of lumbar erectors and derotation of trunk and pelvis against each other. The pelvis of the convex side of the trunk has shifted forward and must be brought backwards.

Katharina Schroth always repeatedly explained: "Rib humps do not occur on their own. They only become obvious when the segments of the trunk above and below shift forwards in the opposite direction. Concavities also do not appear on their own. They become obvious when the trunk segments above and below shift backwards."

Because of this, she developed 'countermovements', exercise movements on the same side and plane.

5. The left (concave) side is being widened, but not by pulling with the raised left arm.
6. A pull upwards and to the right would create a shoulder hump which is already incipient (Fig. 181a). The left shoulder region seems broader than the right.
7. The position of the right arm was kept in the way the patient felt it to be right. She wanted to contract the lateral rib hump by caudal pressure from the right arm. The arm rotates inward, though, and the shoulder is turning far forward.
8. This exercise shifted the shoulder girdle out of the horizontal line. Katharina Schroth also said: "The shoulder girdle is a bit like a clothes hanger. We do not hang our clothes obliquely."

The correct way would be to bring the right arm in an outward rotation to move the shoulder backwards. This also moves the shoulder blade vertically. The rib hump will be pushed forward by the lower scapula angle.

9. During this exercise the head pulls towards the right as well. This increases the shoulder hump on the left and the cervical curvature on the right.

The correct way would be to move the head towards the left side in the direction of the cervical curve. This activates the muscles on the right and derotates this curvature at the same time. Katharina Schroth saw these mistakes by looking at the pictures and she learned how not to do it. She tried to eliminate mistakes because she knew that even one of them would impair achieving the best treatment result or make it impossible. The nine mistakes listed above would negate the result of the five

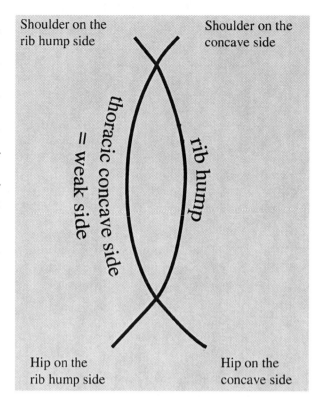

Shoulder on the rib hump side

Shoulder on the concave side

thoracic concave side = weak side

rib hump

Hip on the rib hump side

Hip on the concave side

Fig. 182

correct exercise movements. Katharina Schroth eliminated the mistakes by reversing them.

She developed the "turned sitting position", which moves the right hip backwards and downwards and opens the concavities so they can be ventilated. She eliminated the pull with the left arm and developed 'shoulder countertraction' with the right arm moved obliquely sideways and upwards. This aligns the shoulder girdle. The position of the head was corrected: "One leans the head towards the concave side and turns the chin towards the convex side." She never spoke of a 'hump' but of a 'package', because everybody has to carry their burden. From then on, the head had to be held to elongate the main curvature (thoracic) and an occipital push has to be performed. This flattens the upper ribs on the convexity at the same time.

Katharina Schroth developed the exercises with the utmost accuracy and explained them to the patients. She also watched the patients closely and told them during their group exercises which mistakes were being made and how to change them immediately. The patients also learned by watching each other and they became more confident in what they were doing.

Fig. 181c: Result of three months of treatment. In those days, a three-month course was usual. Katharina Schroth did not treat patients for shorter periods because she believed it was hard to create the feeling for right and wrong in a shorter period of time. This has nothing to do with the intellect of the patient, but rather with body awareness and correct sensibility for the exercises.

79

PART C
Exercise instructions

The causes of scoliosis are still unknown, and there is therefore no alternative but to treat it symptomatically. Each case of scoliosis is different, which also means that there is not a standard treatment. This is why we have developed a very wide range of detailed exercises to meet the requirements of almost all types of scoliosis. The important thing is to change faulty postural stereotypes to avoid further development of misdirected growth and thus ensure that the body adopts a vertical posture.

We must not forget that scoliosis is partly a fixed deformity of the spinal column and that structural changes do exist. At the same time, posture plays an important role. Achieving the best possible posture in the scoliotic patient is the primary aim: this means stabilization of the correction and its incorporation into everyday activities. Postural correction is only possible within the extent of the existing mobility of the patient. Patients must learn to develop a new physical awareness and sense of posture and, when all is said and done, accept and sense as 'straight' what seems to be 'oblique'. Here it is of utmost importance to check posture visually in a mirror.

The following section describes individual components of each postural correction, and mentions the forms of scoliosis for which they are suited.

The explanations should be carefully studied before starting exercises, as they are referred to repeatedly. The explanations are as detailed as possible.

However, to avoid confusion, no details of psychological components are given. During treatment, the therapist explains details repeatedly to help the patient absorb the message and achieve the best success possible. Each exercise description starts with an explanation of the postural changes in the sagittal plane: weakness of the back, kyphosis, Scheuermann's disease, hyperlordosis. These are listed under 'kyphosis' and describe symmetrical trunk movements.

Lateral spinal deformities (scoliosis and kyphoscoliosis) are treated with the exercises listed under 'scoliosis'.

For postural (sagittal) deformities in the sagittal plane, we recommend that the exercises described for scoliosis be performed on both sides of the body, since they have a very beneficial effect on vertebral joints.

Therapists – and indeed patients – may produce variations based on the basic concept outlined.

The exercises require a great deal of effort, and each is followed by a guided resting period in the corrected position, either combined with relaxation or specific breathing, transforming relaxation periods into orthopaedic exercises. It is not necessary to perform the exercises in the order given. During an exercise session, one can vary selections from among the various exercises as needed. It is important to perform each exercise as if it were the sole exercise that is going to lead to success. All available mental power should be invested in it and the aim should be to enjoy the exercise. It should not be a 'Have To' – it should be transformed into a 'Need To'.

I. Breathing exercises

'Breathing exercises' are those which produce an intense exchange of air in the respiratory system and the breathing organs (alveoli and bronchi).

The amount of inhaled air can be determined by a spirometer which measures the volume of exhaled air. There are average readings depending on body size. After a deep inhalation, air is exhaled into a hose connected to the measuring device which displays the volume of exhaled air. A scoliotically deformed trunk with impaired thoracic breathing will not be able to produce a high volume at the beginning. We therefore measure breathing capacity three times, and use the average as a starting figure. The breathing volume is then measured daily. Improvements motivate the patient to intensify breathing movements and to practise. Many scoliotics show unstable measurements at the beginning, depending on their physical state. We often see ambitious patients who try to improve readings quickly, but im-

provement depends not only on the function of the breathing apparatus but also on the overall vital capacity. Naturally, there are ups and downs during treatment. Patients are kept fully informed of their progress, so they understand these deviations, and know why a reading may be low at one point or another. The therapist must also realize that a patient may need longer rest periods during exercises.

After several weeks of treatment, patients experience great pleasure in the increase in their ability to perform everyday activities such as walking, climbing stairs or riding bikes.

The ability to breathe out has to be improved as far as possible, because increased exhalation is followed by increased inhalation and this, in turn, increases the amount of oxygen in the blood. The breathing ability may be stimulated by blowing up a balloon or rubber animals, for example. **The number of breaths needed**

can be quite an incentive. As volume increases, the number of breaths needed decreases. Another motivational aid may be to **measure the circumference of a balloon after one exhalation**. As the force of the breath increases, the circumference increases.

The exhalation capacity may be improved further by **long exhalations**, during which the **chest** is tapped with the palm of the hand to vibrate and activate the inactive alveoli. At the same time, the patient counts the seconds or heartbeats needed to exhale. The goal is a daily increase. It is very motivating to keep a journal of these numbers. **Inhalation** following each exhalation should be guided to the concavities of trunk – the "sunken segments" – and breathing should be guided into them at **"right angles"**.

These breathing movements can be performed in different directions simultaneously, for example, forwards on the right side and backwards on the left, to create an 'oblique breathing pattern' which is very beneficial for scoliosis. To strengthen the intercostal muscles and diaphragm, the **nostrils should be a little compressed during inhalation to make deep breathing necessary.** It is always important to guide breathing mentally and to start in the inactive segments of the trunk. The **diaphragm is lowered** at the same time, even if this is unilateral. Mental guidance and manual stimulation below the thoracic convexity accomplish this.

Training of the voluntary muscles (movement of the diaphragm) can be enhanced by exercises using sound: hissing, blowing, etc., and exhalation exercises using a harmonica or other devices. It is, of course, always important to ensure that incorrect breathing movements are not used.

Measurements of the gas volume in the blood of some of our patients have shown an increase of oxygen, even after 3 or 4 weeks of treatment.

II. Exercises on wall bars

Important warning:
Patients with a spine fusion (Harrington, CD, etc.) are not allowed to do exercises in hanging position on the bars, since they could endanger the implant.

These exercises mainly have an influence on the passive locomotor system of the spinal column (joint capsules and ligaments). They provide the preconditions for physiological muscular activity.

The following exercises are subdivided into 4 groups:

I.   Exercises while hanging: They mainly affect the passive locomotor system, stretch shortened muscles, and flatten the rib hump. After exercising, the hands, arms and legs need to be relaxed thoroughly. These hanging exercises should be omitted in case of rotational slippage of the vertebrae. They can, however, be imagined.

II. Mobilization exercises: These further preserve, restore and improve joint mobility, especially of the spinal column, trunk and shoulder girdle. They do not free up immobilized structures.

III. Shaping exercises: These have a derotating effect on the trunk and shoulder girdle in conjunction with RAB and the appropriate countermovements. They also have a stabilizing effect due to tightening at the end of each correction.

IV. Exercises to stretch and strengthen: These are isometric exercises, strong and forceful, preceded by a shaping exercise and performed in derotation.

The patient must always observe resting periods in the corrected position in between exercises. Exercises from various subgroups should be chosen to avoid overstraining the hands. All exercises are multipurpose exercises and involve several aspects, which means that they have synergistic effects.

They should be done slowly to ensure maximum correction. If not mentioned specifically, the breathing technique may be chosen by the patient. In each case pressing of the larynx must always be avoided!

I. Exercises in hanging position

1. HANGING FROM THE BACK OF THE NECK

(Figs. 183 and 184) – not to be performed in the case of cervical kyphosis or flatback.
Exercise may be done with a special device (neck cradle) or a therapist.

Kyphosis: Standing on the 3rd bar (depending on size of patient); holding the bar at the height of the thighs; arms straight; hands are shoulder width apart; occiput rests in the 'neck cradle' or hand of therapist. The patient presses against it while taking the feet off the bar. A kind of semi-suspension has been created. The head may be turned to the side or pushed up, out of the shoulder girdle. The legs may swing slightly, or circulate, or the knees are pulled towards the chest.
Scoliosis: The hip below the rib hump is brought backwards.

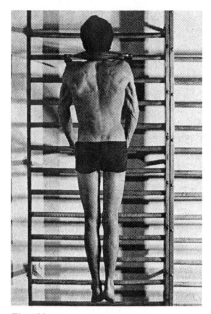

Fig. 183

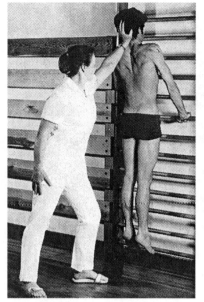

Fig. 184

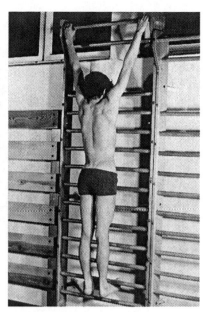

Fig. 185

2. Pulling down the bar (Figs. 185 and 186)

Hanging from highest bar; arms apart.

Kyphosis: During inhalation, the feet push alternately downwards. There is the sensation of a 'heavy lower body' which helps to stretch concave segments of the trunk. Exhale while imagining pulling the bar downward and extending the neck upward. Upright pelvis. No lordosis. Do not do a 'chin-up'.

Scoliosis: The hip below the rib hump is rotated backwards. The head pulls up in a derotated position. Resistance may be felt at the level of the pelvis.

This exercise is not appropriate for patients with cervical kyphosis or flatback.

3. Abducted position (Fig. 187)

Kyphosis: Perform exercise on alternate sides.

Scoliosis: Stand sideways on the 2nd or 3rd bar, concavity towards the wall bars. Hand holds the bar at head level.

Abduct the 'outer' arm and leg, the latter rotated outwards. The hip below the rib hump is brought backwards and downward, so that arms and legs form two crossing diagonals. Maintain this position for some time while using RAB.

The laterally shifted hip on the concave side is brought to the midline by tightening the thigh muscles (3rd and 4th pelvic correction).

Omit in four-curve scoliosis.

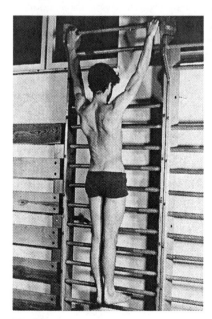

Fig. 186

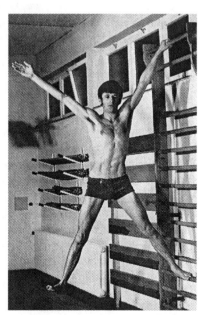

Fig. 187

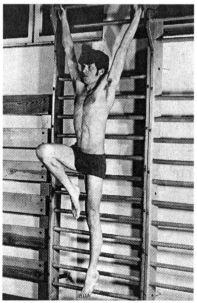

Fig. 188

85

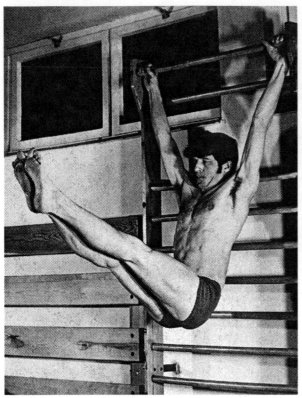

Fig. 189

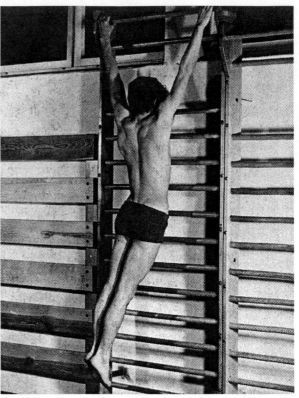

Fig. 190

4. CYCLING (FIG. 188)

Back towards the wall bars, arms apart, hands hold highest bar.

Kyphosis and scoliosis:

a) Both legs perform large cycling movements. The weight of the legs causes passive stretching of oblique abdominal muscles. Caution: avoid lumbar hyperlordosis.

b) Perform the same movements backwards.

c) Same movements obliquely towards right or left side.

d) Breathing: Perform four cycling movements while exhaling; rest while inhaling. Four movements exhaling again. Number of breaths and cyclings may be increased.

5. EXERCISING ABDOMINAL MUSCLES (FIG. 189)

Back towards the wall bars; hands apart, holding on to the highest bar.

Kyphosis: During inhalation, the extended legs are alternately pushed downwards 'out of the pelvis' several times. During exhalation, one or both knees are pulled towards the chest; alternate movements. Avoid a lordosis. The legs may also be in the straddle position; or brought to the left or right side. Circular and swimming movements are also possible. Stretch one or both legs forwards.

Scoliosis: Same procedure. The exercise strengthens abdominal muscles in correct position.

6. SWINGING OF THE LEGS (FIG. 190)

Hanging from the highest bar, arms apart as wide as possible; cushion in front of pelvis.

Kyphosis: The legs are closed and perform small swaying movements to the left and right side. Creates small movements in lumbar spine.

Lumbar scoliosis: Swaying to the dorsal concave side is accentuated to widen the vertex of the wedge below the rib hump. At the same time, the hip below the rib hump is brought backwards. Lateral hip muscles on the concave side are contracted by guided leg movements. Omit in four-curve scoliosis.

Breathing: Inhalation – the feet push downwards; exhalation – the legs are slowly lifted to concave side.

II. Mobilization exercises for the lumbar spine and stretching of the ischiocrural muscles

1. EXTENSION AND FLEXION OF LEGS FROM SQUATTING POSITION (FIGS. 191 AND 192)

Feet on second bar; hands apart on bar at shoulder level; squatting position.

Kyphosis: Extend the legs, buttocks low – rock gently back and forth – back to starting position – repeat rocking movement 5–10 times. Gradually move to lower bars with hands. Bring buttocks as close to the ground as possible (legs extended). Relaxed breathing. Do not strain in the abdomen.

86

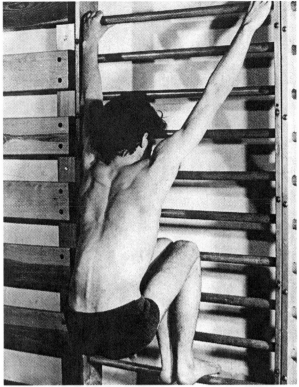

Fig. 191

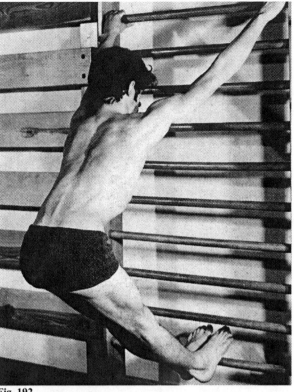

Fig. 192

Scoliosis: Guide the hip below the rib hump laterally, backwards and downwards to move the trunk into an oblique position. Keep this position during movement. This widens the concave side. Ensure that the lumbar hump does not increase in the case of four-curve scoliosis. Do not grasp too low.

2. DIPPING EXERCISE (FIGS. 193 AND 194)

Legs abducted on lowest bar; hands apart at shoulder level.
Kyphosis: Alternate 'dipping' and pulling towards the bars. Hands switch bars every time the body is close to

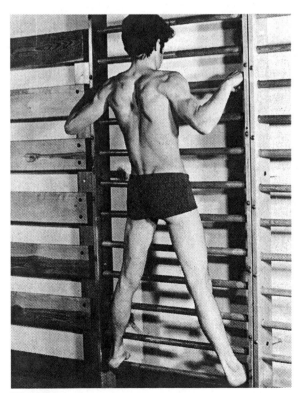

Fig. 193

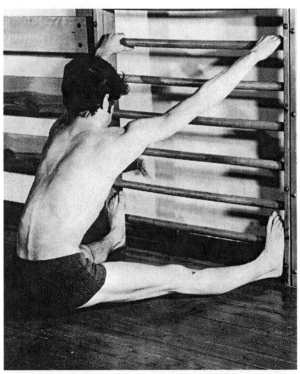

Fig. 194: To be omitted in the case of lumbar kyphosis and a high, protruding lumbar hump.

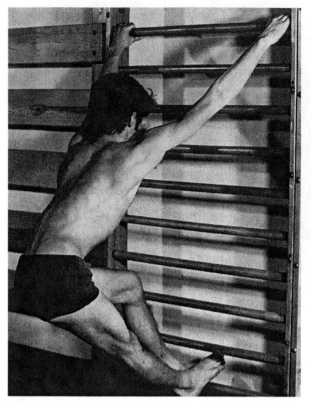

Fig. 195

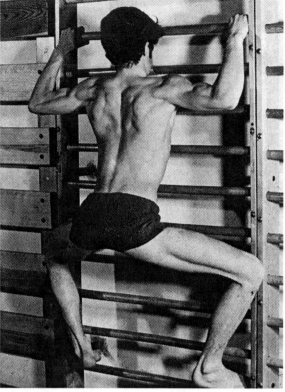

Fig. 196

the bars. Continue until the buttocks are as close to the floor as possible. Come back up the same way. Intensify by starting with feet on second bar.

Scoliosis: The hip below the rib hump is brought backwards, sideways and downwards; the head is held to extend the thoracic curvature. Maintain the corrected position. Four-curve scoliosis: do not dip quite as low, because of the lumbar hump.

Not appropriate for lumbar kyphosis and a high lumbar hump.

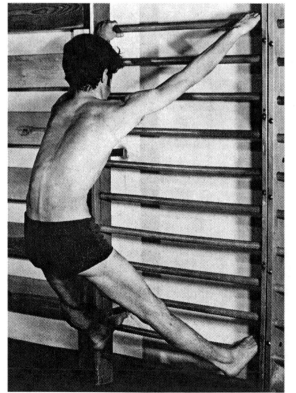

Fig. 197

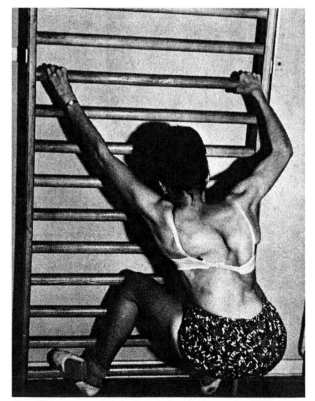

Fig. 198

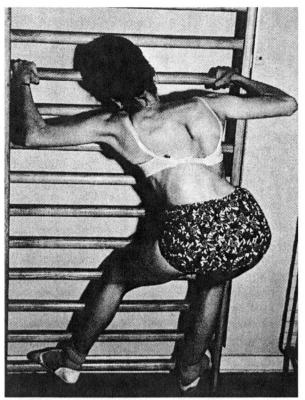

Fig. 199

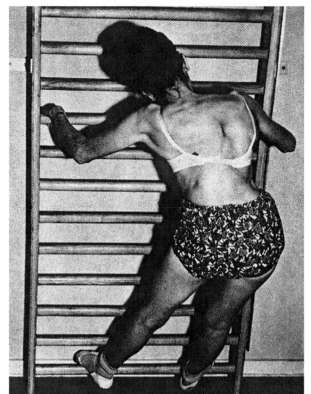

Fig. 200

3. Cycling (Fig. 195)

Standing on lowest bar; feet together; hands at shoulder level; the pelvis moves backwards when the legs are extended.

Kyphosis: Flex legs alternately; 'see-saw' motion. Increases pelvic range of rotation.

Scoliosis: Extend leg on the concave side only once, the other 3, 4, or 5 times. 'Dip' into pelvic corrections 3, 4, and 5 (see section B.I).

Not appropriate for four-curve scoliosis.

4. Sagittal circling with the trunk (Figs. 196 and 197)

Straddle position; feet on second bar; hands at shoulder level. This exercise has three phases:

Kyphosis:

a) Lower the pelvis backwards, lumbar spine showing slight kyphosis; legs straight. In this stretched position, the trunk is elongated even more during inhalation.

b) During exhalation, the knees are flexed and point outwards. While inhaling again, the trunk is brought further down.

c) During the next exhalation, the extended trunk is moved to the upright position while the chest is brought as close as possible to the wall bars. Repeat the sequence in reversed order. In case of flatback, do not move chest towards wall bars.

Scoliosis: The same sequence of movements, but the trunk is leaned towards the concave side. Use RAB; while the thorax pulls upwards, the narrow frontal segment (convex side) is brought forwards and upwards by breathing into it. During the backward movement, breath guides the concave side laterally upwards and backwards.

In cases of four-curve scoliosis without lumbar spinal kyphosis, exercise so that the lumbar hump is not enlarged.

5. Diagonal circling with the trunk (Figs: 198-200)

Starting position same as exercise 4. The hip should touch the vertical side bars with each swing.

Kyphosis: From the upright position, the hip is brought to the right pole, then squatting position and the hip is moved over to the left pole. Back to the starting position. The trunk must not rotate.

Scoliosis: The hip below the rib hump pulls to the pole; then squatting position; from there in oblique position towards opposite pole. The ribs on the concave side spread apart. The head moves to extend the thoracic curve. Not appropriate for four-curve scoliosis.

III. Shaping exercises

1. THE "GREAT ARCH" (FIGS. 201–203).

Omit in case of lumbar kyphosis and lumbar hump. The legs slightly apart under wall bars; feet parallel; hands holding on to the highest bar possible.

Kyphosis: Pelvis upright: the lumbar spine is moved backwards and upwards by RAB. The subsequent exhalation must be accompanied by contraction of the abdominal muscles to bring the frontal rib arch backwards. The head is held straight up.

Scoliosis: First derotate the pelvis (section B.I). Breathe into the thoracic concavity to move the frontal rib arch on the concave side backwards and upwards. During exhalation, contract abdominal muscles. Hold the head so that it extends the curvature.

The same exercise can be done in sitting position (Fig. 203); hip below the rib hump moves backward.

2. OBLIQUE TRACTION (FIGS. 204 AND 205)

Exercise for a high thoracic convexity. Omit in four-curve scoliosis.

Kyphosis: Perform on alternate sides.

Scoliosis: Concave side towards the wall bars; sit on the heels, toes stretched out; the concave-side arm at right angle holds a bar underhanded; convex-side hand guides the hip laterally, backwards, and down till the concave-side buttock meets the heel of the rib hump side. The arm on the concave side resists this movement. While pulling up, the outer hip resists the arm that is pulling the body to the kneeling position. The head is held so that the second spinal curve is extended, the chin turned towards the convex side.

There are two possibilities for guiding the breathing:
a) Use RAB during upward or downward movement (avoid lordosis). Exhale in kneeling or heel position.
b) Use RAB in the kneeling position or on the heels. While resisting, perform the movement exhaling in the firm form that is to be held.

Important: Countertraction of the shoulder girdle is necessary. In the case of a sagittal postural disorder, perform bilaterally to influence ankylosis of the spine.

IV. Stretching and strengthening exercises

1. PULLING TOWARDS THE WALL BARS (FIGS. 206–208)

Legs in straddle position; trunk bent towards wall bars to form a right angle; hands grasp bar. Head straight ahead.

Kyphosis:
a) Strong flexion of arms and pulling of head, move the extended trunk towards the wall bars (exhale). Do not force exhalation.
b) The pelvis may offer resistance to the arms or vice-versa. Breathing: inhale when arms are extended, exhale while pulling towards bars.
c) The therapist may offer resistance by holding onto the hips.

Scoliosis: The hand on the convex side holds onto the next higher bar (derotation of shoulder girdle). The pelvic pull is done mainly with hip below the rib hump (convex side) with the trunk leaning towards the concave side. The latter should stay wide during movement. Semicircular movements with narrow anterior side and (or) subaxillary ribs. This results in thoracic counterrotation (second block). The head leans towards the concave side and the chin rotates to the convex side.

Variation: The therapist puts a belt around the patient's hips and pulls diagonally sideways and backwards.

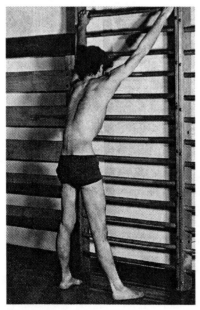

Fig. 201

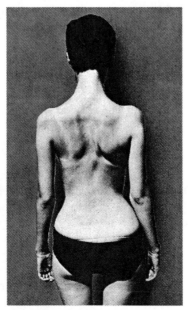

Fig. 202: Without exercise.

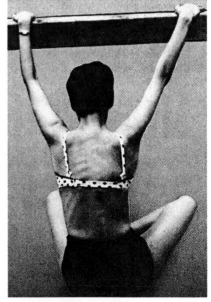

Fig. 203: During exercise.

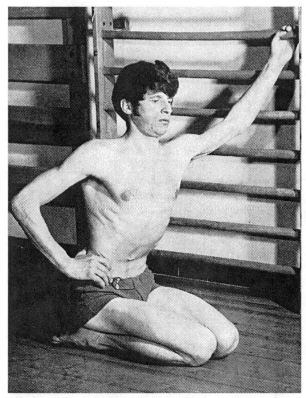

Fig. 204

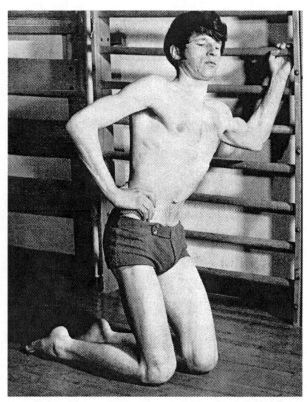

Fig. 205

The therapist's hands provide tactile stimulation in the breathing areas (thoracic concavity and concavity below rib hump). In case of flatback: pull only straight ahead. For four-curve scoliosis, pull the lumbar hump forward and prominent hip in.

d) Basically, the same exercise is possible from a kneeling, prone or supine position. The therapist may give support by holding the waist with his or her legs. The hands are then free to help.

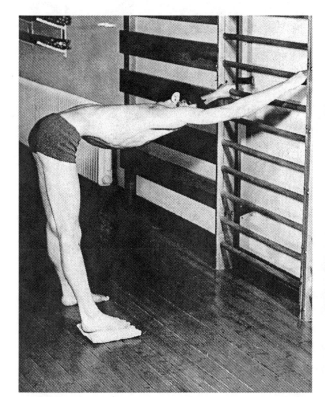

Fig. 206

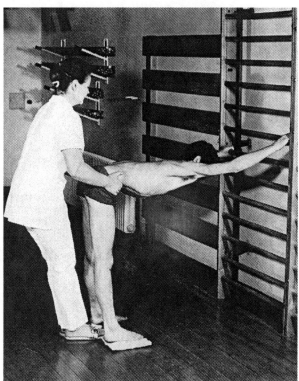

Fig. 207

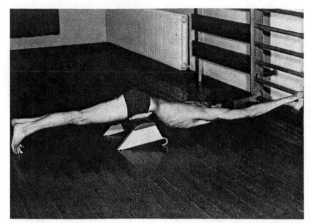

Fig. 208

2. PULLING TOWARDS WALL BARS IN LATERAL POSITION (FIGS. 209 AND 210)

Kyphosis: Perform on alternate sides.
Scoliosis: Concave side towards the floor; hip resting on a footstool or a cushion; hands hold on to bars, vertically above each other. The upper hand may hold on to the bar a little further backwards to widen the narrow front. The therapist fixes the pelvis with his or her legs. During inhalation, the patient stretches the concave side and derotates the trunk. During exhalation, the elbows are bent and the patient pulls towards the wall bars. The head, neck, upper shoulder and hip are drawn backwards. The narrow front turns forwards and upwards, and the concavity widens towards the floor.

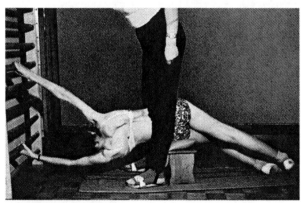

Fig. 209

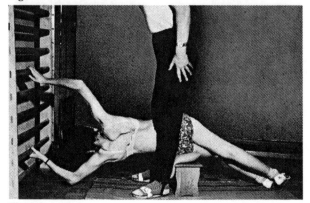

Fig. 210

3. LIFTING THE BODY (FIG. 211)

Abducted position on bar; hands holding at shoulder height; pelvis moves backwards with extended back.
Kyphosis: Elongate the trunk during inhalation. The elbows are flexed and move laterally during exhalation. Meanwhile, the back stays stretched and the neck does not show lordosis. The head meets the bar on which the hands rest. Back to starting position.
Scoliosis: While aligning the pelvis, raise the upper body and head towards the concave side. The hip on the convex side starts a countertraction and the narrow front moves forwards and upwards. Widen the concave side.

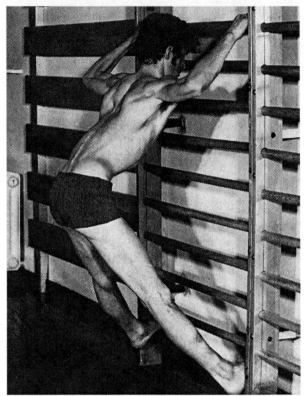

Fig. 211

4. NECK EXERCISE (FIGS. 212A AND 212B)

a) Neck exercise, Fig. 212a:
Sitting cross legged, back towards the wall bars; hands grasping high and far apart; the elbows are slightly bent. Lumbar and cervical lordosis are extended. The head rests against a small board.
Kyphosis: During inhalation, the hands pull strongly downwards while the head is pushed upwards. Stretch the sides. During exhalation, the head pushes backwards while the upper back moves away from the wall bars and the chest moves forwards (intermittent contraction of back muscles).
Scoliosis: Pelvis shifts towards the side of the rib hump; corrective cushions behind and under hip on the concave side (if necessary). Move the upper body in an oblique

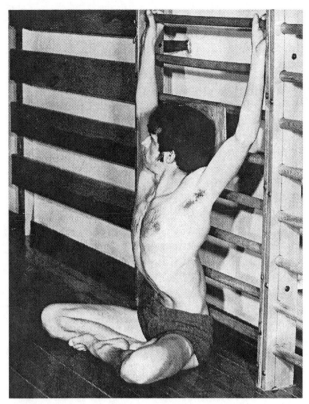

Fig. 212a

way towards the concave side. Breathing: convex side forwards and upwards; posterior concavities sideways, upwards and backwards (RAB). Maintain the resulting position and move the thorax away from the bars during exhalation. Intermittent contraction of the back muscles. Omit this exercise in cases of flatback or cervical kyphosis.

b) Neck exercise variant, Fig. 212b:
Sitting cross-legged, facing the wall bars. Hands grasp a bar at about head height, arms spread wide.
Kyphosis: Perform while inhaling, with elbows spread wide apart. By pulling with the hands, the upper body lifts itself out of the pelvic girdle. Both sides elongate. The spine figuratively grows longer with the help of an occipital push upwards. During exhalation, the chest strives forward, the head and neck backwards, while the rib hump flattens. During this process, make small, intermittent muscle contractions at the crest of the rib hump.
Scoliosis: If necessary, place a corrective cushion in front of one knee and/or under one buttock. Inhale to fill the concavities under the rib hump, the concave side, the narrow front side, and the upper chest. Maintain the length of the trunk during exhalation, and secure it rigorously during the exhalation by strong downward hand pressure in the best corrective position. Feel the tension on both sides, laterally from the arms downwards to the waist.
The therapist, observing from above the head, clearly perceives the derotation of the trunk accompanied by flattening of the rib hump and backwards-rotation of the concave side.

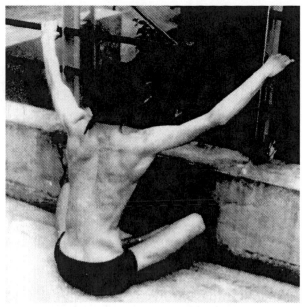

Fig. 212b

It is important that all previously learned details (e.g., occipital push, the derotated head position, shoulder counter-motion if necessary, lateral leaning of the upper trunk if necessary, and RAB) be incorporated into the exercise. There must be no perfunctory exercising. The patient must always be thinking during the exercise, and looking ahead towards the goal. This particular exercise is so effective because the rib hump, which protrudes towards the rear, is flattened from its base upwards.

5. RAISING TRUNK IN SUPINE POSITION (FIG. 213)

Omit in case of lumbar kyphosis, a very prominent lumbar hump, or flatback.
Head pointing to the wall bars; legs bent; hands grasp lower bar. Legs may also be on a chair.
Kyphosis: During inhalation, push the pelvis towards the feet (lumbar spine against the floor). During exhalation, the head and shoulder girdle are lifted off the floor.
Scoliosis: Corrective cushions; trunk leaning towards the concave side. Start with corrective RAB.
Hold all corrections during exhalation.
Reinforcement: pull both knees to the stomach to straighten out the lumbar lordosis even more.

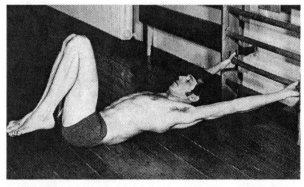

Fig. 213: Raise the upper body

93

III. Exercises using a chair and a table

Here we differentiate between:

I. Mobilization exercises

These exercises improve the mobility of the vertebrae, and the posture of the trunk, shoulder girdle and head.

II. Shaping exercises

These improve the alignment of the trunk, shoulder and head with the aid of RAB. They are performed in a position which makes unobstructed guided breathing possible, thus allowing the breath to reach the trunk segments affected. These exercises require visualization to enhance the derotation.

III. Exercises to stretch and strengthen

These stabilize the derotation results. They mainly consist of forceful isometric tension and follow shaping corrections during exhalation.

Almost all of the following exercises contain two or three of the aspects described above. They should be combined to increase shaping effects. Where no special breathing is required, the patient may choose which exercises to combine. Never force any movements!

Practise slowly to achieve the greatest degree of correction.

Each exercise must be followed by a relaxation period. Use this period for visualization.

I. Mobilization exercises
(These exercises are combined with shaping breathing).

1. SAGITTAL CIRCLING WITH THE CHEST – STRADDLE POSITION ON CHAIR (FIG. 214)

Face back of chair; sit far back; hands hold on to the back of the chair; elbows sideways and upwards (Fig. 214).

Kyphosis: The chest moves forwards and upwards over the back of the chair and the occipital push is added. Back to starting position during exhalation. Spiral-like movements of the spine and chest move the trunk further forwards, while the shoulders, head and neck are moved backwards. Pulling pelvis backwards and downwards.

To increase the effect: Use intermittent contractions of the entire back musculature during exhalation.

Scoliosis: Pelvis derotated (knee on the convex side is held further back). Shoulder girdle derotated. The trunk and head lean towards the concave side; the chin points to the convex side. RAB into the narrow front: forwards and upwards setting off the spiral-like movement. Breathe into the concave side sideways, upwards, and backwards. Omit in the case of flatback.

2. PELVIS IN PRONE POSITION ON A CHAIR (FIG. 215)
(BACK OF CHAIR LATERALLY)

Kyphosis: Pull the trunk forward close to the floor; arms either crossed or straight forward. Very small oscillatory spinal movements. The hip bones must remain on the chair to avoid hyperlordosis of the lumbar spine. The head is held up from the floor and the sides are stretched. This is also a resting position.

During exhalation, intermittent contractions from dorsal to ventral may be performed to bring the sternum closer to the floor. Caution: move the upper sternum and not the frontal rib arches towards the floor.

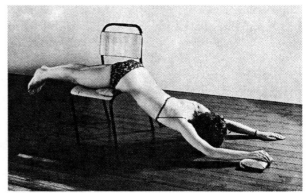

Fig. 215

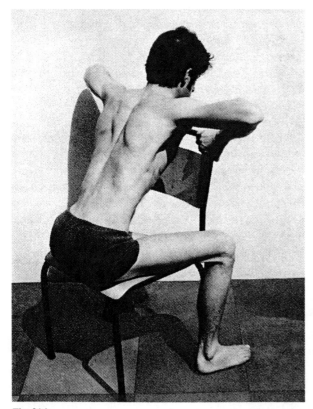

Fig. 214

Scoliosis: A correctional cushion under the hip and wrist on the convex side. The trunk leans towards the concave side. RAB. During exhalation, the thoracic convexity is contracted laterally while the narrow front is widened. In the case of flatback, a strong contraction of the abdominal muscles is needed; never 'sink' towards the floor.

3. STRETCHING BY LEANING OVER THE BACK OF A CHAIR (FIG. 216)

Abducted position behind a slightly tilted chair; the upper trunk is bent over the chair; neck extended; hands grasp the seat to tilt it upwards while the pelvis is pushed backwards by the back of chair. The knees may be slightly bent to decrease tension in the dorsal musculature of the legs.
Kyphosis: The sides of the trunk are stretched by pulling the elbows laterally. The head is pulled forward and oscillatory movements of the spine extend it. During exhalation, the tension can be reduced slightly or the result is stabilized by maintaining the tension and increasing it during the next breath. Intermittent contractions of the intercostal muscles may be used to flatten the back.
Scoliosis: Corrective cushion under the foot and hip on the convex side. Leaning towards the concave side; RAB shapes the trunk; intermittent unilateral contractions of the posterior and lateral rib hump during exhalation. Care should be taken in presence of four-curve scoliosis. Ensure that the lumbar hump is not worsened.

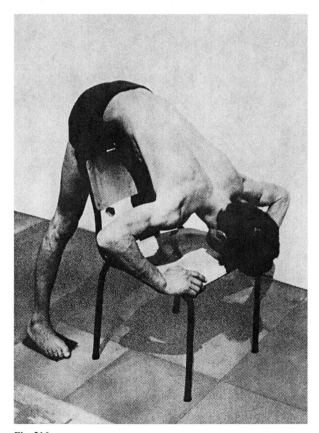

Fig. 216

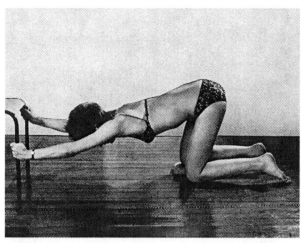

Fig. 217

4. EXERCISE TO STRETCH AND STRENGTHEN THE BACK. (FIG. 217)

Low sliding position; both hands holding on to a leg of the chair.
Kyphosis: The hands move slowly upwards along the legs of the chair. The elbows are kept straight, moving downwards in the same fashion. The chest is kept as close to the floor as possible. Do not force the breathing!
Same starting position: press the legs of chair together or pull them apart isometrically. This exercise may also be done in the supine position.
Scoliosis: Corrective cushion under the knee on the convex side; hand on this side is always further up than on the other side to derotate shoulder girdle. Subaxillary ribs and the narrow front are brought forward. The hip below the rib hump is moved laterally and caudally. Ensure that there is no lordosis. The head is aligned with the oblique position of the trunk. The chin turns slightly towards the convex side. In the case of flatback, keep the trunk horizontal. Use strong contractions of the abdominal muscles.

5. CIRCULAR MOVEMENTS OF THE TRUNK (SAGITTAL PLANE) (FIG. 218)

Sitting in front of the wall bars, back towards the bars; feet parallel; elbows straight, holding onto wall bars from above. Sit back as far as possible.
a) Move the trunk forward as far as possible.
b) Make large, circular movements with sternum upwards and forwards. With each circular movement, the trunk is lifted from the pelvic girdle. Use deep inhalation. Swing back to the starting position during exhalation. Keep the lumbar region straight.
c) Intensification: At the highest point of the circular movement, elbows are bent. This stretches the pectoral muscles and flattens the thoracic hump. The head and neck are moved backwards to increase the effect even further.

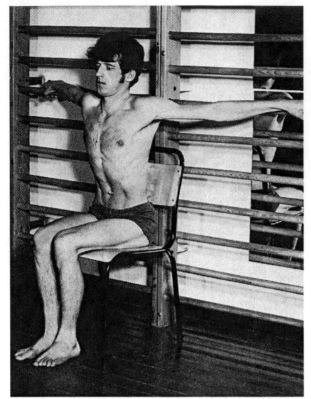

Fig. 218

Scoliosis: Derotation of pelvis and shoulder girdle. Counterrotation of the rib cage using RAB (narrow front forwards and upwards). In the case of flatback, remain in a vertical position. Continue with the 'Great arch' exercise (Figs. 201-203) immediately.

II. Shaping exercises

1. PUSHING AGAINST THE BACK OF A CHAIR (FIG. 219)

Sit upright on the ischial tuberosities. Hands hold onto the back of the chair. Make oscillatory forward movements with the trunk while stretching arms. The head, neck, and back form one line.

There are two possibilities to incorporate breathing:

a) Elongate and move upwards during inhalation, leaning slightly forwards. Back to starting position during exhalation.

b) Remain in forward position, contract back muscles intermittently during exhalation. Keep lumbar region straight.

Scoliosis: Unilateral breathing, RAB, pelvic and shoulder girdle derotated. Strong contraction of abdominal muscles during exhalation. Omit for flatback.

2. CORRECTION FOR THE HYPERKYPHOTIC BACK WITH LUMBAR LORDOSIS (FIGS. 220 AND 221)

Sitting on a chair in straddle position with the back leaning against a table; both elbows rest on the table.

Kyphosis:

a) Extend the back by pressing with elbows against the table during inhalation. This widens the upper chest.

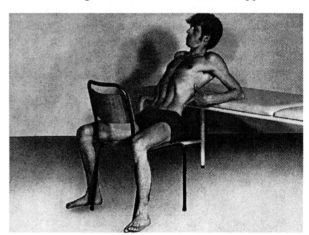

Fig. 220

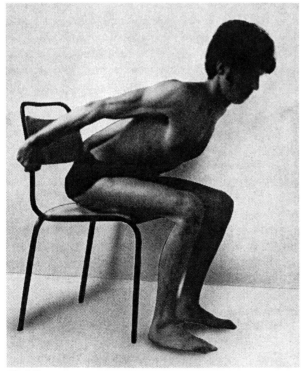

Fig. 219

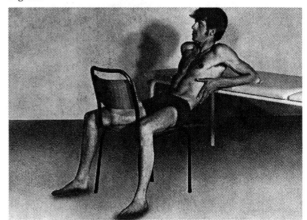

Fig. 221

Contract the back muscles during exhalation: avoid a lordosis. The head and neck are moved backwards as well.

b) During the next inhalation, the chest moves backwards, contract the abdominal muscles during exhalation to further increase lumbar lordosis. The head may be tilted slightly forwards.

Scoliosis:

a) Breathe with RAB into the narrow front during extension. During exhalation the posterior rib hump is contracted forwards and upwards.

b) RAB into the concave side to widen and derotate. At the same time, the frontal rib hump is moved sideways, upwards and backwards.

3. HORIZONTAL ELONGATION ACROSS A TABLE (FIG. 222)

Abducted position; legs straight; feet parallel and slightly under the table. The trunk bends horizontally across the table; the hands grasp the opposite table edge; arms bent.

Kyphosis: The spine and entire back are stretched by strongly pulling the head and elbows. Position is maintained during exhalation and further tension is applied during subsequent breathing. 10 inhalations and exhalations are possible. Then rest.

Scoliosis: Additional corrective cushions under the hip and elbow on the convex side (and frontal rib hump). Pull diagonally towards the concave side. RAB is used, and shoulder countertraction, if needed. After the correction is achieved, stabilization by strong isometric muscle mantle.

4. LATERAL STRETCHING ACROSS A TABLE (FIG. 223)

Kyphosis: Alternate sides. The hip against the table; leg is vertical; the trunk leans across the table; outside leg lifted, extended and rotated outwards. The hand rests on the pelvic brim. The other hand 'pulls' the table edge closer. Widen the side close to the table during inhalation and stabilize by strong tension during exhalation. The head is kept in line with trunk and leg.

Scoliosis: Concave side towards table. RAB widens this side during inhalation, while the opposite shoulder is held backwards. Pushing with the raised foot widens the concavity below the rib hump. Keep this hip backwards. Important: Use RAB also for the narrow front. Push the occiput backwards and upwards. Perform shoulder countertraction to align the cervical curve.

In the case of four-curve scoliosis, position the leg on the convex side very high. Ensure that the hip does not protrude too far.

5. ROTATIONAL MOVEMENT OF THE SHOULDER GIRDLE (FIG. 224)

Sitting on a chair; arms extended; hands on a table; feet parallel; knees bent, lower legs vertical.

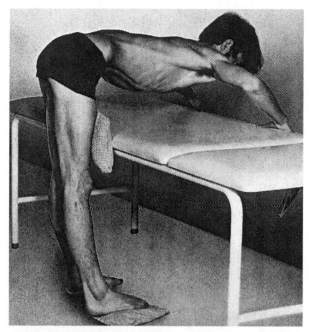

Fig. 222

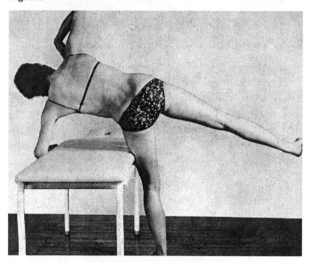

Fig. 223: In the case of a fourth curve, the leg has to be positioned higher.

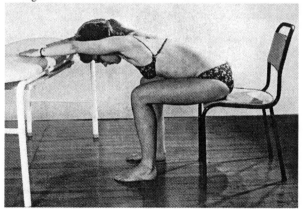

Fig. 224

Kyphosis: Elongate the trunk during inhalation, hands and arms offer support. Small rotational movements of arms and shoulders during exhalation. Head straight; neck extended.

97

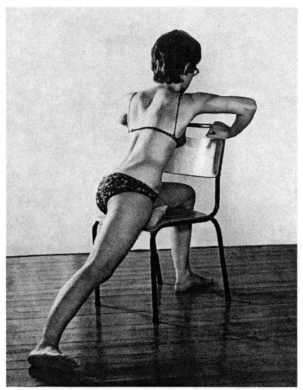

Fig. 225

Scoliosis: Corrective cushion on thigh of the concave side to push back frontal rib hump. Second cushion under hand on the convex side. Incline the trunk towards concave side. Increase rotational movement backwards. More rotational movement with elbow backwards on convex side to move narrow front further forwards and upwards.

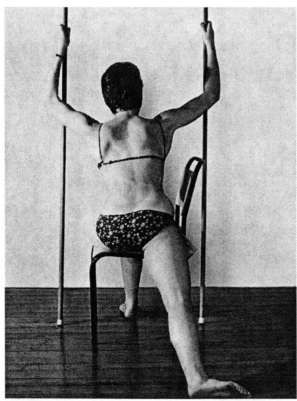

Fig. 226

In the case of lumbar kyphosis or a very prominent lumbar hump, this exercise is performed in the kneeling position with a chair.

6. **ROTATIONAL SITTING (PART B, III, 3 AND FIGS. 225 AND 226)**

Omit in case of four-curve scoliosis.
Kyphosis: Alternate sides.
Scoliosis: Sitting on chair; leg on the convex side extended backwards and rotated outwards; trunk leaning towards concave side and forwards; leg on the concave side bent.

a) The hands point towards each other and hold the back of the chair. The elbows move diagonally outwards and upwards. The head pushes out of the shoulder girdle.

b) The back of the chair is on the convex side and stabilizes the hip backwards (derotation of the pelvis). The hand rests on the back of the chair and this arm performs shoulder countertraction. The hand on the concave side holds a pole.

c) The patient holds two poles. Lift the trunk out of the pelvic girdle by pushing the poles forcefully into the floor.

Breathing: False ribs (11th and 12th) sideways, upwards and backwards, and lower the diaphragm. Thoracic concavity: sideways, upwards and backwards, and lowering the diaphragm. Narrow front: forwards and upwards, and lowering the diaphragm. Subaxillary ribs: forwards and upwards, and lowering the diaphragm.

When the best possible height is reached, all muscles are tensed during exhalation to form a muscle mantle. This prevents collapse of the body and maintains the derotation and widening of the concavities.

7. **WAIST-BELT (FIG. 227)**

Sitting upright; feet parallel.
Kyphosis: Both hands lift the lower abdomen backwards and upwards. The diaphragm lowers during inhalation. The abdominal muscles are strongly tightened during exhalation and the lumbar spine pushes against the back of the chair. The trunk stays upright. The head moves slightly backwards to increase extension. Several repetitions.
Scoliosis: Same procedure but with derotated pelvis.
In the case of lumbar kyphosis, the spine is kept in the middle position. If a lumbar hump is present, ensure that it does not worsen.

8. **RELAXED HANGING OF THE TRUNK BETWEEN TWO POLES AND RAB (FIG. 228)**

Two poles leaning against a table, the lower ends far away from the table. Legs and lower part of pelvis resting on the table. Trunk hanging down; lower arms resting on poles. Hands grasp poles.
Kyphosis: Forearms glide forward along the poles. The head is kept in the middle. The patient feels stretching of

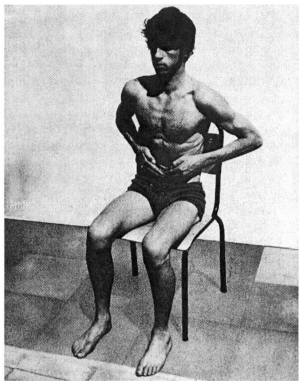

Fig. 227

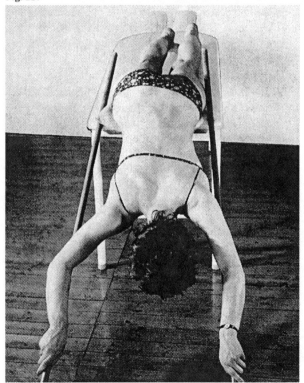

Fig. 228

Corrective cushion under the pole on the convex side to derotate shoulder girdle. Corrective cushion under hip on the convex side.

a) Stretching the upper trunk widens the concave side and the area below the rib hump. These areas are filled and tightened during lowering of the diaphragm.

b) The ribs on the concave side are moved sideways, upwards and backwards during the next inhalation. Maintain the correction during exhalation.

c) Another inhalation moves the narrow front towards the floor and cranially. The subsequent exhalation phase includes a unilateral contraction of the intercostal muscles on the convex side to flatten the rib hump and move the ribs forwards in the narrow front.

d) The next inhalation is guided towards the subaxillary ribs to bring them forwards and upwards. This moves the scapula against the rib cage and the lateral top of the shoulder backwards. The rib hump is then no longer visible.

e) The next inhalation phase moves the false ribs below the thoracic convexity sideways and backwards and towards the head. The head and neck are guided backwards during the next exhalation, and all corrective results are "engraved" deeply by strong contraction of all muscles forming a muscle mantle – isometric tension. Do not let the sternum sag in the case of flatback.

9. HEAD UNDER THE TABLE (FIGS. 229 AND 230)

Omit in case of flatback and cervical kyphosis.

a) Kneeling or sitting on a chair in front of table; elbows on top of table; head under the table.

Kyphosis: During inhalation, the pelvis pushes backwards and the lumbar area is kept straight. The clavicles move downwards and cranially. The rib arches are kept backwards. The diaphragm is consciously lowered. During exhalation, the head pushes strongly against table. This causes the upper back to flatten. The neck is kept straight.

Scoliosis: The head is in a rotated position under the table and has to push and to activate and strengthen weak neck muscles above the rib hump. The trunk is in an oblique position, leaning towards the concave side. Corrective cushions are placed under the knee and elbow on the convex side. The hip on the convex side pulls downwards. The same RAB movements as under No. 8 are now applied.

b) This exercise may also be done with a chair. In this case, the trunk is in a more horizontal position, a better compensation for hollow back (Fig. 231).

The following is an exercise to stretch the pectoral muscles: omit in case of cervical kyphosis or flatback.

10. ROTATION OF ELBOWS IN PRONE POSITION
(FIG. 232; OMIT IN CASE OF FLATBACK)

Roll or footstool under pelvis; arms in V position, hands resting on seat of chair. The upper chest is directed to-

trunk and deeper breathing, which is now possible. The rib cage moves further down and forward during exhalation and is kept in this position for some time. Short muscle contraction may be performed at the vertex of the rib hump. Direction: downwards and towards the head.

Scoliosis: The poles are put in a slight oblique position towards the concave side. The trunk leans towards that side, but the hands are kept an equal distance from floor.

99

wards the floor. The head is held so as to extend the spine. The heels are pushed down.

Kyphosis: The pectoral muscles are stretched while pushing the sternum towards floor during inhalation.

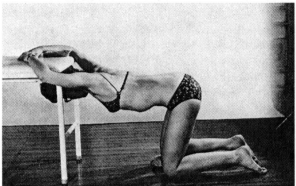
Fig. 229

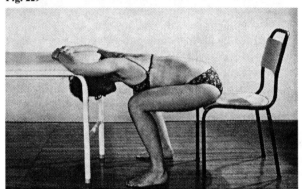
Fig. 230

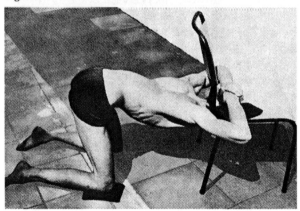
Fig. 231 In the case of flatback, there is only an isometric push of the head to strengthen the neck and upper back muscles without ventralisation of the trunk.

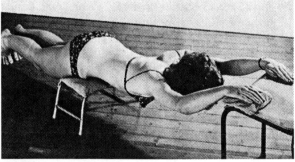
Fig. 232

The elbows are rolled backwards quickly and forcefully. This brings the shoulder blades close to the rib cage and flattens the back. The lower rib arches must not be widened during this action.

Scoliosis: The trunk is in an oblique position, leaning towards the concave side. Corrective cushions are in place. The head is in a derotated position. The narrow chest pushes forwards towards floor. Pronation of the elbow is emphasized on the convex side. Additionally, the heel is pushed down on the convex side.

III. Elongating strengthening exercises

1. RAISING THE TRUNK TO A HORIZONTAL POSITION (FIGS. 233 TO 236).

Omit in the case of rotational slippage of vertebrae, a very prominent lumbar hump, or four-curve scoliosis. The legs and pelvis rest on a table; the feet are tied down; the upper body hangs down straight; the arms are crossed.

Kyphosis:

a) The elbows are moved down towards the floor with small stretching movements. The head also pulls. Both sides are stretched and allow room for the ribs to fan out.

b) The elongated position is maintained while the trunk is raised to an almost horizontal position during exhalation. Do not raise above the horizontal, so as to avoid hyperlordosis of the lumbar spine. Activation of the lumbar muscles aims at length and strength.

c) The therapist may pull on the elbows during the inhalation phase to reinforce the length correction. The trunk is lowered slowly during exhalation. Stretch again while taking several breaths.

Scoliosis: Corrective cushions under the hip on the convex side. During extension, all narrow areas are widened and breathing is directed to them. The therapist supports corrective movements from above. The patient holds on to the therapist around the waist. The therapist's hands are now free to assist with derotation by tactile stimulation in the specific areas and they pull the patient into the oblique position to activate the lumbar erectors below the rib hump. The goal here is also length and strength. If the patient is not able to keep the acquired length during horizontal position, the therapist assists by pulling correctively.

1. Variation: With the trunk in a horizontal position, the therapist can fixate the arms while the patient tries to lower them forcefully, maintaining derotation of the shoulder girdle.

2. Variation: With the trunk in horizontal position; the patient's hands are folded behind the therapist's lumbar area. Now, the therapist moves softly backwards and stretches in this way the sides of the patient, who bends the elbows and tries to overcome the resistance of the therapist. The therapist pushes with the hands the patient's back forwards. (Fig. 236).

Never move above the horizontal!

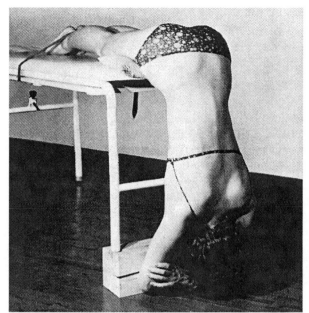

Fig. 233

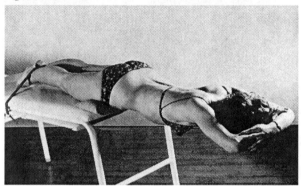

Fig. 234

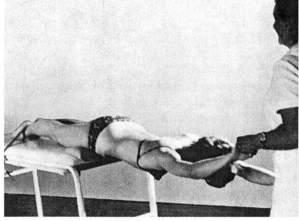

Fig. 235 Never above the horizontal!

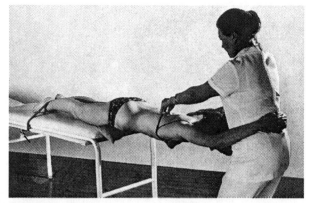

Fig. 236

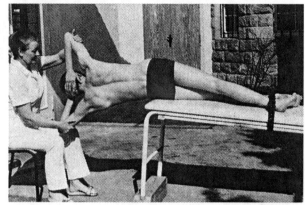

Fig. 237

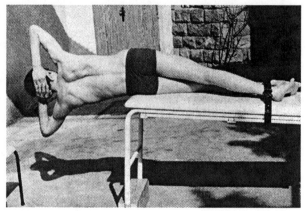

Fig. 238

2. Lateral suspended position with an aid (see Figs. 237 and 238).

Alternative for four-curve scoliosis: see Fig. 386.
Pelvis and legs in lateral position on a table; feet fastened to the table.
Kyphosis: The patient folds the hands behind the neck, the elbows pointing backwards. They try to stay in this position with the trunk and legs in a straight line. The therapist assists with corrective traction while patient tries to correct the lumbar spine. The chest is pushed forwards and the neck and head backwards. The therapist's hands let go during the exhalation phase and hold and support again during the inhalation phase. Alternate sides.
Scoliosis: The hip of the concave side rests on a table; the therapist assists corrections with vocal and tactile instructions. Important: the shoulder on the convex side has to stay back (derotation of shoulder girdle) and the narrow front has to be brought forward by RAB.
Variation: Manual assistance of a second therapist who applies tactile stimulation during RAB and ensures fixation of the result during exhalation.

101

I. Mobilization exercises to gain flexibility

II. Formative or shaping exercises starting from the optimal position to allow effective RAB.

III. Stretching and strengthening exercises to keep correction and derotation of the body segments in position.

At this point, it must be mentioned that these exercises cannot be separated entirely. Indeed, a much better result can be expected if exercises from different subgroups are combined.

I. Mobilization exercises

1. FORWARD AND UPWARD DIPPING OF THE TRUNK (FIG. 239).

Omit in the case of lumbar kyphosis and a marked lumbar hump.

Legs abducted, back extended, sitting on ischial tuberosities.

Kyphosis: Arms above head in a V-position. Pulling the arms upwards pulls the upper trunk from the pelvis upwards and forwards during inhalation. It is not necessary to reach the feet since the front must not be narrowed. During exhalation, the body swings back to starting position (vertical position). This creates a 'dipping forwards and upwards, and back-to-starting movement'. The waist is stretched each time.

Scoliosis: Extending upwards, the patient pays close attention to the narrow body segments: the area below the rib hump; the concave side and the narrow front. Dipping forwards, the body must be in an oblique position, aiming towards the concave side. Never lean or bend towards convex side! The shoulder girdle is used as a counterhold.

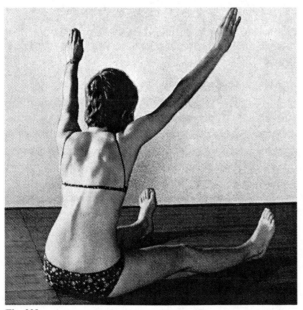

Fig. 239

2. ROCKING CRADLE (FIG. 240).

Omit in the case of lumbar kyphosis. Supine position; hands clasped around the knees, pulling them over the abdomen.

Kyphosis: Alternate lifting of the head with the shoulder girdle and pelvis. This results in a rocking movement. Restrict movement to the lumbar area of the spine.

Scoliosis: Corrective cushions to secure straight rocking movement.

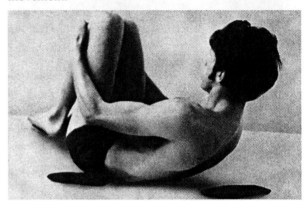

Fig. 240

3. 'FEATHERING' AND TENDER MANUAL CORRECTIONS BY THE THERAPIST, WHILE THE PATIENT IS KEPT IN A DEEP GLIDING POSITION (FIGS. 241-247)

Kneeling position; thighs vertical; trunk leaning forwards; arms extended in V-position; clavicles close to the floor.

a) Effective position during relaxation as well as an orthopaedic exercise by itself. The weight of the rib hump pushes the sternum down and forward. This, in turn, creates a contraction at the vertex of the rib hump. In the case of hyperlordosis, the pelvis is brought further back and the thighs form an acute angle (Fig. 241).

b) *Kyphosis*: Sternum or narrow front moves towards floor with spiral-like circular movements. This increases the sensation of contraction in the back.

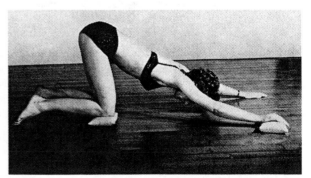

Fig. 241

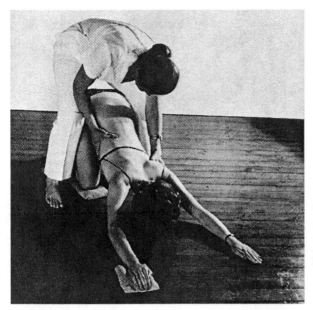

Fig. 242

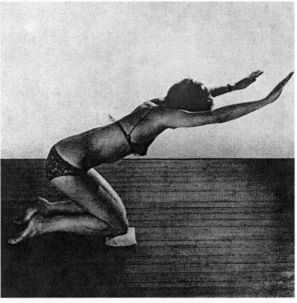

Fig. 244

c) The therapist fixates the pelvis (Fig. 242) with the lower legs and lifts the trunk out of the pelvis simultaneously with forwards and upwards pulling movements. The hands are below the elevation of the back.

d) The therapist's thumbs are placed on the sides of the transverse processes of the lumbar spine. Each vertebra is now pushed gently and firmly forwards and upwards (Fig. 243). Omit in the case of flatback.

e) After the best possible alignment is reached, a strong and forceful contraction to the count of 12 follows. The patient's hands push forcefully against the floor. The head and neck are aligned with extended back. This results in tensing of all the muscles which fixates the optimal results of the exercise and thus, a new shape.

f) Elongation and derotation of the upper trunk during inhalation.

The patient then pushes off the floor while exhaling, and his or her back and arms form a horizontal line (Fig. 244). If necessary, the feet are stabilized by the therapist or anchored under a piece of furniture. *Scoliosis*: Corrective cushions in place; oblique position of trunk; hip below rib hump backwards; head derotated. Unilateral circular movement with most narrow front. Be aware of the sensation of contraction and flattening effect on the rib hump.

The therapist can apply a range of aids:

1. See above (also Fig. 243): Thumbs on the sides of the spine; pushing each transverse process towards the floor and towards the head.

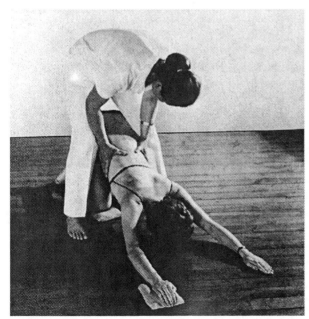

Fig. 243

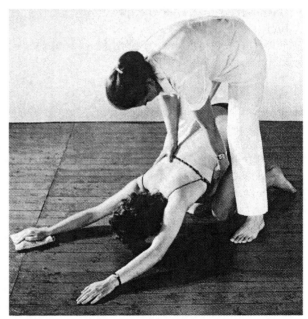

Fig. 245

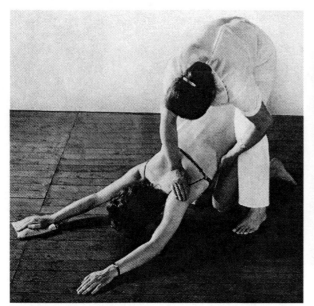

Fig. 246

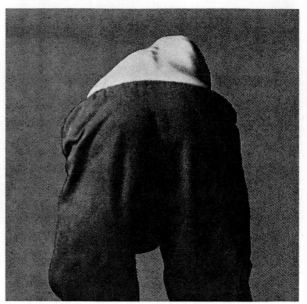

Fig. 249

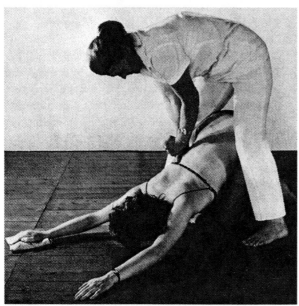

Fig. 247

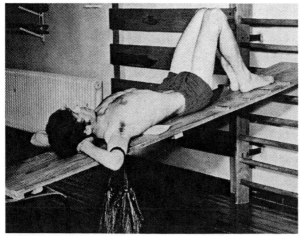

Fig. 248

2. Counterrotation (Fig. 245): Concave side sideways, upwards, and backwards, rib hump forwards and upwards.
3. Counterrotation (Fig. 246): The concave side moves sideways, upwards and backwards; the concave-side shoulder moves forward.
4. Selective rotational pressure with the thumb (Fig. 247): the thumb is placed on the rib that should be moved forwards. The other hand puts weight on the thumb and produces a derotational movement in the desired direction.

4. STRETCHING SHORTENED (UNILATERAL) PECTORAL MUSCLES LYING ON THE OBLIQUE BOARD (Fig. 248)

Relaxation in between exercises as well.

Supine position on a board which has one side raised; head hanging down; hands folded behind the neck.

Kyphosis:
a) A weight (a shopping bag in which the weight can be increased every day) hangs from each elbow. Add one minute of exercise time daily. Effect: stretching stimulus for the pectoral muscles and the shoulder blades are pressed in towards the rib cage more and more due to the weight.
b) First contraction phase: elbows raise the weight, little by little.
c) Second contraction phase: extension and pressure of head and neck against the board.

Scoliosis: The weight is carried by the elbow on the convex side. Corrective cushions are positioned.

The weight may also be in the form of a sand bag, positioned on the upper part of the shoulder on the convex side.

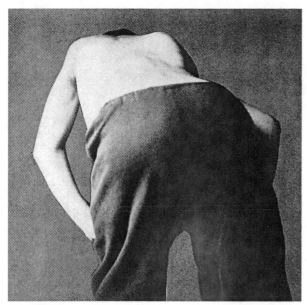

Fig. 250

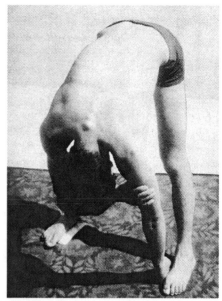

Fig. 251

5. TRUNK HANGING FORWARD IN THE STANDING POSITION (FIGS. 249–251)

Abducted position; upper trunk hanging forward as vertically as possible; arms crossed.

Kyphosis: The elbows are gradually moved towards the floor. The head serves as a weight pulling on the spine. The spine performs small oscillatory movements, getting larger and larger while the elbows approach the floor. The knees may bend at times to change the stretching effect from one area of the trunk to the other. Concentration is necessary, as is RAB.

Scoliosis: In this position, the dorsal convexity is more obvious. Breathing into the concavity sideways and upwards and backwards and upwards. That will even out the back (derotation). The shoulder on the concave side is forcefully held forward to achieve a levelling effect on the rib hump. The hand on the concave side stabilizes the exercise by being held under the toes or at the ankle level (Fig. 251). Several phases of RAB may be necessary.

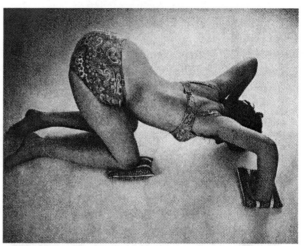

Fig. 252: Omit corrective cushion underneath the knee in the case of four-curve scoliosis.

6. THE MACHINE (FIGS. 252 AND 253)

On all fours.
Kyphosis:
a) Preliminary exercise: raising and lowering anterior pelvic crest while concentrating on lumbar spine. The latter alternately adopts a kyphotic and lordotic position.
b) In connection with breathing: lifting and inhalation; lowering and exhalation. Another possibility: Contracting abdominal musculature during exhalation (omit cushion under the knee in case of four-curve scoliosis).
c) Sitting on heels is starting position. The trunk moves forwards in a semicircle with the arms bent.

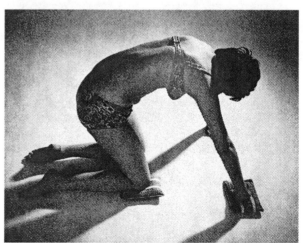

Fig. 253

105

Return to the starting position in the same manner. In case of flatback, move only into elongation – no lowering of the sternum.

d) Starting position: sitting on the heels. The upper body is moved forwards above the horizontal and comes back the same way. The head serves as resistance, as does the pelvis. Inhalation during the semicircular movement. Breath is directed into narrow lumbar region.

e) Complete circular movement: Starting as above. During inhalation, the chest moves towards the floor, and the head pulls forward. Then exhalation and straightening of arms. During following inhalation, the lumbar spine is arched and the patient returns to the heel position. Exhalation. This may be repeated in the opposite order as well.

f) To gain flexibility, this movement is done more rapidly and in a larger radius.

g) The same sideways: the hands and knees a little further apart to allow shifting of balance. Practise as follows: from right along the floor to left and back. Deep breathing . Do not force breathing or hold the breath.

Scoliosis:

a) During preliminary exercise: raising and lowering of anterior pelvic crest; derotation of shoulder girdle and pelvic girdle with corrective cushions. Upper body in oblique position towards the concave side. Head derotated extending the second curvature. Raise anterior pelvic crest: the head swings forward. Lowering of the pelvic crest, the head swings backwards. The concave side and frontal rib arch are brought backwards while the pelvic crest is raised. The dorsal rib hump and narrow front are brought forwards and upwards while the pelvic crest is lowered.

b) Include breathing: inhalation during raising phase. During exhalation, the abdominal muscles are tightened. The intercostal muscles of the frontal rib arch are also contracted (the shoulder on the concave side pushes forwards). Next inhalation: lowering of frontal pelvic crest, and narrow front is widened. During exhalation, the intercostal muscles of rib hump are contracted.

c) During the semicircular movement towards the floor, the anterior narrow front is carried closely along the floor while special attention is paid to counterrotation of the shoulder. During the movement upwards, the ribs on the concave side and those below the rib hump fan out. The head pulls obliquely away. Keep the body in an oblique position at all times.

d) Faster movements for flexibility may be performed, but correction is always the priority. Rapid mental adaptation is required.

e) Perform lateral circles only up to the midline. For example: a thoracic-right scoliosis needs movement from right to low to left. The concave side is important during the sideways and backwards phase. it has to be kept wide. No movement to the right.

II. Shaping exercises

1. DOUBLE TWIST IN SUPINE POSITION (FIG. 254)

Knees bent; feet on the floor.
Kyphosis:

a) Preliminary exercise: both knees are brought to the ground. Alternate sides. Trunk stays flat on the ground.

b) Both knees remain on the right side. The ribs on the left are spread out by breathing and raised sideways and upwards. An oblique pull should be felt from the right hip across the umbilicus to the left costal arch. This oblique pull continues to the spine, which also rotates. Same on the other side.

Scoliosis:

a) Corrective cushions; the pelvis is shifted to the convex side; both knees on that side, or just slightly leaning. In the case of a large lumbar hump, only the knee on the convex side may lean over to avoid stretching of the lumbar hump. Hand pushes hip below rib hump towards the feet. The pelvis is now derotated and fixated, and forms a fixed point for the counterrotation of the trunk.

b) Inhalation: RAB
   1. Into the thoracic concavity
   2. Into the lumbar concavity with lowering of the diaphragm and occipital push
   3. Into the narrow front

When corrections are complete, stabilize during exhalation. Then elongation again with inhalation and another strong exhalation with muscle contraction. May be increased and held to a count of 12.

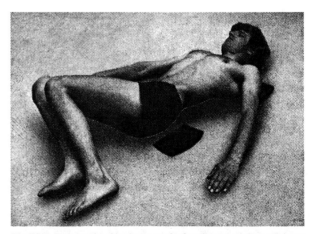

Fig. 254: To be omitted in the case of a fourth curve and a prominent lumbar hump.

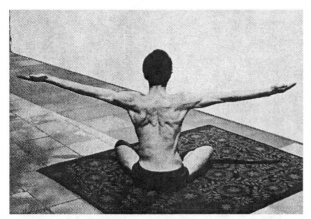

Fig. 255

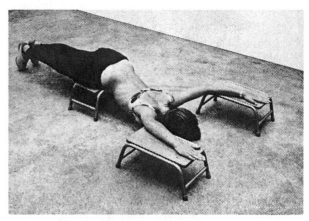

Fig. 256: To be omitted in the case of flatback.

2. Funnel circles with arms (Fig. 255)

Sitting cross legged, on ischial tuberosities. The upper body leans slightly forwards; arms in horizontal position and turned with the palms upwards.

Kyphosis: Both arms describe a circle starting forwards and upwards. During the backwards and downwards movement, the clavicles are brought forward and the neck and head backwards. This is the inhalation phase. During exhalation, the arms swing back to starting position. Increase the circles and breathing. Some discomfort may be felt in the rib hump: this is due to the forceful pull on the shoulders downwards.

Scoliosis: Stronger movements on the convex side with special attention to derotation of the shoulder girdle and correct position of the head. Oblique position of trunk. Manual checking whether the lumbar erector spinae below the rib hump is activated.

In flatback, move the circles forward. The upper body should be upright and not arch forward.

3. Stretching the pectoral muscles in the prone position (Fig. 256)

Omit in the case of flatback.
The pelvis rests on a footstool; roll under costal arches if necessary; left and right elbow abducted and placed on corrective cushions.

Kyphosis: Circular movements of subaxillary ribs and clavicles towards the floor. Pectoral muscles stay relaxed as much as possible, even when it is a little painful. Attempt to continue working with that feeling of stretching.

Scoliosis: Additional corrective cushion under elbow on the convex side. Emphasis is on the subaxillary ribs on this side. Contraction of rib hump during exhalation.

4. 'Shovelling,' or correction of the shoulder blades, for scapula alata (Figs. 257–259)

Sitting upright or standing; upper body slightly leaning forward, head held back.

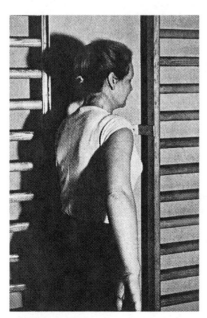

Fig. 257

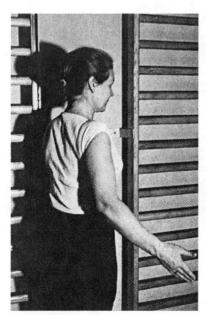

Fig. 258

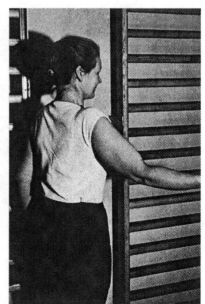

Fig. 259

107

Kyphosis: The hands and shoulders perform shovelling movements: backwards, downwards and forwards. The patient should feel the lower shoulder blade pressing firmly against the rib cage. The movement may be done first with one shoulder and then the other. While the scapula pushes the ribs forward, the rib cage must move forwards and upwards. The shoulder blades should rotate about their frontal axis, i.e., the longitudinal axis of the clavicles.

Do not press the shoulder blades against the spine.

Scoliosis: Oblique position of trunk; concave side widened. Movement is only performed on the convex side. In the case of flatback, the frontal rib arch needs to be brought backwards first, then held in position.

5. ROTATION OF SHOULDER GIRDLE IN KNEELING POSITION (FIG. 260)

Kneeling; upper trunk leaning forwards; left arm on the floor – extended or bent; right arm on a chair.

Kyphosis: Right chest performs circular movements forwards and upwards during inhalation. This pulls on the ribs of the rib hump. During exhalation, these intercostal muscles are further contracted by intermittent muscle contractions. Alternate sides after three exhalation phases.

Scoliosis: Corrective cushions under the knee on the convex side. The arm on the same side rests on the chair. The narrow front is moved forwards and upwards by directing breathing. The concave side is arched by breathing sideways-upwards and backwards-upwards into it. The therapist may assist manually. It is necessary to pay close attention to the sensation of derotation.

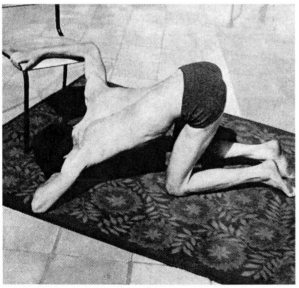

Fig. 260

6. "KNEE IN THE BACK" (FIG. 261)

Omit in case of flatback.

The patient is on the concave side; corrective cushion under hip or lumbar hump (derotate first). Lower knee

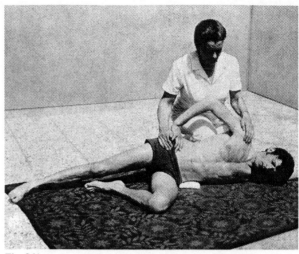

Fig. 261

bent; the upper leg rests extended on the floor; outward rotation. No lumbar lordosis should occur. The upper trunk is slightly inclined forwards; the frontal pelvic crest is raised. In four-curve scoliosis, the upper leg rests on a footstool: the upper hip in the resting position; the arm on the floor is extended; the therapist kneels behind patient.

Kyphosis: The therapist's knee is a little below the rib hump and pushes forwards and cranially. The hands pull the lateral top of shoulder and upper hip backwards. The goal is the patient's awareness of both countermovements. Appropriate breathing: inhalation brings the narrow chest forwards while the diaphragm is lowered. The frontal pelvic crest is raised. The therapist assists during exhalation. Both the abdominal and overstretched intercostal muscles are contracted. Alternate sides after 5 exhalations.

Scoliosis: Patient on concave side; corrective cushion under lumbar curvature; the arm on the floor is extended even more to widen the thoracic concavity. RAB during the inhalation phase and stabilization during exhalation. The effect is increased by pushing the extended hand to the floor and pressing the knee to the same.

Note: The pressure of the knee and pull of the hands must be balanced to avoid forward or backward movement of the body. Patient should stay vertically on the side.

A fellow patient may assist as well. The knee on the concave side is used to push while the narrow front is pulled across the partner. The breathing must be the opposite of that of the exercising patient.

7. ALIGNING THE FRONTAL RIB HUMP (FIG. 262), LYING ON CONCAVE SIDE, WITH ASSISTANCE

Only for patients with scoliosis.

Patient on concave side; corrective cushions; lower leg bent; upper leg straight and rotated outwards.

a) The therapist kneels behind the patient. One hand is under the patient to pull the frontal rib hump gently backwards and upwards, while the other hand push-

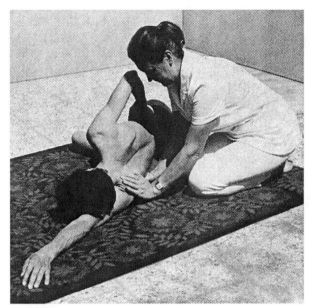

Fig. 262

es the shoulder forwards. This must happen during inhalation to apply counter-pressure from inside against the ribs of the concavity. This way, the ribs are not pressed or bent. Exhalation is a relaxation phase. Then the patient tries to visualize the procedure before repeating it.

b) During exhalation, the patient tries to maintain the alignment tensing all muscles to form a muscle mantle.

8. ASSISTED ELONGATION OF THE TRUNK IN PRONE POSITION (FIG. 263)

Omit in the case of flatback.
Prone position; pelvis elevated by a footstool; forehead rests on the hands.
Kyphosis: The therapist's hands glide laterally during inhalation from the spine to the hollow lumbar region. After these areas have filled with air, the therapist moves the rib hump gently forwards and upwards during exhalation. The patient is aware of the elbows gliding further forward, stretching the sides and bringing relief to the hollow lumbar region. The movement is supported by the patient moving the head even further into elongation.

Scoliosis: Corrective cushions under the hip and elbow on the convex side and the frontal rib hump on the concave side. The legs are closed and slightly moved towards the concave side (do not narrow this side). The helping hands are positioned below the dorsal rib hump and on the shoulder of the concave side. The fingers are spread and push these areas gently cranially and towards the floor. The patient directs his/her awareness towards these areas and the sensation of opening up. The following inhalation increases these sensations even more. The therapist then pushes the lateral rib hump inwards and upwards during exhalation. Attention! The area below the dorsal rib hump must not become smaller.

After several of these assisted corrections, the patient gets up and tries to recreate the sensations and corrections in front of a mirror.

9. PELVIC DEROTATION (FIG. 264)

Omit in the case of four-curve scoliosis and lumbar kyphosis.
Supine position; legs raised; hands on hips.
Kyphosis: The sides are stretched by pushing the hips and widening the waist during inhalation. During exhalation, the right heel pushes against a chair and thus brings the hip on the same side forwards and upwards. Repeat 3 times, then switch sides.
Scoliosis: Corrective cushions; the leg on the concave side turned inwards; the leg on the convex side turned outwards. During exhalation, the heel on concave side pushes strongly against the chair. The hip is contracted intermittently forwards. The lumbar hump is contracted forwards and upwards as well. Use hands to check the result.

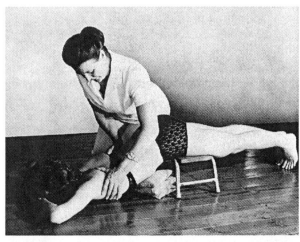

Fig. 263

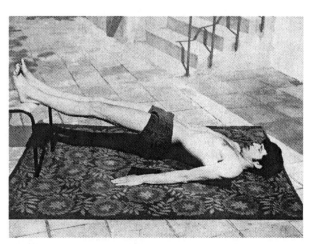

Fig. 264

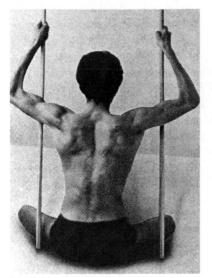
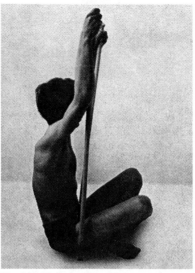
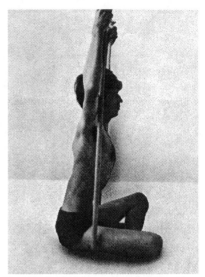

Fig. 265

Fig. 266: Unfavourable: Sitting on coccyx.

Fig. 267: Good! Sitting on ischial tuberosities.

10. STRETCHING UPWARDS BETWEEN TWO POLES (FIGS. 265, 60 AND 61)

Sitting upright in front of a mirror; two poles on right and left side; elbows spread wide above shoulder height.

Kyphosis:

a) The spine is moved upwards in small serpentine movements, and the head is also pulled upwards. The trunk is lifted out of the pelvis.

b) Once the best possible height is reached, RAB is guided into the narrow areas and the diaphragm is lowered. Directions of breathing are: the sides – laterally and upwards; the lumbar area – backwards and upwards. the clavicles forwards and upwards.

c) During the exhalation phase, the results are stabilized and should be improved with each following breath.

d) Before ending the exercise, push both poles strongly against the floor while tensing all muscles to form a muscle mantle. Attention! Keep shoulder blades far apart and downwards, and move the head and neck backwards. Tensing all the muscles concerned may only be performed after all possible corrections have been completed and the body is in best possible corrected position.

Scoliosis:

Bodyweight on the concave side; pelvis and shoulder girdle derotated. Perform oscillatory movements, incorporating RAB. Pay special attention to weak musculature below the rib hump. Incline the head toward the concave side and turn the chin to the convex side, combined with an occipital push.

Before tensing all muscles to form a muscle mantle, the concave side must be arched as far as possible across the hip and rotated backwards. Contraction during exhalation must be strong enough to lift body from floor.

III. Stretching and strengthening exercises

1. LEARNING TO SIT ON EITHER THE COCCYX OR ISCHIAL TUBEROSITIES (FIGS. 266, 267)

Starting position cross-legged.

Kyphosis: The pelvis is lifted off the floor while the poles are strongly pushed into the ground. In suspension, the pelvis is rotated around its horizontal axis and then put down on either the coccyx (forming a round back) or the ischial tuberosities (forming a lordosis). Feel the different sensations in the back. Be aware that you must 'rethink' because when standing, the anterior iliac crest should be lifted to bring the pelvis into a horizontal position, but in sitting position it must be lowered to achieve the same effect.

Scoliosis: During the rolling movement around the horizontal axis, the pelvis must also be rotated around the longitudinal axis: the hip below rib hump must be moved backwards. Nevertheless, the weight has to be kept on the concave side. Feel how the atrophied muscles below rib hump are activated.

2. RAISING ARMS IN THE PRONE POSITION (FIG. 268)

Omit in the case of flatback. Prone position; hips on a soft roll cushion; arms extended in V-position.

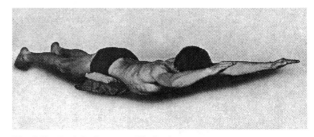

Fig. 268: Omit in the case of flatback.

110

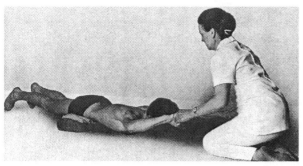

Fig. 269

Kyphosis:
a) Both arms are alternately lifted off the floor and moved forwards while the head is raised (occipital push). Counter-push of the heels to correct lumbar lordosis. Breathing: inhale and stretch, exhale and lift the head and arms off the floor. Inhale and stretch again; during exhalation return to the starting position on the floor.
b) The arms may be held above the floor alternately, if it is too difficult to raise both at the same time.
c) The therapist may support the movement. Breathing is used as described above. Again, the patients must be made aware of the bodily sensations so they can repeat the exercise later without assistance.
d) The height to which the arms are lifted may vary with assistance of the therapist. The upper chest should stay on the floor during small lifts (Fig. 269).

Scoliosis: Corrective cushions. The arm on the convex side is raised higher (derotation of shoulder girdle), the chest performs counterrotation. This exercise is primarily for patients with a high dorsal rib hump. In the case of lumbar kyphosis, the legs may be raised as well.

3. LIFTING THE PELVIS IN LATERAL POSITION (FIG. 270)

Omit in the case of four-curve scoliosis.
Lateral position; arm supports weight; elbow bent; upper arm in vertical position; hip on a corrective roll cushion; legs extended.
Kyphosis: During inhalation, the body stretches and the head also pulls. During exhalation, the pelvis is lifted off the support with intermittent contractions. After three repetitions, switch sides.
Scoliosis: The concave side faces the floor. This side is widened first by RAB and stays wide while the pelvis is

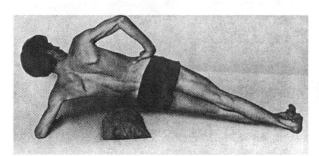

Fig. 270: Omit in the case of four-curve scoliosis..

lifted. The upper hip is rotated backwards and the narrow front forwards.

4. LIFTING WEIGHT WITH SHOULDER ON CONCAVE SIDE (FIG. 271)

Only in the case of scoliosis: supine position; corrective cushions in place. Heavy dumbbell or sack filled with sand on top of the shoulder of the concave side. This shoulder is lifted off the floor. Breathing: corrective inhalation; lifting during exhalation. This aligns the distorted shoulder and unilaterally regulates the stretched pectoral muscles.

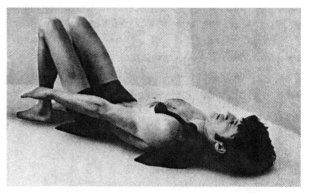

Fig. 271

5. ISOMETRIC RESISTANCE EXERCISES COMBINED WITH VISUALIZATION (FIG. 272)

Legs bent; arms raised above head; lumbar area on the floor.
Kyphosis: During inhalation, the arms are further extended to stretch the sides. The lumbar spine stays on the floor. During exhalation, both fists pull down an imaginary weight, while the elbows remain on the floor and the head is pulled upwards. This is accompanied by forceful contractions of the lateral muscles.
Scoliosis: Corrective cushions. The exercise concentrates on the concave side and the narrow lumbar area below the rib hump during inhalation. The arched dorsal concavity and widened lumbar concavity are stabilized during exhalation. The concavities should approach the floor.

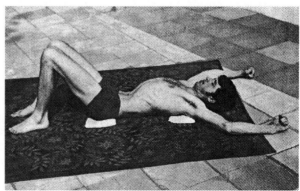

Fig. 272

6. Isometric resistance exercise in prone position (Fig. 273)

Pelvis resting on a roll; arms extended in V-position on the floor.

Kyphosis: The hands and feet push away from the body during inhalation. During exhalation, the fists pull an imaginary weight towards the body. Both shoulders also pull caudally. The elbows are bent and brought backwards while the upper chest is kept close to the floor. The head is held backwards and also pushes against imaginary resistance.

Scoliosis: Corrective cushions; upper body in oblique position. Preparatory RAB to widen the concave side and stabilize it during exhalation. Contraction of the lateral and posterior rib hump. The head stays derotated. Heel-push with the foot on the convex side.

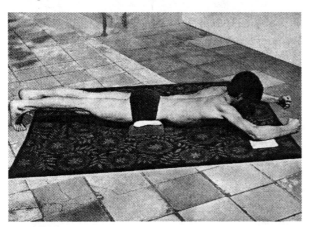

Fig. 273

7. Isometric exercise with belt (Fig. 274)

If no wall bar is available, a piece of wood is put through one side of the strap, then the strap is guided underneath a door and the door is closed (Fig. 579). Poles are pushed against the door.

To avoid damage to the door, the poles should be rubber tipped. See section C.IX on corrective aids.

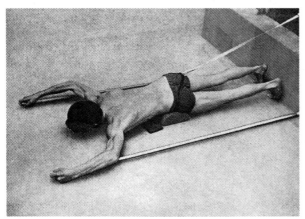

Fig. 274

Prone position; feet towards the wall; corrective roll cushion under pelvis; the belt is put around the hips and attached to the strap. The belt fixates the pelvis during exercise. The arms rest on poles, which should be pushed against the wall at right angles.

Kyphosis: The spine performs minute oscillatory sideways movements during inhalation to reach full extension. The clavicles remain close to the floor. A heel push prevents a lordosis. The head is lifted. During exhalation, the poles are pushed against the wall.

Scoliosis: Corrective cushions; the strap is slightly pushed over to the convex side of the pelvis to stretch the narrow waist musculature on this side. The body leans towards the concave side to open it. During exhalation, push the poles against the wall and lift the upper body out of the pelvis. The shoulders must not be pulled upwards. The head and neck are in elongation, lifted off the ground and pushed backwards: rib hump should flatten.

If the pelvis is straight and there is no prominent hip, the strap is put over the middle of pelvis. The same is done in cases of four-curve scoliosis.

Two straps on either side are used for lumbar kyphosis and a very prominent lumbar hump.

The exercise is performed without a fastened belt in patients with rotational slippage of the vertebrae.

8. Isometric exercise with a belt in the supine position (Figs. 275 and 276)

The strap is fastened to the lowest bar; the belt is tightened around the hips and attached to the strap; two poles at right angles to the wall bars are held at shoulder height (lower arms below the poles). The knees are bent.

Kyphosis: The lumbar and cervical spine are close to the floor; the head pulls out of the shoulder girdle while the shoulders are pulled downwards. Small oscillatory movements of the spine are performed to reach full elongation during inhalation. While exhaling, the poles are strongly pushed against the wall; the head pushes against the floor and the round back is flattened by intermittent muscle contractions.

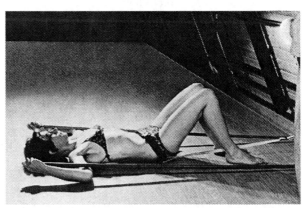

Fig. 275 Exercise for kyphosis and scoliosis, but not in the presence of rotational sliding vertebrae.

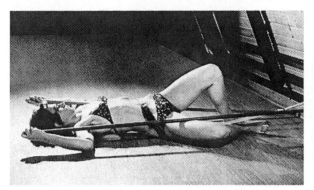

Fig. 276 Exercise for scoliosis while derotating pelvis.

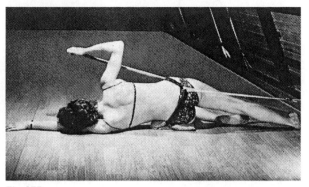

Fig. 277

Scoliosis: Corrective cushions; the knee on the convex side is brought towards the ground; the strap is moved a little towards the convex side to widen the lumbar area on this side. The pole fixates this pelvic derotation (Fig. 276). Omit in the case of four-curve scoliosis. All hollow areas are moved towards the floor during RAB. During exhalation, the shoulder on the convex side pushes towards the floor, which contracts the rib hump forwards. The concave side must remain wide.

9. ISOMETRIC EXERCISE WITH THE BELT IN LATERAL POSITION (FIG. 277)

The belt is fastened to the lowest bar; corrective cushions are put in place; the lower leg is bent to 90°; the upper leg is extended and slightly rolled outwards; the lower arm is extended with the head resting on it; the upper body leans slightly forwards; the upper hand grasps the pole and pushes it against the wall.
Kyphosis: All following movements may be performed on either side three to five times.
Scoliosis: Corrective cushions; the concave side is on the floor: the extended arm pulls and stretches this side; small serpentine movements of the spine are performed to elongate and bring the concavity closer to the floor. Additional push of the pole against the wall. RAB is performed to move the concave side backwards and upwards and the narrow front forwards and upwards. Pulling the pole backwards keeps the shoulder and hip backwards (derotation of shoulder and pelvic girdle). During exhalation, these corrections are stabilized by firmly pushing the pole atainst the wall. In four-curve scoliosis, the strap stays in the middle of the pelvis and the upper leg rests on the pole. There is only a corrective cushioning under the lumbar hump.

10. ON ALL FOURS (FIG. 278)

On all fours; feet towards the wall bars; belt around hips; arms in V-position; hands on the floor; upper body towards floor; the head is kept off the floor.
Kyphosis: The hands pull forwards to stretch the sides of the trunk. The strap prevents the pelvis from gliding forwards. The thighs are in a 90° position. The upper body performs small oscillatory movements. Breathing: inhale during stretching. During exhalation, the chest moves towards floor and stays there as long as possible. Both hands push against the floor to increase the contractions of back muscles and widening of the front. In case of flatback, work only straight ahead.
Scoliosis: Strap on convex side (to widen the area below the rib hump). The upper body pulls obliquely to the concave side. The knee and wrist on the convex side rest on corrective cushions (derotation of shoulder and pelvic girdle). In the case of four-curve scoliosis, the strap runs in the middle of the pelvis.
Breathing: RAB while pulling towards the concave side – sideways, upwards and backwards. Attention: in cases of four-curve scoliosis, the breathing is guided into the area above the lumbar hump, which has first been derotated forwards and upwards. During exhalation, the correction results are stabilized. The next inhalation moves the narrow front forwards and upwards (the dorsal rib hump is contracted forwards, upwards and inwards). During exhalation, the results are stabilized. A few deep breaths are performed in the corrected position.

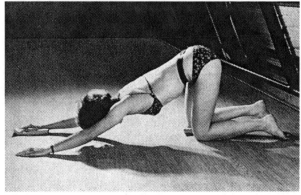

Fig. 278

113

V. Neck Exercises

In the case of scoliosis, these exercises may also be done on both sides at first. In this case, the body has to be aligned and corrected from the pelvis to the shoulders. The best starting position is sitting upright on a chair or on the floor in front of a mirror. The best exercise position of the head activates the posterior ligaments of the neck (Fig. 279). Care should be taken in the case of cervical kyphosis or the absence of lordosis. In such cases, the head pushes upwards in a middle position. See also Figs. 568 and 569 on cervical kyphosis.

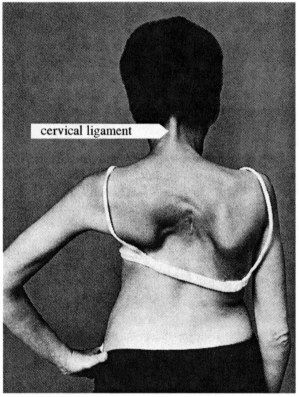

cervical ligament

Fig. 279

1. Awareness of correct and incorrect head position (Figs. 280 and 281)

a) The chin pushes forwards horizontally and pulls back. The patient observes the neck and shoulder line. Exercising quickly mobilizes the cervical spine.
b) With breathing: during inhalation, the chin is brought backwards and upwards, and is pushed forwards during exhalation to the beginning position.

2. Neck exercise with resistance (Fig. 282)

a) The hands are folded behind head and pull it forwards. This stretches the neck.

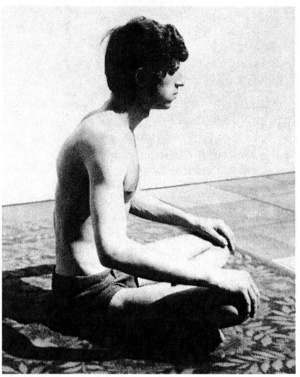

Fig. 280

b) The head pushes against the hands. Elbows are spread as far apart as possible to permit optimal widening of chest. In the case of scoliosis, the narrow front is turned forwards and upwards (Fig. 283).
c) The hands are removed suddenly. The head jumps further backwards (Fig. 284).
d) The head pushes against a table, chair or similar object (Fig. 212).

3. Inclining the head laterally (Figs. 286 and 287)

During inhalation, the head pushes upwards and the spine is elongated. Be aware of the pulling feeling that elongates all the way down to the lumbar spine. During exhalation, the head is inclined towards the shoulder without rotation. Be aware of the stretching on the opposite side. During the next inhalation, the head is brought to the middle position. During the next exhalation, the head is inclined to the other side. Preference is given to the side with greater restriction. For example: 5 times to the left and 3 times to the right side. In the case of torticollis, the exercise is unilateral. Ensure that the shoulders are kept horizontal and never bend the trunk! The breathing can also be changed: inhale while inclining the head. Exhale while returning to the middle position.

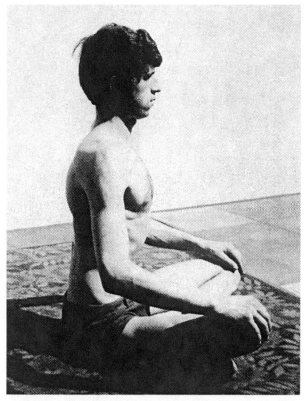

Fig. 281

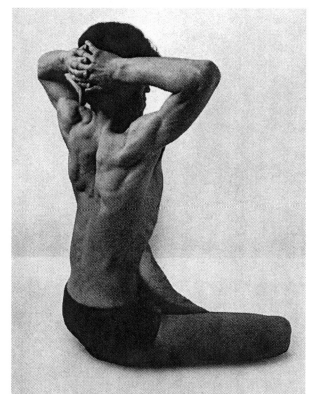

Fig. 283

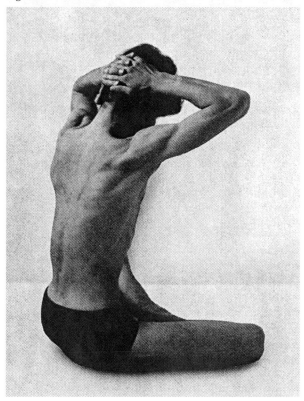

Fig. 282

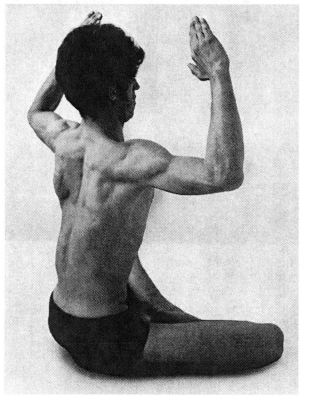

Fig. 284

115

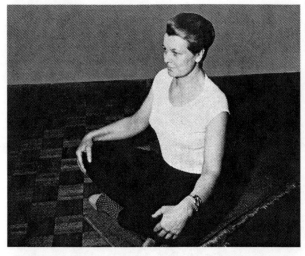

Fig. 285

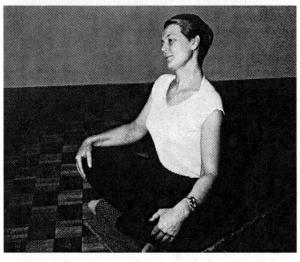

Fig. 286

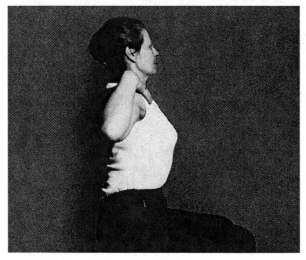

Fig. 287

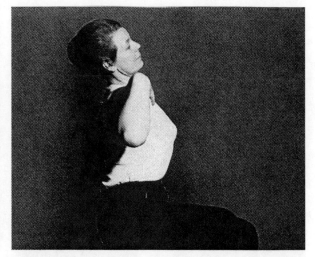

Fig. 288

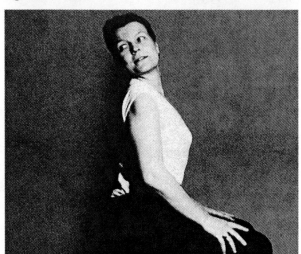

Fig. 289

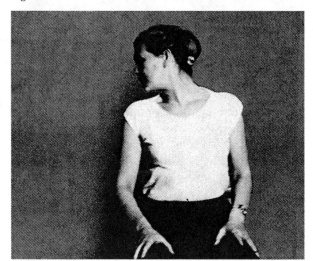

Fig. 290

4. Inclining the head (Fig. 288)

This exercise achieves the greatest degree of elongation during inhalation (with the occipital push). During exhalation, guide the head obliquely backwards. The neck should be in the most elongated position and the shoulders must not rotate. They may be stabilized by the hands. The upper trunk should be held straight as well. This exercise is combined with RAB into the narrow front. In the case of flatback, move only to the midline.

5. Turning the head (Figs. 289 and 290)

a) Occipital push during inhalation. During exhalation, turn the chin towards the shoulder without turning the shoulder girdle or trunk.
b) During exhalation, the chin is turned sharply towards the shoulder four times. During inhalation, head is pulled straight upwards again. Repeat on the other side.
c) After turning the head, it is pushed backwards against a real or imaginary wall. Omit in case of flatback.

6. Carriage driver's position on a chair (Fig. 291)

Sit on a hard chair, knees flexed.
Lower legs vertical; elbows resting on knees; upper arms in vertical position; chest sagging forwards.
a) The head sinks between shoulders during exhalation. During inhalation, it is pulled strongly upwards while the shoulders are pushed downwards in a countermovement.

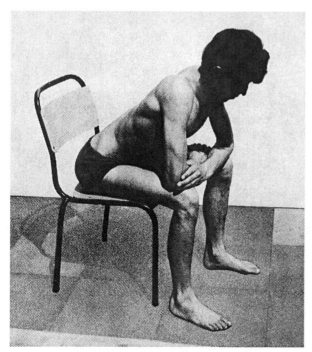

Fig. 291

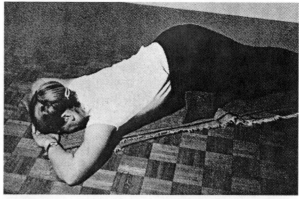

Fig. 292

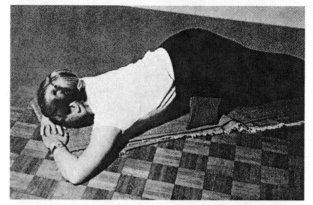

Fig. 293

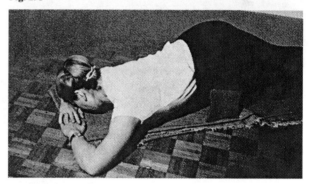

Fig. 294

b) The head sinks forwards during exhalation. It is guided forwards, upwards and backwards during inhalation, and stays extended. The head, neck and back should form a straight line. Care should be taken with this exercise in the presence of cervical kyphosis or flatback.
c) Several breaths are taken while the head is moved further backwards. Be aware of the sensation of contraction in the upper back. Omit in case of flatback.

7. Various movements of the head in the prone position (Figs. 292–294)

Corrected prone position, corrective cushions included; forehead rests on hands; shoulders are abducted; chin points towards sternum; clavicles close to the floor.

117

a) During inhalation, the head pushes forward from the shoulder girdle. The shoulder girdle is pushed towards the feet. During exhalation, the head and neck are lifted off the floor. The chest remains close to the floor.

b) The head is inclined to one side.

c) The head is turned to perform a figure-eight movement.

8. Head and neck strengthening in supine position (Fig. 295)

Omit in case of cervical kyphosis or flatback.

a) Corrective cushions; knees bent and moved towards convex side (spiral position). The ribcage, assisted by elbow pressure, is rotated against the derotated pelvis. The shoulder girdle is counter-rotated and provides a point of resistance. By applying pressure with the head and intermittent contractions of back muscles, the rib hump is lifted off the floor. Take care: compensate for possible lordosis. For the purposes of extension, the neck is lifted only very slightly, for a precise corrective effect.

b) Head and neck elongation and rotation: the same as above, but the head turns once to the left and then to the right, and is lowered to the floor.

c) In case of an extreme cervical curve (the shoulder on the concave side may resemble a rib hump), intermittent contractions are performed (including intercostal musculature), once on the rib hump, then the high shoulder. Each person has to perform this exercise in a slightly different way, even if ten people are exercising at the same time.

d) Enhancement: the shoulder girdle is suspended and the knees are pulled towards the abdomen, in compensation for lumbar hyperlordosis.

9. Lateral fanning exercise (Fig. 296)

This exercise is for an atrophied or overstretched trapezius muscle on the concave side and is an effective exercise against a faulty head position, i.e., inclination of the head towards the convex side.

Resting on a roll and corrective cushions on the concave side; lower leg on the floor, knee bent; knee pulled towards chest; upper leg extended, rolled outwards and guided backwards. Arm on the floor extended horizontally forward; the head rests above the shoulder on the floor. If this is not possible, a cushion may be placed underneath the head.

Now, the concave side is widened during inhalation and rotated backwards. During exhalation, the head pushes against the floor, assisted by pushing the palm of the hand on the floor. This lifts the shoulder on the concave side off the floor. The trapezius muscle is activated, forming a 'fan'. Activation and strengthening of this muscle will finally help to fill out the concavity.

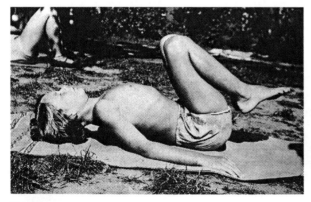

Fig. 295:
To flatten the lumbar hump, the hand of the concave side pushes against the floor. To decrease the rib hump, the elbow of the convex side also pushes against the floor. In the case of a shoulder hump, both elbows push while the patient concentrates on contracting the elevated body areas.

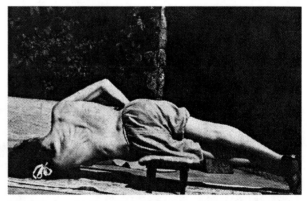

Fig. 296: see also Fig. 370. The left m. trapezius seems to be fan-shaped.

118

VI. Exercises with a resistance band

The 'Deuser-Band', available in German stores, is an excellent device to assist with Schroth exercises. Elsewhere look for 'Thera-band', exercise band, or resistance band. The following exercises are suitable for malposture, kyphosis and scoliosis.

These exercises may also be done with one or more Thera-Bands. They exert different degrees of resistance and are marked accordingly with different colours.

A belt may also be used, but this changes the nature of the exercises to more isometric exercises.

We follow the same principles as before: shaping exercises are always done during inhalation; strengthening exercises are done during exhalation. It takes some time before these exercises can be performed correctly, and a mirror should be used to observe them. There should be appropriate relaxation periods between exercises, during which time the patient is in either the prone, supine or lateral position with corrective cushions in place. Patients who suffer from Scheuermann's disease or malposture do the same exercises on alternate sides and exercise straight upwards. Scoliotics must follow the instructions below. Supporting devices are small cushions tacked on boards which can be hung on the wall bars. For example: to derotate the pelvis in the squatting position, the knee of the convex side is placed against such a cushion to derotate the pelvis. The other knee stays against the wall bar. It is helpful to attach a mirror behind the wall bars to be able to check the posture during exercises. From time to time, though, patients should close their eyes, to be guided by body-awareness and physical sensations.

> **Fasten band to the highest bar**

1. Strap-holding exercise (Figs. 297 and 298)

Face the wall bars, feet parallel and slightly apart; corrective cushion at knee height on the convex side.

a) The left and right hand are guided through the loops and hold tightly; the knees are bent. The body pulls downwards, thus stretching the sides.
b) To increase elasticity, bring the buttocks downwards four times using dipping movements. Bring the narrow chest to the wall bars, elbows bent. In case of flatback, maintain the middle position.

2. Exercise with rod (Figs. 299 and 300)

a) The rod is threaded through both loops. Face the wall bars.
b) Hold the two ends of the rod, with the feet parallel and slightly apart and the knees bent. During inhalation, widen the lumbar area and dorsal concavity. Maintain this position for a short period. RAB is

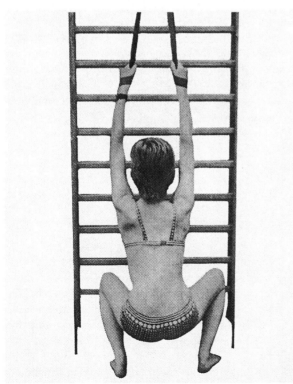

Fig. 297

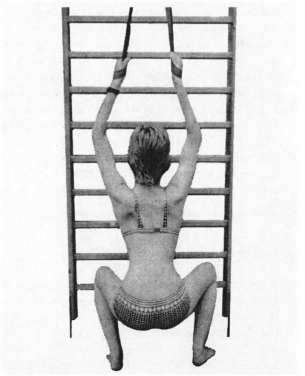

Fig. 298

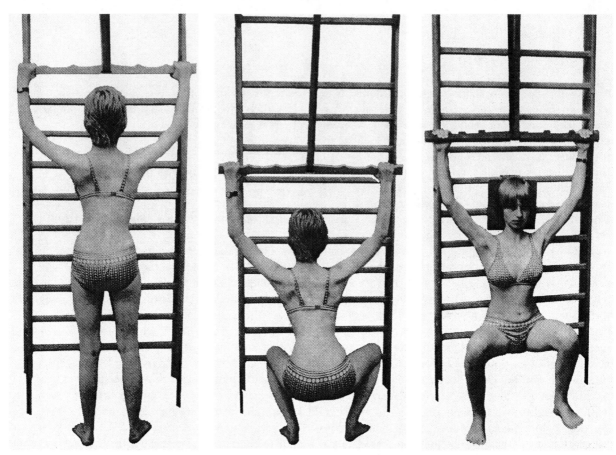

Fig. 299   Fig. 300   Fig. 301

used during the next inhalation. Contract the abdomen and bring the frontal rib arch backwards and
upwards during exhalation. Try to maintain this position a little longer. Concentrate more on the hip
below the rib hump and move it downwards with
the next inhalation. Observe that the diaphragm is
moved downwards.. During the next exhalation,
move the elbows sideways and downwards and turn
the narrow chest forwards and upwards. Extend the
head further and move the neck and head backwards.

c) Same exercise with the back towards the wall bars
    (Fig. 301). Corrective cushions against the shoulder
    and hip on the concave side.

During each exercise it is most important to adopt the
correct starting position and to correct the pelvic position properly before strengthening during the exhalation
phase.

3. Pulling the band apart (Figs. 302–304)

a) Straddle position, back to wall bars, resistance band
    is held with both hands and pulled apart. Perform
    necessary pelvic corrections. Stay close to wall bars.
    While using RAB stretch upwards. During exhala-
    tion, the band is pushed firmly sideways and down-
    wards along the wall bars. Feel the strength all the
    way to the waist line. The narrow front is turned for-

wards and upwards and frontal rib arch is brought
backwards.

b) Place the spacer against the wall bars (Fig. 303).
    Face the wall bars, with the feet slightly apart and
    parallel; corrective cushion is attached to the spacer.
    Incorporate pelvic corrections. Watch corrections
    while using RAB. During exhalation, tighten the
    abdominal muscles and move the frontal rib arch
    backwards.

c) Exercise without the spacer and feel the corrections
    in your body.

4. Band around chin (Figs. 305 and 306)

a) Face the wall bars; the resistance band is placed
    around the chin, with the hands at shoulder height.
    Slowly bend the knees, dipping downwards with the
    pelvis. Take the next lower bar with each dip. Take
    care to move the chin towards the sternum to avoid
    the band slipping off. The neck is straight; occipital
    push.

b) Incorporate pelvic corrections. Buttocks should al-
    most touch the floor (Fig. 299).

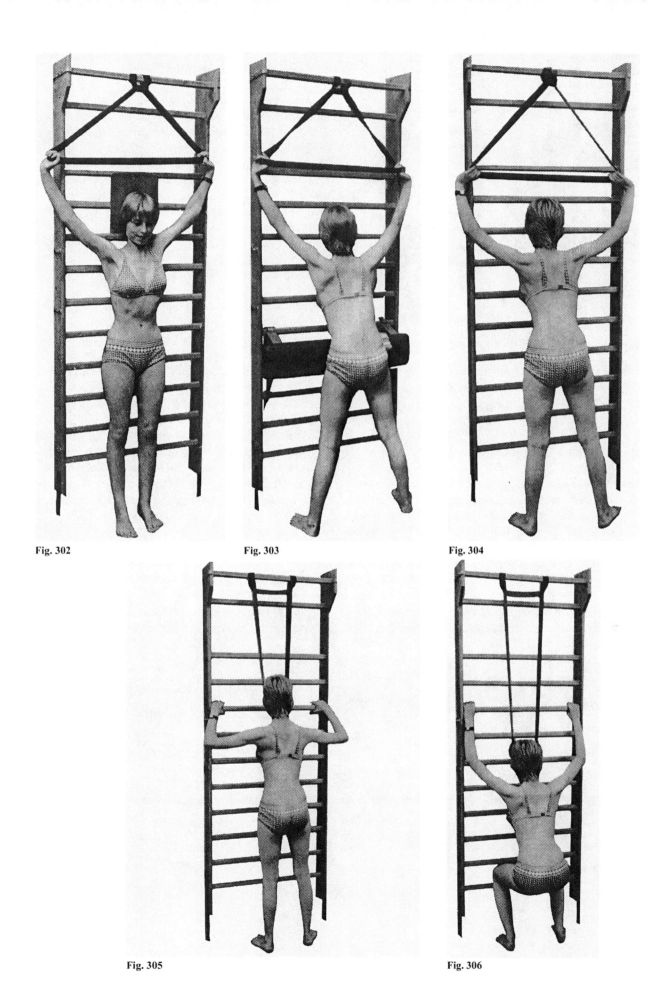

Fig. 302

Fig. 303

Fig. 304

Fig. 305

Fig. 306

121

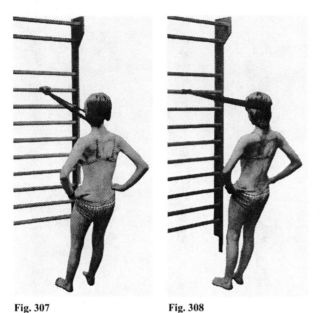

Fig. 307   **Fig. 308**

Rubber band at head level

---

6. Band around forehead (Fig. 309)

Back to the wall bars; slight straddle position, hands on the pelvic crest, one step away from the wall bars. The head is kept back and the narrow front is turned forwards. Widen the concave side! The chin is brought towards sternum. Derotate the shoulder girdle. Occipital push. Guide the frontal rib arches backwards and upwards. RAB. Also derotate the pelvis. Balance, and maintain the corrected position. Increase the time the position is held.

7. Band around shoulder joint (Fig. 310)

Back to the wall bars; feet one stride apart; weight on anterior (concave-sided) leg.
a) Resistance band is placed around the shoulder joint of the convex side. If necessary, hold the band or stretch the arm sideways. Support the concave side with one hand. The narrow chest is pushed forwards. RAB. Feel how the concavities widen and convexities flatten. Pelvic corrections.
b) Band around elbow of convex side. Arm is extended horizontally. Guide it upwards and feel the position that stretches the pectoral muscles the most. Note: the pelvic corrections need to be maintained while the narrow front pushes forwards by guided breathing (Fig. 311).

5. "Dead man" (Fig. 307)

Omit in case of cervical kyphosis. Face the wall bars.
a) Resistance band placed around neck, feet straddled, one step away from wall bars, hands resting on hips. The entire body is lowered backwards. Keep hip joints straight! Only the neck and feet are supporting. The anterior pelvic crest is raised. Derotate the pelvic girdle, bring the frontal rib arch backwards. RAB.
b) Band around occiput. Same exercise as before. Do not let the head be pulled towards the wall bars (Fig. 308).

8. Back-Pack (Figs. 312–314)

Back to the wall bars; loops around shoulder joints; one step away from the wall bars.
a) Lean forwards keeping the body straight. Raise the anterior pelvic rim and keep the lower costal arches

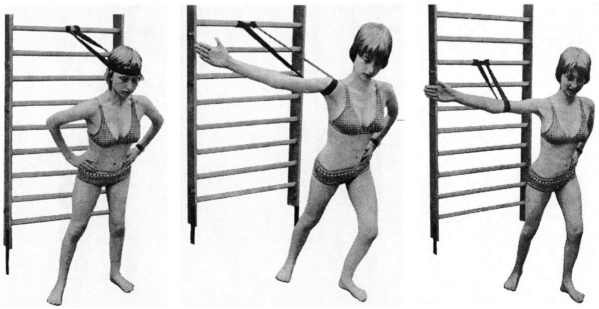

Fig. 309   **Fig. 310**   **Fig. 311**

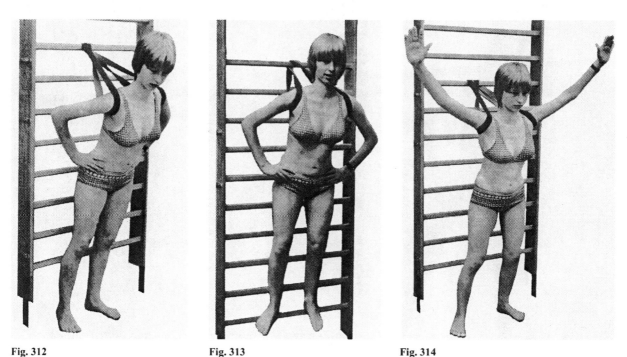

Fig. 312   Fig. 313   Fig. 314

pointing backwards. Feel how the pectoral muscles widen. Full head and neck stretching and occipital push. RAB. The abdominal muscles are tightened during exhalation.

b) A little more difficult: heels on the lowest bar, hands on the hips or hold the band, keep the abdomen firm.

c) The arms are stretched obliquely upwards and the body sinks forwards. Try to reach the point at which maximum extension of the pectoral muscles is achieved.

d) A second band around the hip. Feet in the walking position; derotation of pelvis with counterrotation of the narrow front forwards and upwards (Fig. 315).

9. Resistance band laterally (Fig. 316)

Convex side to the wall bars, feet in front of one another, the weight rests on the anterior leg and the leg on the convex side is turned outwards, the band is above the ear.

a) The head pushes against the resistance of the band towards the concave side. The hand supports the elongation of the concave side.

b) Hold the band with the fingers if necessary (Fig. 317). Derotate the shoulder and pelvic girdles.

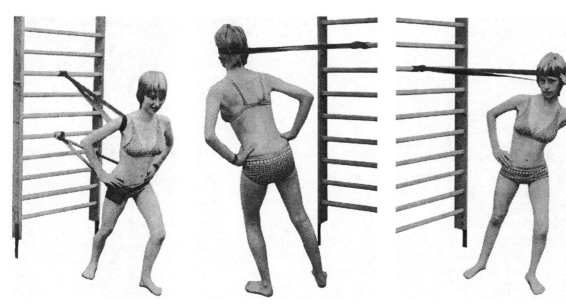

Fig. 315: Omit in the case of four-curve scoliosis.

Fig. 316: Omit in the case of four-curve scoliosis.

Fig. 317: Omit in the case of four-curve scoliosis.

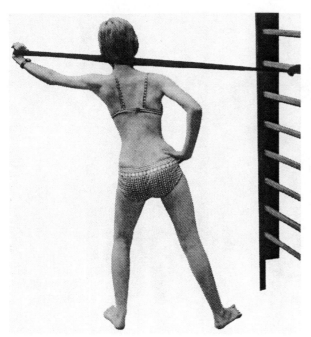

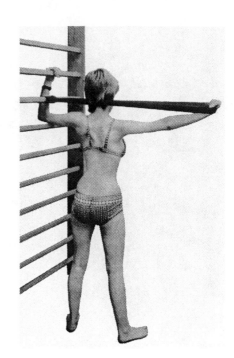

Fig. 319

Fig. 318: Omit in the case of four-curve scoliosis.

Band fastened at shoulder height

10. Stretching band with arm on concave side (Fig. 318)

Convex side to the wall bars. Convex side loop behind the back at shoulder level. Move the arm slowly diagonally sideways and upwards. Incline the entire trunk towards the concave side.

The other hand checks the area below the rib hump to see whether the muscles are activated. RAB. Head and neck extension. Derotation of pelvis. The head also pulls to the concave side, to activate the weak cervical muscles above the rib hump.

11. Shoulder countertraction (Figs. 319 and 320)

Concave side towards the wall bars; slight straddle position; forearm resting behind the bar.

a) Guide the band behind the back. Push with the hand of the convex side outwards and upwards. At the beginning of the exercise, to improve flexibility, you can extend and contract the shoulder above the rib hump several times. Watch yourself in the mirror.

b) Note: never arch the rib hump outwards, but bring it forwards, upwards and inwards. Continue pushing the arm obliquely upwards, but incline the head towards the concave side. Total head and neck elongation. Watch the protruding hip carefully in the presence of a fourth curve, and ensure it does not glide too far.

12. Pulling the band apart (Fig. 321)

Back towards the wall bars; feet in slight straddle position; hands inside loops. Use RAB to move upwards. During exhalation, extend the arms slowly outwards = push the loops to the right and left. The head pushes upwards against the bar. Move the lumbar spine backwards. Contract the abdominal muscles and bring the frontal rib arches backwards.

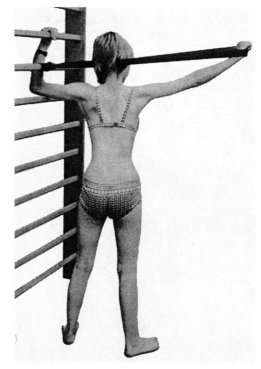

Fig. 320

124

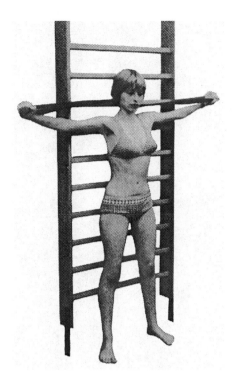

Fig. 321

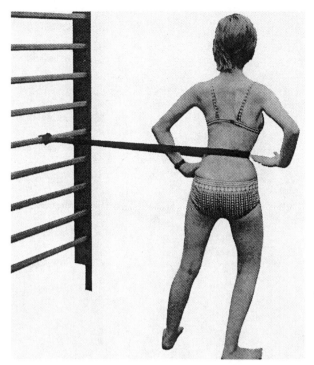

Fig. 323

13. Muscle cylinder with blockage of lumbar hump (Fig. 322)

Convex side towards the wall bars; band around the lumbar convexity. Stretch the band a little in front before putting it on (derotational effect). Stand on the leg on the concave side. The other leg rests on an appropriate

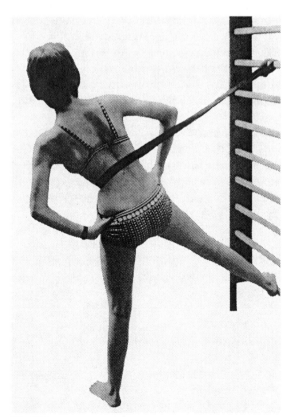

Fig. 322

bar. The trunk leans towards the concave side and forms a straight line with the leg. Use your hand to check the area below the rib hump. Visualise the breathing movements: sideways and upwards and backwards. Feel the sensation of lowering the diaphragm. At the end of the exercise, push the extended leg down onto the bar to stabilize the results and contract the abdominal muscles during exhalation.

Band at hip level

---

14. Moving floating ribs outwards (Fig. 323)

If the hip on the convex side protrudes (as in four-curve scoliosis), the band is placed around the waist to prevent false ribs being 'breathed out'. These ribs should be expanded at right angles outwards and upwards. The diaphragm supports this expansion from inside by being lowered both physically and mentally.

15. Keeping the hip on the concave side aligned (Fig. 324)

Omit in case of four curves.
Convex side to the wall bars; band around the hip on the concave side.
a) Feet in front of one another. Incline the upper body towards the concave side. Derotate the pelvis. Place the hand on the hip to stretch the concave side. RAB.

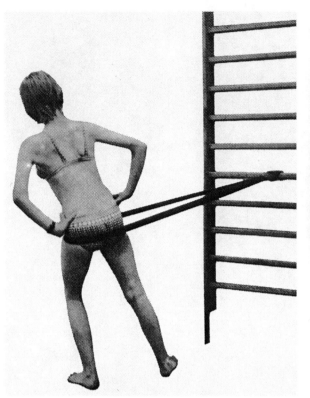

Fig. 324: Omit in the case of four-curve scoliosis

Stabilize best correction during exhalation using the muscle mantle. Count in your mind and try to increase time of contraction.

b) Quarter turn. Now the band is in front of the hips. Stretch the arm of the concave side upwards and forwards. RAB. Stabilize the result during exhalation (Fig. 325).

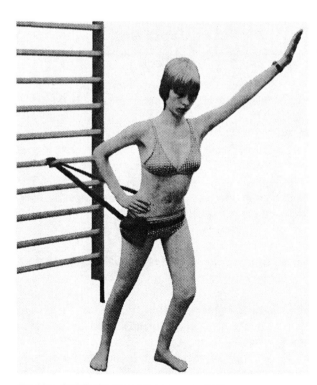

Fig. 325: Omit in the case of four-curve scoliosis

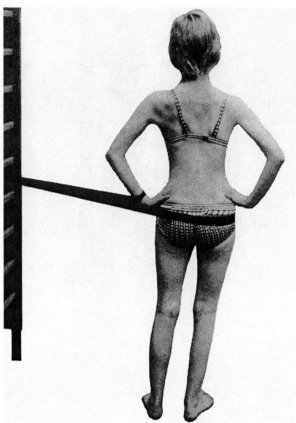

Fig. 326: Omit in the case of four-curve scoliosis

16. Swing the hip sideways

Omit in case of a lumbosacral curve. Concave side to the wall bars. Place the band around the hips.

a) Slight abducted position. Swing the hip below the rib hump outwards and backwards (Fig. 326).

b) Maintain the position for a short time and add RAB. Use the hand on the hip to stretch the concave side (Fig. 327).

c) If the concave side is very narrow, shorten the band by winding it several times around the wall bar. The hand holds on to the bar with the elbow straight. This stretches the concavity, and it can be better ventilated.

d) To align shoulders use shoulder countertraction (Figs. 328, 329)

e) The hand may hold an additional band (Fig. 330)

f) Once the corrections have been performed, integrate RAB. If necessary, add shoulder countertraction and stabilize the results with a strong muscle mantle (Fig. 331)

17. Upper trunk hanging forwards

Back to the wall bars; band around the pelvis; one step away from the wall bars.

a) Abducted position, arms slightly raised, then bring the upper body to the floor. Stretch the trunk for-

126

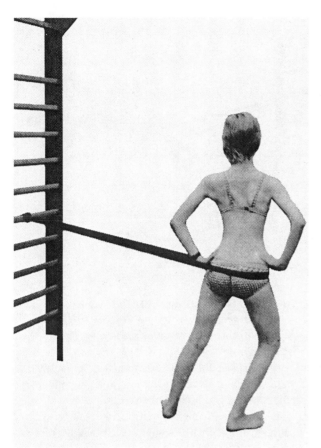

Fig. 327: Omit in the case of four-curve scoliosis

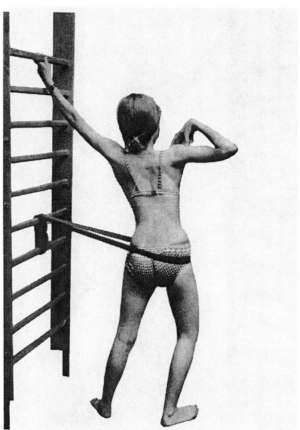

Fig. 329

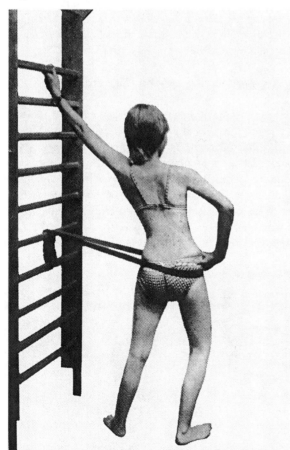

Fig. 328: Omit in the case of four-curve scoliosis

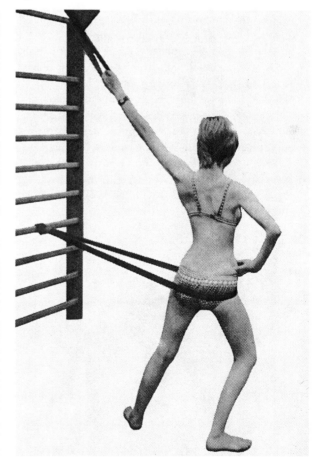

Fig. 330

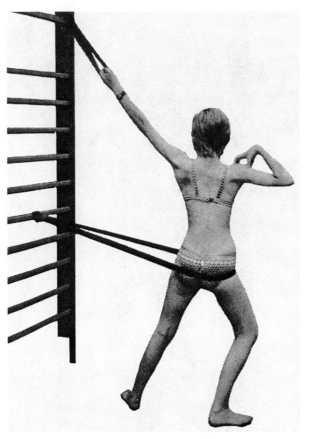

Fig. 331: Omit in the case of four-curve scoliosis

wards and downwards with little oscillatory movements. Then raise the stretched upper body to the horizontal, stretch it once more and bring it to the floor again. Stretch the trunk forwards and downwards to the floor. The arms form a "V." Dip downwards. Continue dipping and moving your arms further and further forward. Step forwards as well and keep the legs straight. The trunk is inclined to the concave side. RAB. Keep heels on the floor (Fig. 332).

b) Raise the arms slowly during exhalation until they are horizontal (Fig. 333) with the back flat; the nar-

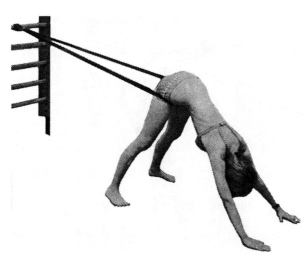

Fig. 332

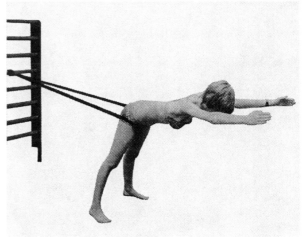

Fig. 333

row front is moved forwards and upwards; the arm on the convex side is held a little higher. The head is held in line with the upper body. Tighten the abdominal muscles. Keep the body in this position for a few seconds and keep breathing deeply. Stretch the upper body again and lower it again. Try to increase the time the position is maintained.

c) Swimming movements with arms. Inhale during circular movements; exhale while pushing the arms forwards (Fig. 334).

d) Therapist holds the hands to give support. Patient tries to bend the elbows against this resistance. During inhalation, elongate the trunk; during exhalation try to bend arms, but keep trunk elongated (Fig. 335).

18. Abducted sitting position (Fig. 336)

The feet are placed against the lowest bar. The foot on the convex side is held backwards by a corrective cushion. The band is around the rib hump and the knees are straight. Sit on the ischial tuberosities. Both arms extend obliquely forwards and upwards and the trunk inclines slightly to the concave side. Muscle contractions flatten the back. Try to reach a bar above the head. Keep the neck straight. Push the fingers forwards bit by bit. Elongate during inhalation and dip forwards during ex-

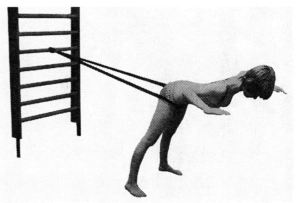

Fig. 334

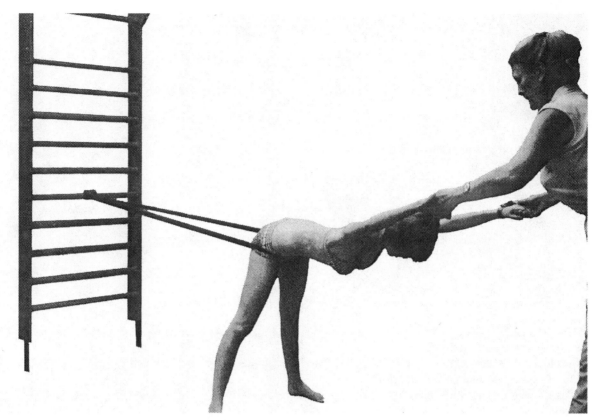

Fig. 335

halation. Repeat 4–5 times. Ensure that the lumbar hump does not worsen. Omit in case of lumbar kyphosis.

19. Sitting cross-legged; pull band apart (Fig. 337)

Back to the wall bars. Hold the band with the hands far apart. The arms and lumbar spine remain in contact with wall bars.

a) The head pushes against a small board. RAB while moving upwards. During exhalation, pull the band apart and perform total extension of the head and neck with the arms straight. The abdominal muscles are tightened. Feel the strength all the way to the waist.

b) Incline the upper body obliquely forwards.

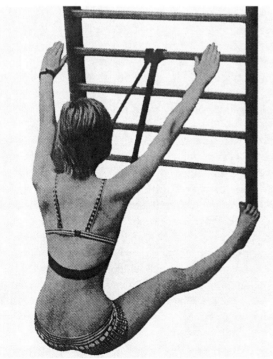

Fig. 336

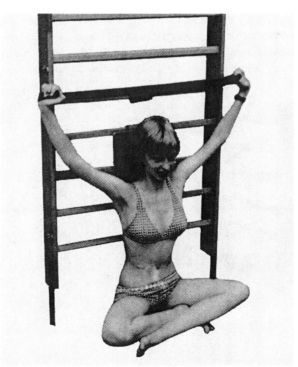

Fig. 337

129

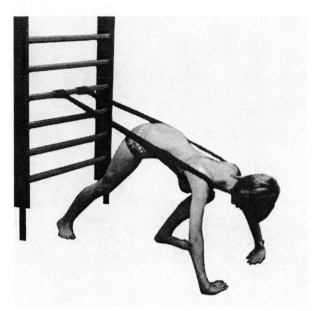

Fig. 338

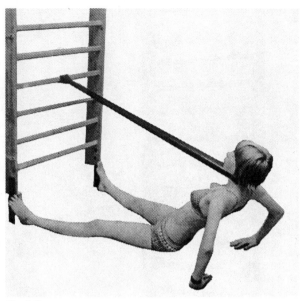

Fig. 340

20. Push-ups with two bands

Place the bands around the shoulder joints.
a) Begin with one foot in front of the other. The upper body is inclined forwards with the hands on the floor (Fig. 338)
b) The legs are straight; bend and straighten the arms alternately. Try to keep the entire body straight (Fig. 339).

21. Backwards push-ups

Straddle position in front of the wall bars with the feet against lowest bar and the band around the neck and the hands next to the buttocks (Fig. 340). RAB. Lift the pelvis during exhalation. The entire body should be in one straight line (Fig. 341). Omit in case of flatback.

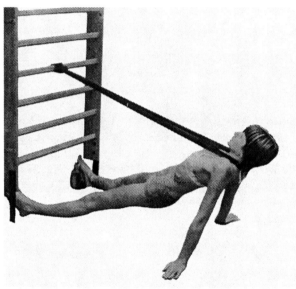

Fig. 341

22. Kneeling position, band around hips

Back to the wall bars; low-sliding position with the chest towards the floor. In case of flatback, stretch only forwards (Fig. 342).
a) Move slowly forwards with the hands and knees; then position the corrective cushions as in Fig. 343.
b) Do "The machine" (Figs. 252-53): arms slightly bent; the upper body performs circular movements backwards or forwards. Perform in slow motion, so that targeted RAB can be incorporated (Fig. 343).
c) Inhale; pull over to the concave side with the arms. Raise the upper trunk to horizontal during exhalation. If possible, maintain this position for a short while and continue RAB (Fig. 344).
d) Swimming movements with arms while maintaining the corrected position of the trunk (Fig. 345).

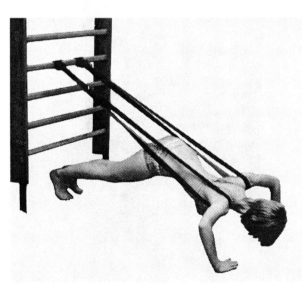

Fig. 339

130

e) The therapist fixes the patient's pelvis between her knees. With a rotating grip, the therapist then first moves the rib hump slowly downwards-cranially and inwards. The patient pulls forward and stretches more and more. Feel the sensations of correction, and stabilize by pushing your hands against the floor and tightening the abdominal muscles (Fig. 346).

23. Horizontal balancing

Back to the wall bars; knees hip-width apart; corrective cushion underneath knee on convex side. Hold the band in front of chest, shoulder-width apart. The toes may be placed under the bar.

a) Extend the arms forward and bring the upper body into a horizontal position, while the arms, neck, back and pelvis form a straight line. Keep the lumbar spine horizontal. Push the arm on the concave side a little further forward. RAB. Stay in this position for a few seconds and continue breathing (Fig. 347).

b) Push the upper trunk further and further forward until the thighs are in an oblique position. Tighten the

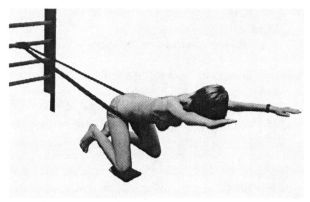

Fig. 344

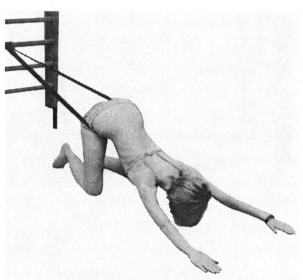

Fig. 342

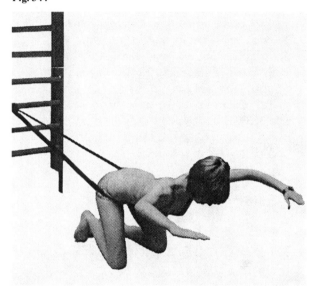

Fig. 345: Take care in case of flatback..

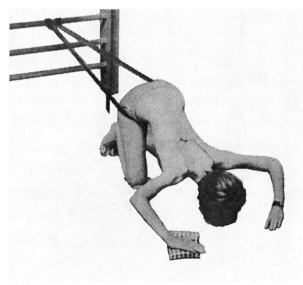

Fig. 343

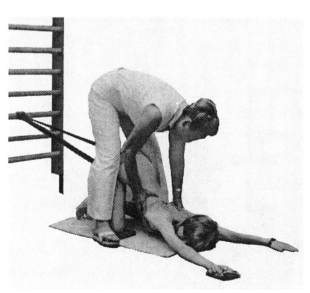

Fig. 346

131

abdominal muscles and bring the frontal rib arches backwards. Raise the arm on the convex side higher than horizontal (Fig. 348).

c) When in the best corrected position, try to pull the arms apart: during inhalation, align the body, and during exhalation, tighten the muscles to stabilize corrections.

24. Abdominal muscles and leg exercise (Fig. 349)

Supine position; head towards the wall bars with corrective cushions in place.

a) Feet in the loop. The legs are straight and vertical. Hold on to the lowest bar with the arms wide apart and the lumbar spine touching the floor (Fig. 350).

b) During inhalation, move the legs straight down to an angle of 45°. Take care that hyperlordosis does not occur. Work slowly so that you can incorporate the correction of the pelvis and the occipital push. During exhalation, the legs bounce back into the starting position, the legs a little to the concave side to widen the area below the rib hump (Fig. 350).

c) Straight legs are lowered. During exhalation, bring both knees to the chest. This stretches the lumbar lordosis (Fig. 351).

d) and e) Cycling with two resistance bands (Figs. 352 and 353).

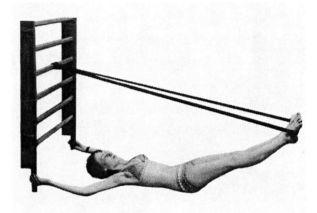

Fig. 349

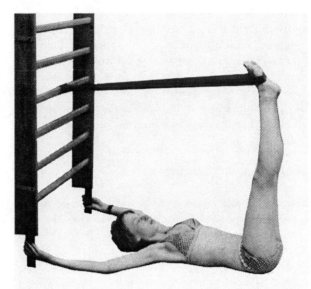

Fig. 350: Try to spread the feet in this position.

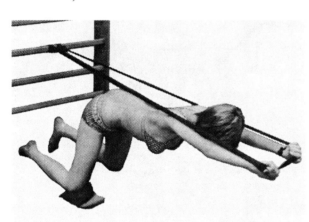

Fig. 347

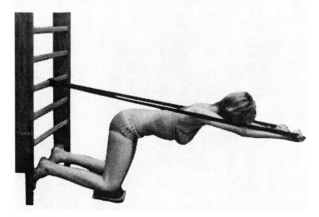

Fig. 348

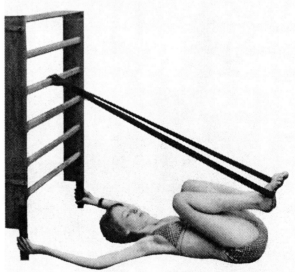

Fig. 351

132

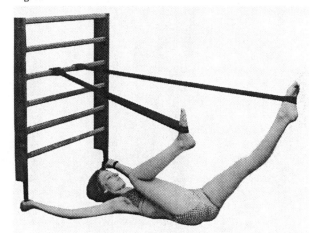

Fig. 352

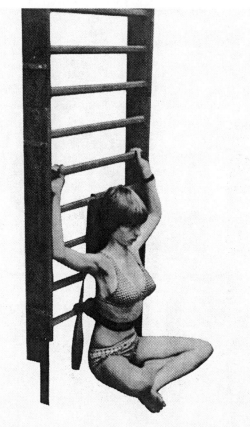

Fig. 353

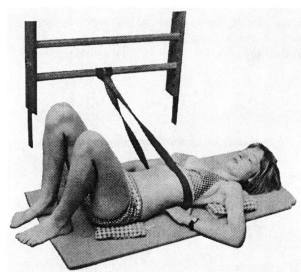

25. Sitting cross-legged, total elongation of head and neck with fixed rib arches (Fig. 354)

The band is placed around the rib arches and attached to wall bars with a piece of wood. Position corrective cushions to bring the hip on the concave side forward. The hip on the convex side stays in contact with the wall bars. Align the head; occipital push. The hands hold the bar above the head. RAB and pulling on the bar moves the trunk into the best possible extension. The elbows are bent. During exhalation, the entire trunk is tightened by pushing the head very strongly against the bar.

26. Resistance exercise for concavity

Supine position parallel to wall bars; corrective cushions.
a) The band is positioned tightly around the concave ribs. These ribs are now widened sideways and up-

Fig. 354

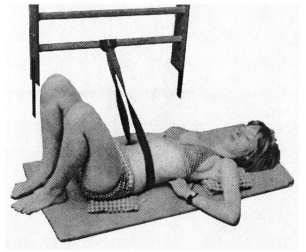

Fig. 355

Fig. 356

133

wards against the resistance and are ventilated by lowering the diaphragm. RAB of the same ribs to backwards and upwards. Check the results with your hand (Fig. 355).

b) In the case of a marked lumbar hump, the band is placed further down around the lumbar convexity to block it while the superimposed concave ribs above it are widened and ventilated sideways, upwards and backwards (Fig. 356).

Exercises standing without devices, legs slightly apart (Fig. 357)

---

27. Pulling the band apart

Guide straight arms upwards while holding the stretched band. Use RAB. During exhalation, pull band apart in corrected posture.

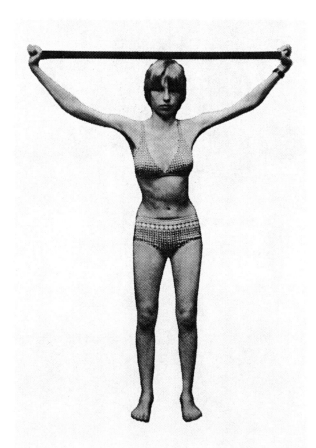

Fig. 357

28. Pushing the band apart (Fig. 358)

Band in front of or behind the body. RAB. During exhalation, push the band forcefully apart and tighten the entire body.

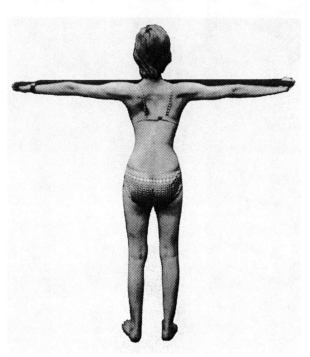

Fig. 358

29. Neck resistance (Fig. 359)

Straddle position on top of the band. Place the loop around the neck. Use RAB to correct the trunk. During exhalation, push the head and neck backwards and bring the narrow front forwards.

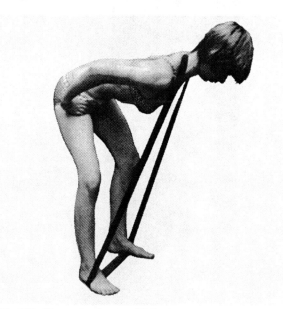

Fig. 359: Use caution in case of flatback.

134

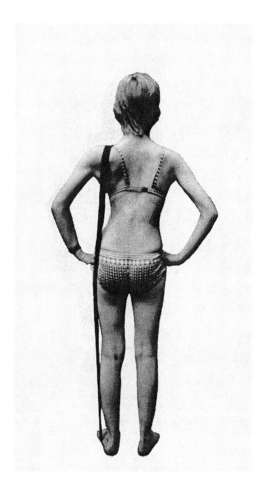

Fig. 360

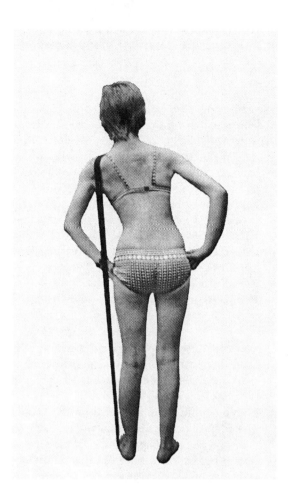

Fig. 361

30. Resistance against shoulder on the concave side

a) The foot on the concave side steps on the band. Place the loop over the shoulder. Use RAB to fill the concavity (Fig. 360).

b) **During exhalation, stay in this position, but push the band with the shoulder diagonally upwards and sideways (Fig. 361).**

VII. Exercises to correct the lumbosacral curvature and scoliotic pelvis (the 4th curve)

The following explanations refer to the corresponding illustrations, thus for the sake of simplicity, we use the terms right and left.

Slightly abducted position; standing upright between two mirrors. The left thigh is rotated backwards.

1. Use strong pressure with the hand against the lateral area of the right thigh (region of trochanter major) to move the pelvis in the opposite direction, to a position above the centre of gravity. The thumb of the left hand pushes the left lumbar hump forwards, upwards and inwards as in Fig. 362. The same effect can be achieved by pushing laterally against a table or hip bar, or manually counter-pulling at the level of the lumbar spine as in Fig. 363. The hip bar (Figs. 555 and 591) placed against the wall bars is also used for resistance. The patient watches the corrections in the mirrors. When the maximum correction is reached, the results are stabilized by performing the muscle mantle.

2. Starting position as above. Now the breathing is guided: the floating ribs on the right side are brought sideways and the diaphragm is lowered unilaterally on the right while visualizing this widening of the right side of the waist. Countermovement to this: the hip is brought in. After completed correction of the entire pelvis and waistline, the muscles are tightened during exhalation.

3. Manual countermovement between the two caudal

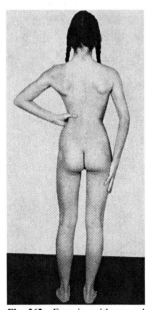 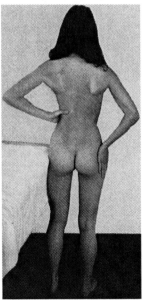

Fig. 362: Exercise with manual support: Countermovement of the pelvis and waist area.

Fig. 363: Exercise performed as in Fig. 362; however, additional isometric pressure is applied laterally by a table at the level of the left femur. This intensifies the pelvic correction. The scoliotic pelvis seems to be compensated.

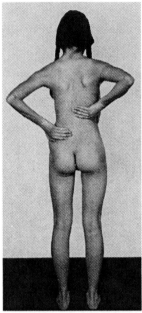 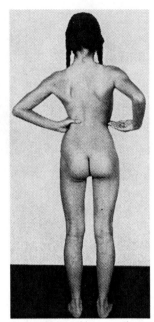

Fig. 364: Manual countertraction between the lumbar and lumbosacral curvature.

Fig. 365: Breathing exercise at 'right angles' for the floating ribs on the right; manual guidance.

curvatures (Fig. 364): right fingers on the spinous processes of the lumbar curvature. Left fingers on the spinous processes of the lumbosacral curvature. The lumbar curvature is now being pulled to the right, the lumbosacral curvature to the left. Both hands add a movement upwards which initiates the elongation of the trunk and continues in an active movement, the occipital push. The patient follows the movement mentally and watches it in the mirror. The diaphragm has to be lowered during the lifting movement of hands.

Using manual guidance in this way means that the necessary countermovements can be more easily understood (Fig. 365). Such refined exercises have to be practiced first between the mirrors. Then the patient has to combine seeing and feeling. It is important to develop a perception for muscles and joints. At the end of the corrections, again, all the pelvic and waist muscles are tightened with simultaneous isometric tightening of the legs, as if both feet (in particular the right foot) were being pushed into the ground. This tightening of legs should complete any exercise in the upright position.

4. It is especially necessary to strengthen the inactive lumbar musculature. To avoid pulling the lumbar curve in the wrong direction, the patient derotates the lumbar convexity manually forwards, upwards and inwards. The right leg is placed fairly high (Fig. 368). Standing upright, it might be placed on a chair or a bar of the wall bars so it creates a push against the lumbosacral curvature. In the kneeling position,

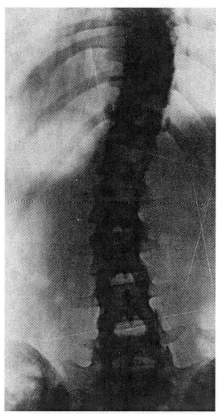

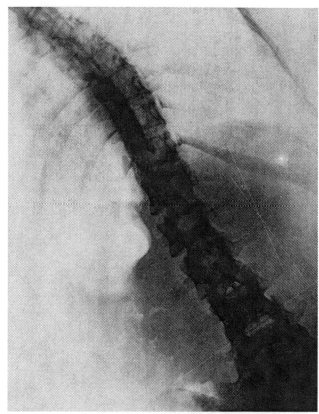

Fig. 366: X-ray of a 21-year-old patient with idiopathic scoliosis. The spinous processes of the lumbar spine point to the right, the inside of the curvature.

Fig. 367: Schroth exercise to strengthen the weak lumbar muscles on the right. Elongation of the lumbar spine. Lifting the floating ribs on the right. Widening the depressed waist area (Fig. 368). The spinous processes of the lumbar spine are in the middle, which shows the derotation.

the leg might be placed on a footstool. The optimum position brings the trunk and leg into a straight line. The lumbar spine is derotated and shifts to the middle. Under no circumstances should the trunk hang or bend down at the hip of the convex side. It should be held by the weak lumbar musculature which is now working in elongation and with force. The patient must discover how far forward to incline the upper trunk to stimulate the dorsal lumbar musculature. During manual derotation of the lumbar hump, the left thigh may be rotated outwards to raise the hip, which is in a ventral and caudal position, and to form a countermovement to the lumbar hump.

This is followed by firm tightening of the right leg – all the way up to the waist – by pressing the right foot against the chair or other support.

A special strengthening stimulus is applied when the upper trunk is inclined diagonally forwards and sideways to create instability. This results in a reflex tightening of the muscles below the rib hump – which in turn leads to increased strength. The tight musculature of the lumbar hump is then released and relaxed.

An added increase in strengthening is achieved by not giving support with the hands on the pelvic rim.

For a further increase, the right leg is lifted and the patient puts all weight on the leg on the concave side.

Variation: The upper body moves forwards and backwards in very small (1 cm) oblique movements; this adds a further effect below the rib hump.

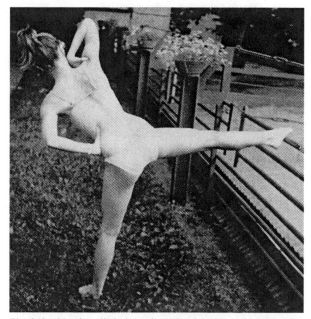

Fig. 368: 'Muscle cylinder' standing: the right leg is lifted hip-high to keep the right hip from moving outwards. The weight of the trunk is carried by the atrophic musculature of the right lumbar region. This strengthens these muscles. Derotation and guided breathing of the corresponding body segments with additional manual support.

137

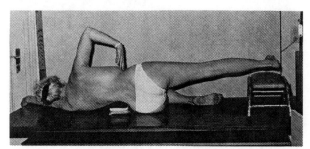

Fig. 369: Positioning on the thoracic concave side is only of advantage after the lumbar hump has been derotated and placed on corrective cushions. The right leg is positioned higher than the hip. Placing a sandbag on the ankle joint will increase the work performed by the lumbar muscles.

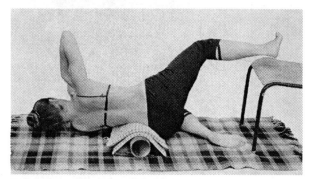

Fig. 370

5. Strengthening of the weak lumbar musculature in lateral position (Figs. 369 and 370 for the four curve scoliosis):
   Never rest on the convex side presuming that the fold below the rib hump will widen or the protruding hip will be pushed in. This would only increase the thoracic rib hump.

a) The patient rests on the left side. Two or three corrective cushions are placed underneath the lumbar

convexity. The lumbar hump is rotated forwards manually before being placed on the cushion. This straightens the lumbar curvature passively. The left leg is placed at an angle of 90° and the right leg is extended on a footstool. This position straightens the lateral shifting of the hip and normalizes the waist area. The thoracic concavity is widened and the thoracic spine can drop towards middle position.

b) RAB is then added on the right, just above the hip. The patient registers by touch any movements in this region. Conscious unilateral lowering of the diaphragm on other side and visualization of widening leads to filling of this area.

c) During the subsequent exhalation, the upper leg is lifted about 2 cm, and the weak muscles are therefore activated and stimulated (Figs. 369 and 370).

d) You may push against the support as well.

e) The upper leg may also push from below against a bar.

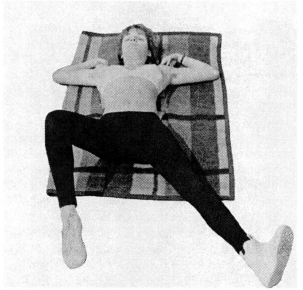

Fig. 372

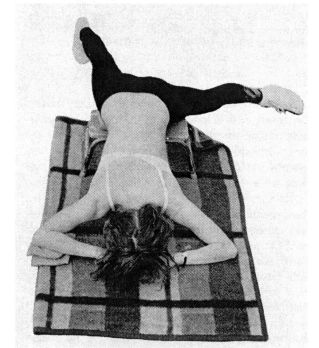

Fig. 371

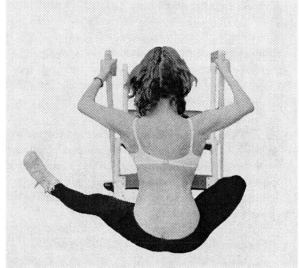

Fig. 373

138

Prone position; pelvis elevated. The left leg is extended in abducted position and the inside of the foot touches the floor (backward rotation of the leg). Corrective cushions are placed under the right hip (Fig. 371), and under the right elbow and left frontal rib arch. This position may be used to exercise with a strap or belt. The strap runs exactly along the middle of pelvis. Guide the breathing as usual: into the concavity below the rib hump and on the left side laterally, cranially and dorsally – including guidance downwards of the diaphragm.
Note:
If the starting position is prone, supine, low-sliding or sitting, the leg on the side of the lumbar hump is straddled and rotated outwards. The entire caudal part of the pelvis is shifted in the frontal plane to the concave side (Fig. 371).

The higher the leg, the more the lumbar hump is compressed. During manual derotation, the hip on the same side may push slightly against the floor to create a countermovement (Fig. 372). There are no cushions under the pelvis in the supine position because of the flexed leg.
When the leg on the side of the lumbar hump is abducted in the prone position, care should be taken to ensure that the pelvis is horizontal. It might be necessary to put a cushion under the hip on the convex side.

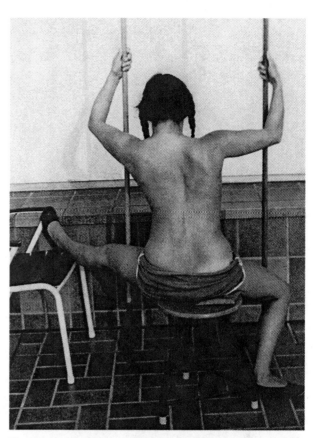

Fig. 375: In order to compensate for the lumbosacral curvature which shifts to the right, the left leg is extended sideways and lifted horizontally. By pushing the leg outwards (to the left), the pelvis is moved from right to left and thus brings the lowest curve to the middle. The pressure on the poles provides optimum stretching of the sides and the spine. This makes it easier to fill out the sunken trunk segments.
Now the upper body is lifted over to the left, across the lumbar hump. This takes pressure off the weak area below the thoracic right convexity. The atrophic muscles are activated and start to perform a load-bearing function. The force that has created the scoliosis is removed. It is not enough to simply stretch the leg out. It has to be rotated outwards as well to pull pelvis, sacrum, and the lowest portion of the spine into the correct position. RAB is performed in this favourable starting position. The higher sections of the trunk are ventilated and corrected at the same time. At the end, all the muscles are tightened to stabilize the correction.

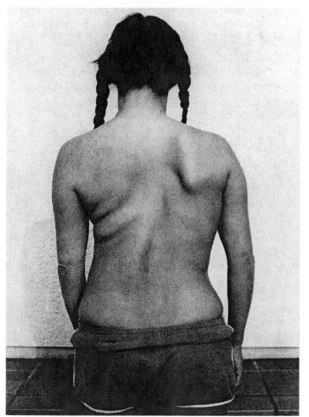

Fig. 374: 24-year-old patient with idiopathic scoliosis: thoracic 71°, lumbar 58°, lumbosacral 22°. The lumbosacral curvature cannot be detected on clinical observation. During exercise, however, the right hip shifts laterally to the right. This is a symptom demonstrating the existence of this curvature. It starts at L4 and deviates by as much as 22°.

To keep the pelvis horizontal while sitting, it might be necessary to put a cushion under the buttock on the convex side (Fig. 375).
With some imagination, it is possible to keep the leg in this position, even during exercises in the kneeling position or hanging from the wall bars.

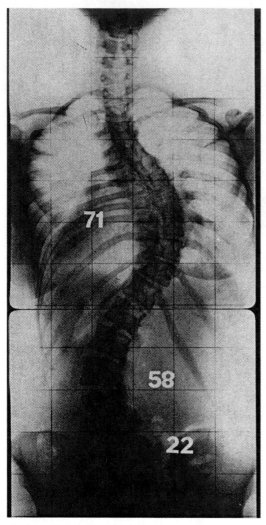

Fig. 376: Comparison of X-rays: Patient in upright position.

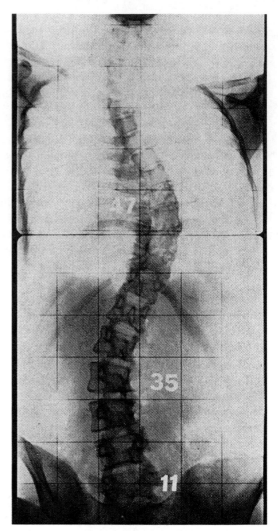

Fig. 377: During the exercise described above: reduction of thoracic convexity from 71° to 47°, lumbar from 58° to 35°, and lumbosacral from 22° to 11°.

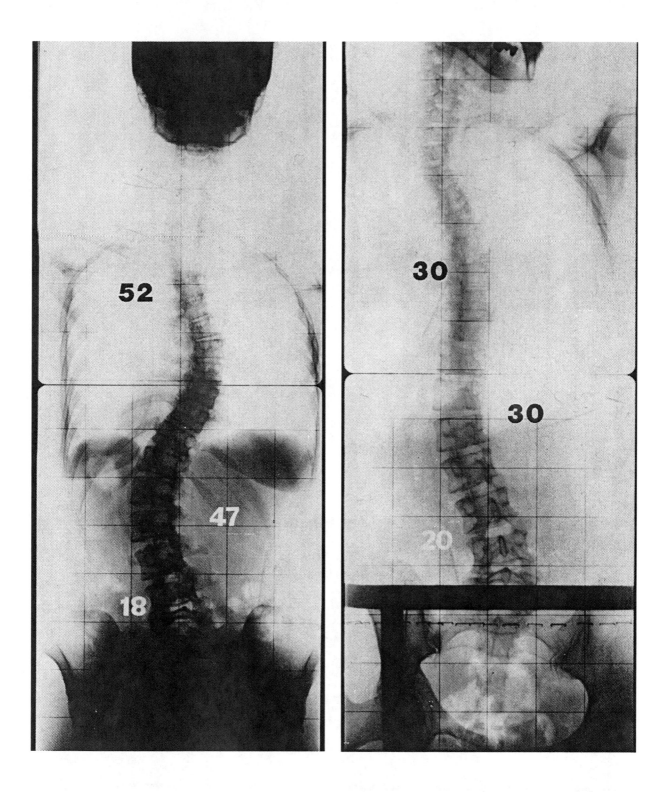

Fig. 378: X-ray of a 37-year-old patient with four-curve scoliosis.

Fig. 379:
The same patient during exercise in the prone position, with the leg on the lumbar convex side in abduction. This reduces the lumbar curvature from 47° to 30°. The thoracic curve straightens from 52° to 30°. The cervical curvature does not appear when the patient positions the head in the correct manner: head leaning towards the concave side, turning the chin to the convex side.

The increase in the lumbosacral curve from 18° to 20° is due to raising the left hip. Such mistakes inspire learning. It has to be decided carefully in which way the leg on the side of the lumbar hump has to be guided to ensure a positive effect on the lumbosacral curve. The following photos demonstrate that the principles of the method are correct.

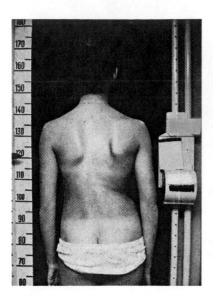 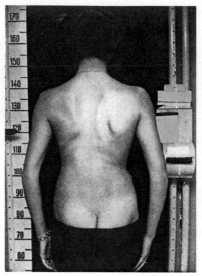

Fig. 380 (left):
14-year-old girl with idiopathic scoliosis.

Fig. 381 (right):
Correction result after in-patient treatment. The pelvis which had shifted to the right and had caused severe indentation of the waist has returned to an aligned position after six weeks. The waist is now even. All four spinal curvatures appear much straighter.

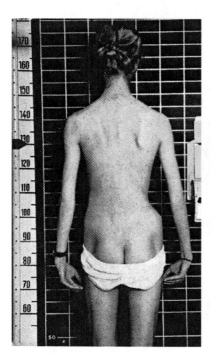 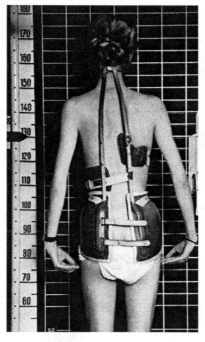 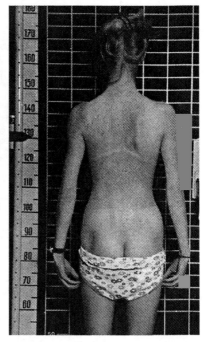

Fig. 382:
14-year-old girl with idiopathic scoliosis.

Fig. 383:
The same girl at the beginning of treatment in a Milwaukee brace which she wore during exercise-free periods. Unfortunately, the pelvic harness of the brace does not correct the right-protruding hip.

Fig. 384:
The same girl after five weeks of active in-patient treatment. Brace treatment should consider the same principles as well. When fitting the pelvic cage, the hip should be aligned on both sides and there should be enough room to allow filling and strengthening of the waist musculature on the right.

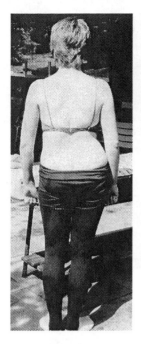

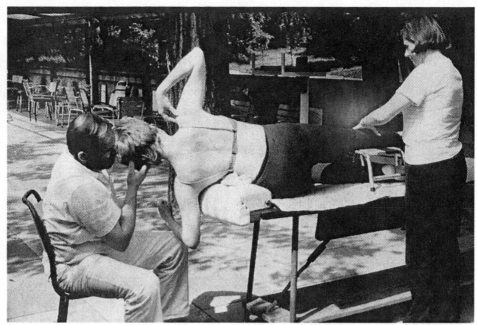

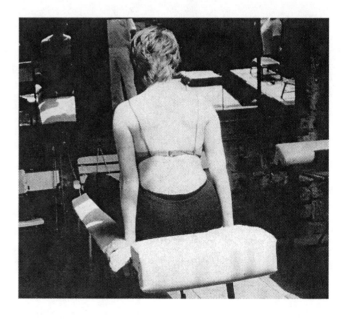

Fig. 385 (top left):
Patient with a severely shifted pelvis and a lumbosacral curvature.

Fig. 386 (top right):
The upper trunk hangs down due to the weak lumbar musculature on the right.

Fig. 387 (right):
Stabilising the correction in an upright position.

Figs. 385–387 demonstrate how it is possible to achieve correction of the lumbar and lumbosacral curvature using simple aids. This exercise is perfect for use in individual therapy. The feet may be fixed with a strap as well. It is very important that the patient derotate the lumbar hump forwards before lying down on the corrective cushion. It is also important that breathing continue calmly (i.e., RAB is performed in the right waist area), gradually increasing the period for which the position is maintained (Fig. 386).

The therapist assists by applying tactile stimulation or pulling the head or arms. At the end of exercises, the patient should do the correction once more in the upright position and stabilize the effect by pushing the arm strongly against the support (Fig. 387).

Note:
If the X-ray shows a lumbosacral curvature, but there is a protruding hip on the thoracic concave side, the appropriate exercises are those for three-curve scoliosis (Fig. 86 [on p. 43], about 40° lumbosacral).

A table against a wall is a perfect resistance aid to exercise the pelvis. Fig. 363 shows that it is not always necessary to use leg-length compensation once the patient knows how to correct the laterally shifted pelvis. Exercise: Standing position, left thigh rotated outwards; weight on both legs. Tightening the lateral musculature of the right thigh shifts the pelvis to the left and pushes it against the table (or hip bar at the wall bars). At the same time, the lumbar hump counterrotates forwards, upwards and inwards (with the help of RAB), and thus creates even waist triangles on both sides. Now the entire pelvic, abdominal and waist musculature is tightened forcefully to stabilize the result of the correction.

143

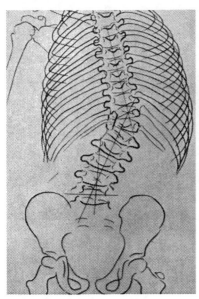

Fig. 388

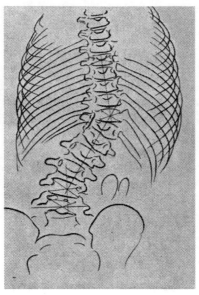

Fig. 389

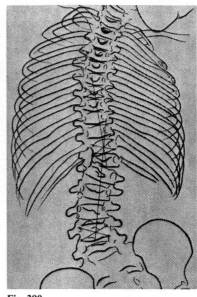

Fig. 390

VIII. Problems in the treatment of scoliosis

"Never underestimate the value of making an error.
Errors which lead us to look for the causes
and make corrections improve."

Alexander von Willers

"We must not do anything without
knowing the risks we are taking."

Hans A. Pestalozzi

Note: To distinguish clearly between suitable and unsuitable
exercises, the latter have been marked as such.

1. Retroflexion, lateral flexion and distortion of trunk

Each case of scoliosis is a sum of malpostures which
have developed into one wrong shape. For this reason,
it is not enough to correct only one specific malposture,
since those remaining spoil the overall result. **Avoid
bending the rib cage,** whether forwards, sideways or
backwards, since it would worsen the existing scoliotic

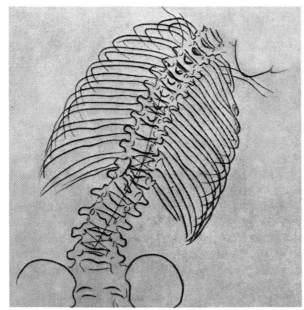

Fig. 391

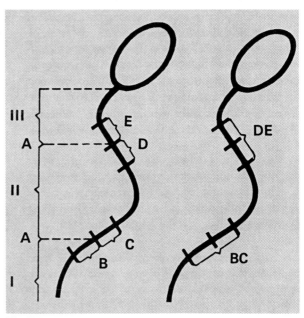

Fig. 392

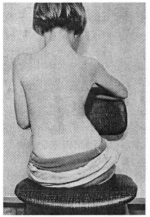
Fig. 393

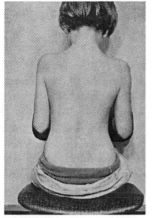
Fig. 394

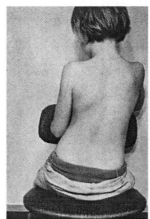
Fig. 395

Fig. 393: 8-year-old girl with a right thoracic convexity. The bodyweight is resting on the left hip. The lumbar spine is shifted to the left.

Fig. 394: Bodyweight is in the middle. Minor right thoracic scoliosis with a lumbar counter-curvature.

Fig. 395: Bodyweight on the right hip. The thoracic spine deviates to the side which carries the weight.

form of the spine: Fig. 388 shows an X-ray of a four-year-old girl with wedging vertebrae T10 to L1 and the resultant low main scoliotic curve. The lumbar spine deviates from the vertical line by 19°. Fig. 389 shows a follow-up X-ray after one and a half years. The lumbar spine now deviates 30° from the vertical. The deviation has increased by 11°, which represents a significant

deterioration. Both X-rays were taken in the resting position.

Fig. 390, which was taken on the same day as Fig. 389, but during exercise, shows a very distinct flattening of the main scoliotic curve. If the pelvis were not visible, one might imagine that the spine might have been straightened up by this exercise. However, turning the

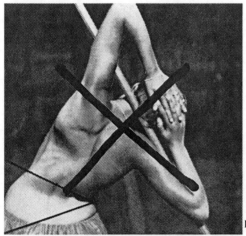
Fig. 396

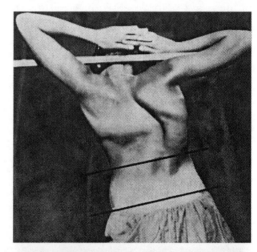
Fig. 398

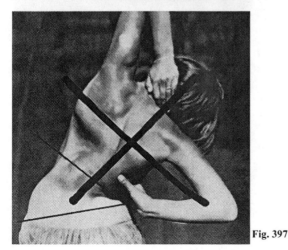
Fig. 397

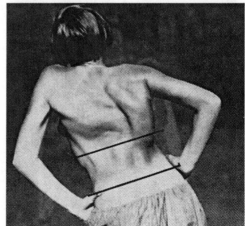
Fig. 399

Figs. 396, 397:
18-year-old girl. Unfavourable exercise: Bending of the upper body to the convex side results in a wedge-shaped lumbar segment. The bodyweight is on the right leg. The thoracic spine shifts to the right.

Figs. 398, 399:
Favourable exercise: Leaning the trunk to the concave side creates a rectangular lumbar segment (done with or without a pole). The lines on the pictures represent the imaginary borders of the body segments, see part A.

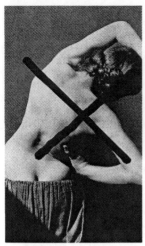
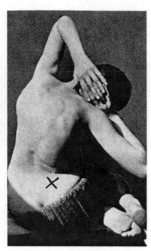

Fig. 400: Unfavourable exercise, description in text.　　**Fig. 401**

An exercise aiming at reversal of curvature (Fig. 396, 397) concentrated on the main curve (thoracic). The connecting segment remained in the wrong direction and was also forced to carry even more weight. Since the thoracic curve seemed to be flattened, this exercise is often regarded as appropriate. But this is not the case, since bending over to the right shifts weight to the right as well. In dorsal right scoliosis, the weight is already on this side. If the pelvis is not moved to the left at this point during the reversal exercise, the body sags to the right. The consequence would be to worsen the lower (lumbar) curve. If the upper trunk is bent to the right and the pelvis is moved to the left, the trunk is balanced over the centre of gravity. This is why the bodyweight rests more on the right leg while standing and on the right buttock while sitting. This position represents quite a disadvantage for scoliosis patients. See Part A.

X-ray so that the pelvis is horizontal (Fig. 391) shows that the body has been unbalanced even further by this exercise. The floating ribs on the right have moved even closer to the pelvic crest than in Fig. 388. Trying to open up the main scoliotic curve between the thoracic and lumbar spine will push the upper trunk in the same direction that is due to the lumbar curvature. The caudal part of the thoracic curve goes in the same direction as the cranial part of the lumbar curve. Thus, the two spinal curves lead into one another and form one line which has *an oblique direction to the right* (Fig. 392).

One can verify this: sitting on the left hip brings the trunk out of balance; weight is taken from the right hip, the upper trunk bends to the right, the left ribs arch sideways. Putting weight on the right hip results in the opposite postural changes. Figs. 393–395 show these changes in an 8-year-old girl with dorsal left scoliosis. These observations taught us that the pure reversal of a cranial curve is ineffective, or even wrong, when the caudal curve is enlarged during this process. Movements to the side must never be bending movements: the body must be inclined but always held straight (figs. 398 and

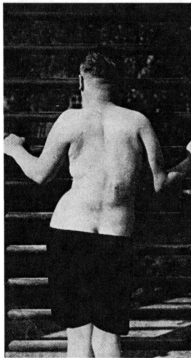

Fig. 402:
18 year- old patient with scoliosis resulting from polio.

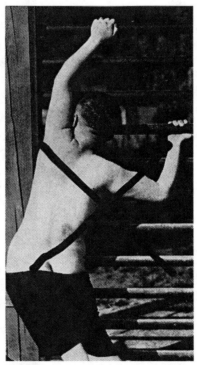

Fig. 403:
The same patient during an unfavourable exercise. He is using his bodyweight to 'stretch' the concave side. The body shifts from the vertical and the lumbar segment becomes wedge-like.

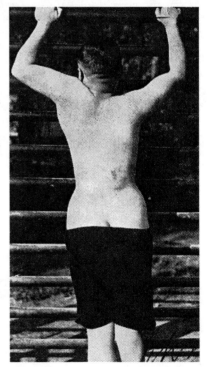

Fig. 404:
Favourable exercise: the lumbar segment is straight.

146

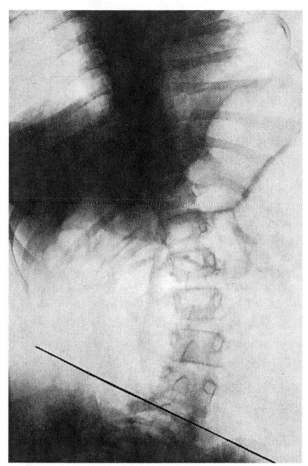

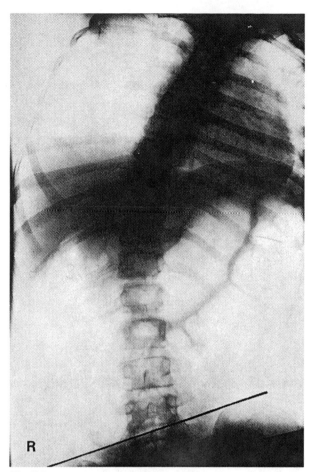

Fig. 405:
Bending the trunk to the right. The lumbar spinous processes point to the right.

Fig. 406:
Bending the trunk to the left. The lumbar spinous processes realign. Figs. 405 and 406 are functional X-rays.

399), starting at the hip in combination with the guided RAB.

Katharina Schroth pointed out this fact as early as 1929 in her prospectus.

Bending backwards of the upper trunk (Fig. 408) is strictly forbidden from all starting positions, since it will increase lumbar lordosis as well as thoracic lordosis in almost all cases. However, the rib hump is not affected. The same applies to bending backwards from a sitting-on-heels position (Fig. 409), as well as the forceful lifting of the upper trunk starting from a hanging position (Fig. 411), struggling up from sitting, reading in the prone position without an elevated pelvis (Fig. 410), and the "bridge" (Fig. 412). These positions increase the lumbar lordosis and thus, the anterior lumbar wedge without provoking a contracting effect on the rib hump.

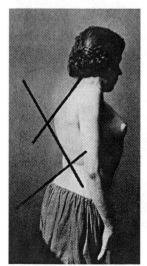

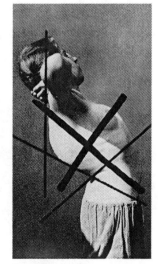

Fig. 407: 20-year-old girl with kyphoscoliosis.

Fig. 408:
The same girl bending backwards. This exercise increases the lumbar lordosis and overstretches the stomach muscles.

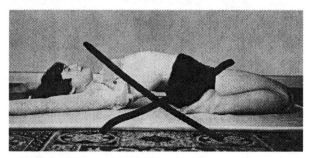

Fig. 409: Unfavourable exercise.

147

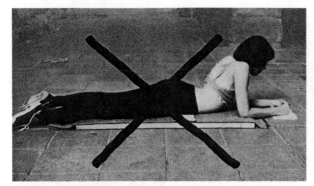

Fig. 410: Unfavourable exercise.

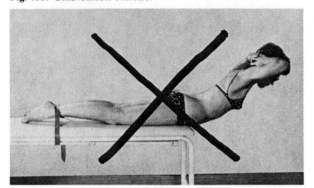

Fig. 411: Unfavourable exercise.

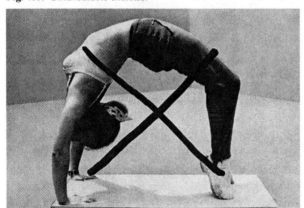

Fig. 412: Unfavourable exercise.

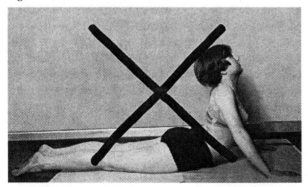

Fig. 413: Unfavourable exercise.

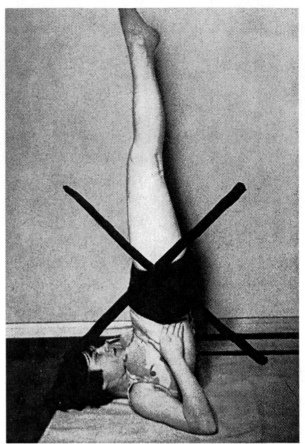

Fig. 414: Unfavourable exercise.

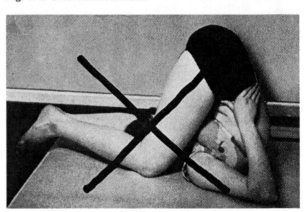

Fig. 415: Unfavourable exercise.

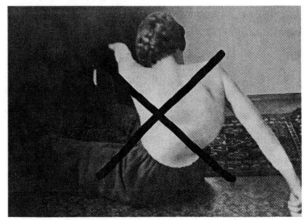

Fig. 416: Unfavourable exercise.

The neck balance (Fig. 414) and the gradual lowering of legs above the head (Fig. 415) are very disadvantageous flexing movements, because the weight of the legs and pelvis rest on the rib hump and increase it. To achieve a real correction of the spine, one has to start at the lowest spinal curve (caudal).

148

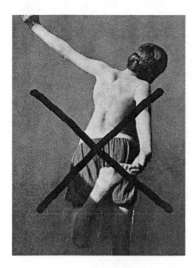

Fig. 417:
Unfavourable exercise.

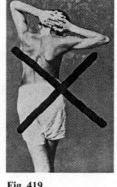 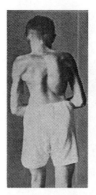 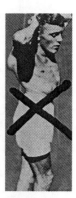

Fig. 418   **Fig. 419**   **Fig. 420**

Fig. 418: 17-year-old patient with a marked lumbar hump.
Fig. 419: The same patient during an unfavourable rotatory-lateral
     bending of the trunk: the lumbar curvature increases.
Fig. 420: Rib hump increases.

All rotations of the shoulder girdle and rib cage against the pelvic girdle are unsuitable and must be avoided (Figs. 416–420). The central segment, the rib hump, is enlarged as it rotates backwards into the existing curvature, regardless of whether the rotation is to the left or right side.

As we have explained before, scoliosis involves *three* distortions of the individual trunk segments: the distortion of the pelvic girdle, the rib cage in the opposite direction, and the shoulder girdle, again in the opposite direction, but the same direction as the pelvis. It is of great importance to pay attention to all *three* distortions at the same time. Simple counterrotation of the chest against the pelvis moves the shoulder girdle in the same direction and bends it at the same time. This increases the kyphotic changes in the trunk. Rotating the kyphotic side of the rib cage backwards, including the shoulder girdle, does not bring about a correction. This is because the kyphosis makes the rib cage tend to move backwards and the pelvis on the same side moves forwards automatically, thus increasing the existing distortions.

It is of fundamental importance that the rib cage always be aligned in the opposite direction to the pelvic girdle and the shoulder girdle. There are always *three* existing distortions. And these *three* distorted body segments have to be derotated as follows:

On the convex side: hip backwards, rib cage forwards, shoulder girdle backwards.
On the concave side: hip forwards, rib cage backwards, shoulder girdle forwards.
Figs. 425-426 show the importance of corrective cushions in the supine position.

a) Distorted shoulder girdle without cushions. Due to this shoulder distortion, the rib hump is turned outwards. The pressure of the floor supports the distortion and lateral shifting (Fig. 425).
b) Corrective cushions correct the shoulder girdle and bring the shoulders into one line. Now the floor pushes the rib hump straight forwards (Fig. 426).

As each scoliosis is three-dimensionally deformed (in the sagittal, transverse and frontal plane), it has to be treated three-dimensionally. In each exercise, elongation is of the utmost importance, since each elongation also results in a certain degree of spinal derotation.

All spinal exercises are performed from the caudal to the cranial against the pelvis, and should contain derotatory moments. These three directions (dorsoventral, lateral, and cranial) usually lead into one another. They should, however, be learned separately, and be performed very precisely to bring about derotation. It is very important that both therapist and patient be aware of the anatomical and physiological conditions and the effects of each exercise. Patients must learn about the anatomical changes in scoliosis. The exercises are explained to the parents of very young patients so they can practise with their child at home. Older children are instructed in a way that makes it possible for them to exercise at home without constant supervision.

Katharina Schroth said: "The essential point is to widen narrow parts and thus cause the weak and atrophied muscles in these areas to be supplied with blood and fluid (lymph), and be strengthened. This is the only way to re-establish a harmonic balance within the musculature. At the same time, this creates space and length necessary to lift the sunken ribs and to rotate them to the proper place – the latter being visible in X-rays. However, the effort of raising the depressed ribs is in vain if patients and therapists do not have the necessary body awareness. A patient (thoracic right scoliosis) who sits on the right buttock will have a protruding left hip to balance the weight. You may observe this in the mirror. In this case the ribs on the concave side are firmly wedged in, and it is not possible to perform an aligning rotational breathing movement. But as soon as the patient moves in the hip area against the scoliotic pattern, it will be easy to achieve the desired result because a free space and width has been created. This is decisive in treatment.

"For example: If the heel is inclined outwards and the

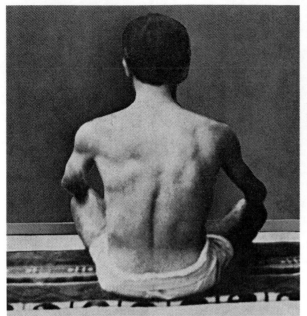

Fig. 421: 24-year-old male with scoliosis.

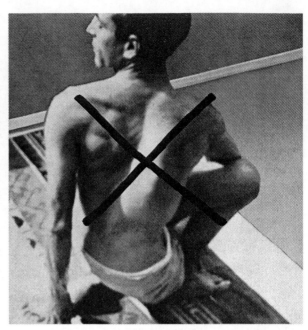

Fig. 423: Unsuitable. Noteic the further rotation of the body blocks.

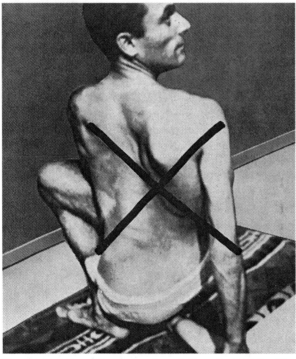

Fig. 422: Twisting of the trunk, pelvic girdle against the shoulder girdle. Unsuitable.

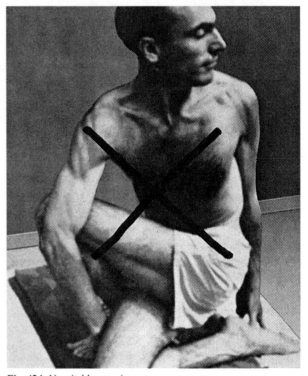

Fig. 424: Unsuitable exercise.

Note the further turning of the three blocks of the body during the exercise!

inner ankle tries to compensate for this by deviating inwards, even this is important in scoliosis. The faulty posture of the feet creates a first curve, then continues up the body in the form of one valgus-knee (valgus position), and then through the hip, all the way to the head. Once patients have learned to see and to be aware of their bodies, they will recognize the middle curvature (main curvature) in the thoracic spine, and will know that this is only one of several curves compensating for the lowest one. It is interesting that in the above case the hip curve begins in the middle of the left thigh and may

only be corrected by making changes in the feet and lowest origin. Taking these facts into consideration, it is easy to obtain correct natural balance and to remove pathological forces leading to scoliosis. The knowledge of all these facts leads to the conclusion that we can overcome the compensatory imbalance to activate the musculature of the hip to produce a shifting of the pelvis across the midline. Only then do we have the guarantee that the muscles are really activated in this area. The natural alignment and straightening of the body is achieved faster than by just exercising towards the

150

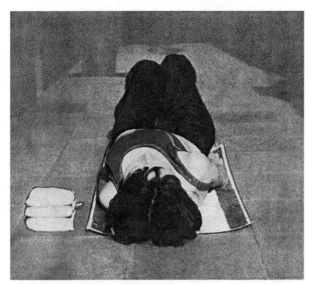

Fig. 425: Kyphoscoliosis: supine position without corrective cushions under the shoulder girdle.

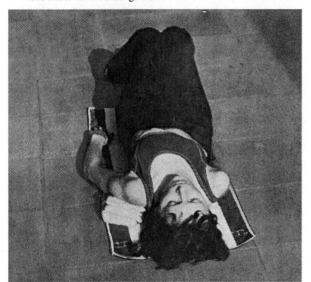

Fig. 426: With corrective cushion. For explanation see text.

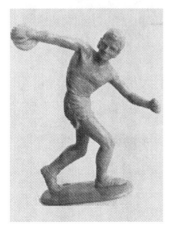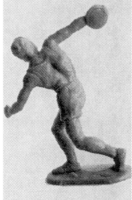

Fig. 427:
This model of a discus thrower was found in a toy store. The artist has observed closely how the trunk twists when the shoulder girdle turns backwards to the right and the pelvic girdle forwards to the right. The middle part, the rib cage, (block B), turns backwards in this case. Here, in this model, it creates a rib hump. If a scoliotic chose this sport, the rib hump would certainly increase.

vertical axis. The latter would only activate part of the weak and atrophied musculature. A certain restrictive disharmony would remain.

"We must consider these facts especially with regard to the middle (main) curvature. Correction of the lateral overhanging trunk and the posterior protrusion are only possible at the point where it begins. An arch cannot be removed in any other way, even in bracing. Considering this fact, the correction is easy, otherwise it is hopeless. Training patients in body awareness is the start of treatment. The newly-gained knowledge, the new perception, and the capabilities are applied in everyday life and thus result in improving the scoliosis by changed habits. Breathing is the most powerful force that can affect the distorted trunk, but only after observing and keeping in mind the above-mentioned conditions."

Scoliotic deformities take different forms. We can treat them according to the same principles. We must strive for an artistic, sensitive way of working, with no rigid exercise regime. It cannot be rigid, because each body is different, though the basic principles will always be helpful.

The abdominal muscles make a significant contribution to obtaining correct posture. They must be trained separately and with care. During exercise, the laterally shifted parts of the trunk (lateral rib hump, lumbar hump, protruding hip) must first be shifted towards the

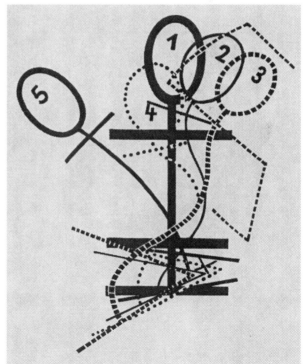

Fig. 428:
1 Upright trunk; statically compensated.
2 Scoliotic malposture with "scoliotic balance" or static decompensation.
3 'Swedish bending exercises' which increase the scoliotic balance.
4 Therefore they lead to increased scoliotic malposture.
5 Direction of movement according to Schroth, which resolves the 'scoliotic balance' by overcorrection.

151

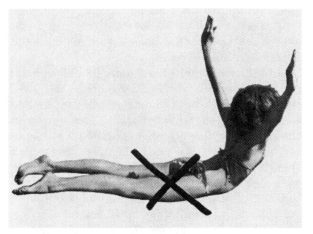

Fig. 429: Stretching exercise (unsuitable).

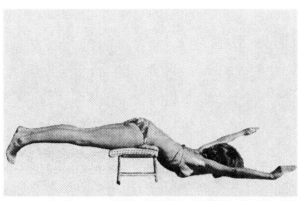

Fig. 430: Suitable positioning according to Schroth for exercises with the arms and head. This exercise strengthens the cranial dorsal musculature and helps reduce the cranial rib hump once the RAB is used as a corrective component against the dorsal concavity.
Omit in case of flatback.

middle. Then the abdominal muscles will work in their physiological way.

We never lift legs in extension (for instance in supine position or hanging on wall bars), as this would increase an existing lumbar lordosis. One part of the quadriceps, the rectus femoris, extends to the anterior superior iliac spine. Raising the extended legs will pull the spinae caudally, which will create a lordosis.

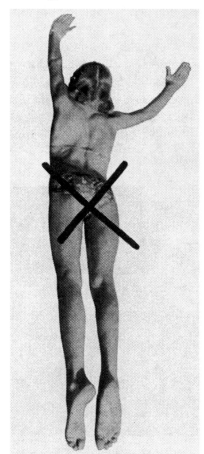

Fig. 431: Stretching exercise for scoliosis (unsuitable).

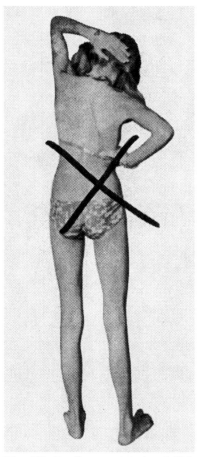

Fig. 432: Bending exercises (unsuitable). Creates the "scoliotic imbalance", the static decompensation.

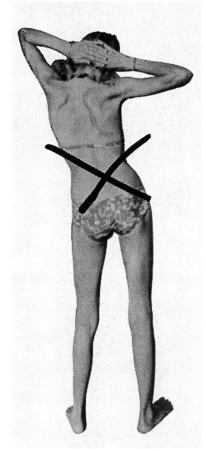

Fig. 433: Bending exercise with shifting of the hip, thus favouring the malposture.

152

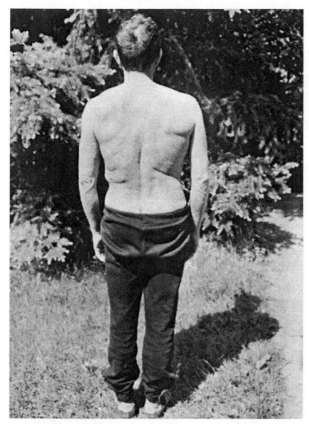

Fig. 434 (Case A):
This 52-year-old patient was suffering from rotational slipping vertebrae L 2/3 which caused him much pain. He had surgery (fusion of L 2/3) which then caused L4 to slip laterally as well. Follow-up surgery may be necessary. The picture shows him after the first operation..

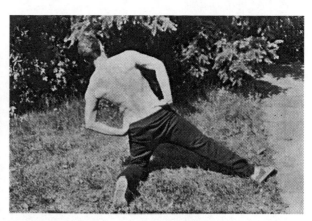

Fig. 435 (Case A):
'Muscle cylinder'. In the case of rotational slipping vertebrae, this exercise may only be performed lying down. This patient likes this exercise because it trains the musculature beneath the rib hump. He can feel the spine moving towards the midline.

2. Problem cases

CASE A: ROTATIONAL SLIPPAGE OF VERTEBRAE

If the Schroth exercises are performed correctly it is possible to make corrections, even beyond the age of sixty years. Most important is always that the lumbar curve move towards the middle of the spine and straighten

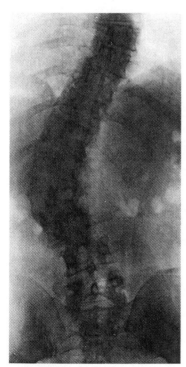

Fig. 436, 437:
We had X-rays made to find out if this exercise is suitable for the patient. You can see that by inclining the trunk to the left, L4 and L5 move further over to the right and that they show a strong distortion, which is not the case in the upright position. If there had not been the X-ray, the patient would not have agreed to omit this exercise. This shows clearly the ability of this exercise to derotate the lumbar spinal curve, as can be seen in X-rays or so-called bending pictures.

Fig. 436 (Case A)

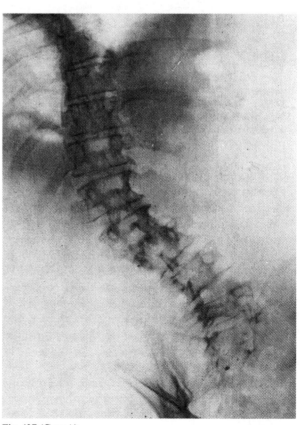

Fig. 437 (Case A)

153

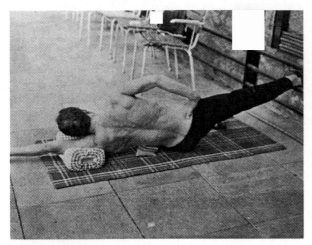

Fig. 438 (Case A):
When exercising in lateral position, the leg has to be placed horizontally from the beginning to prevent an increase in the lumbosacral curvature. After corrective inhalation, the right leg presses firmly against the upper bar during exhalation. Goal: strengthening of the lateral lumbar musculature.

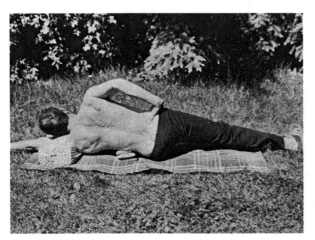

Fig. 439 (Case A):
In this lateral position – during sleep for example – the patient should derotate the lumbar region forwards before lying on the corrective cushion. The three lowest ribs which create the lumbar hump have to be moved forwards and inwards. This lateral position then corrects the lumbosacral curvature as well.

out. This is also the reason for starting corrections at the lowest point. A straightened (vertical) lumbosacral curvature also causes the caudal segment of the lumbar curve to move to the middle. The laterally extended right leg pulls the pelvis to the right and induces a passive contraction of the lateral lumbar hump, which then must be rotated and breathed (with RAB) simultaneously forwards, upwards and inwards. Assistance of a therapist may be required. Once the lumbar curve is straightened, its cranial part will follow. This in turn causes the caudal segment of the thoracic segment to move towards the middle. The occipital push has an effect all the way down to the cranial part of the thoracic curve. It is most important to stabilize the correction obtained during exhalation by tensing all the muscles involved, in order to engrave the changed pattern in the mind as well as the body.

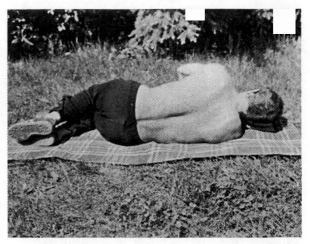

Fig. 440 (Case A):
Although this patient does not show very pronounced vertebral and rib distortion in the thoracic region, he should not rest on the right side. This posture pushes the right protruding hip in, straightens the lumbar curvature (it can drop downwards), and breathing into the right waist area is possible, BUT nevertheless, the thoracic spine and rib distortion increases. Therefore the right rib area has to be derotated forwards and a corrective cushion has to be placed underneath.

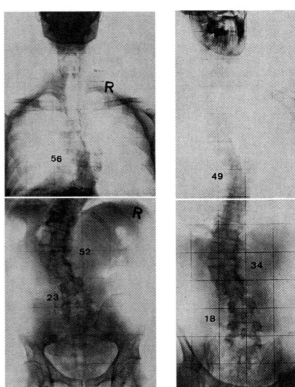

Fig. 441 (Case A)   **Fig. 442 (Case A)**

Fig. 441:
X-rays of the now 63-year-old patient (upright standing position); thoracic curve 56°, lumbar curve 52°, and lumbosacral curve 23°.

Fig. 442:
During exercise in the supine position. The left leg abducted. The trunk area above the lumbar hump is inclined towards the left; occipital push and RAB. Flattening of the convexities: thoracic curve 7°, lumbar curve 18°, and lumbosacral curve 5°.

154

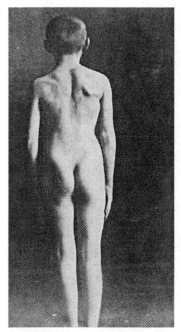

Fig. 443 a

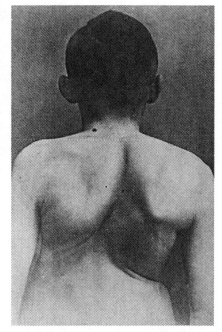

Fig. 443 b

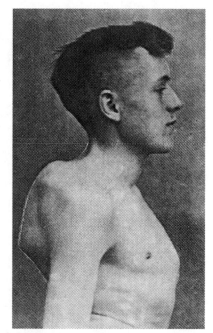

Fig. 443 c

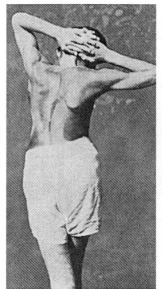

Fig. 443 d

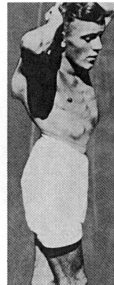

Fig. 443 e

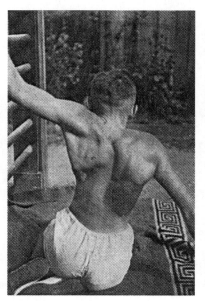

Fig. 443 f

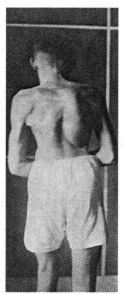

Fig. 443 g

Figs. 443 a - g (Case B): Results of Schroth exercise treatment

a: 12-year-old patient who has improved his muscles within two months of in-patient treatment at the Schroth clinic.
b and c: The same patient aged 16. This is the result of a popular treatment in former times (bending exercises).
d and e: The patient demonstrates one of the (old, traditional) exercises during which the upper trunk is turned and twisted against the pelvis.
f: Schroth exercise to restore body balance. The exercise shows other possibilities for positive development. The isometric muscle-traction may
   be performed only after RAB has started.
g: The patient after 10 weeks of in-patient treatment and Schroth exercises. A balanced body has almost been achieved.

155

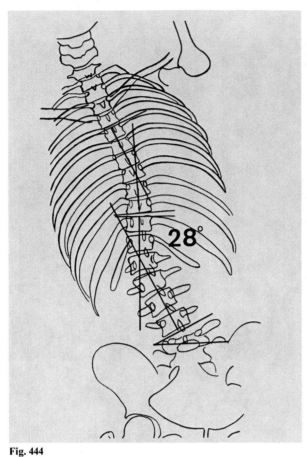

Fig. 444

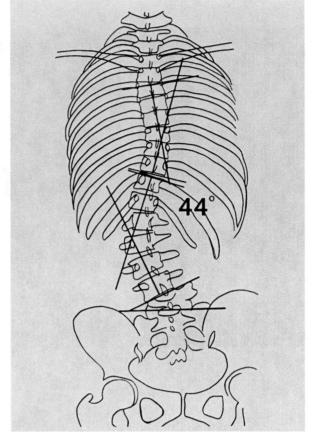

Fig. 445

Fig. 446 (right):

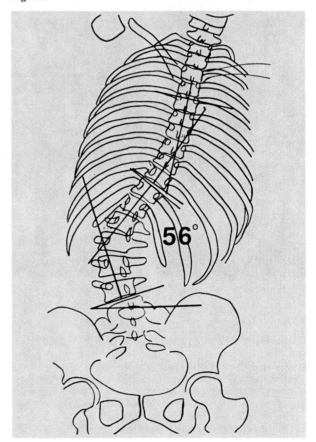

Figs. 444-446, CASE C:

Fig. 444: Drawings of the X-rays of a 16-year-old girl with idiopathic scoliosis: thoracic right, lumbar left. Inclination of the thorax to the left reduces the thoracic and lumbar curvature and derotates the lumbar spine.

Fig. 445: Upright standing position.

Fig. 446: Inclination to the right elongates the thoracic curvature, however it increases curvature and rotation of the lumbar spine.

156

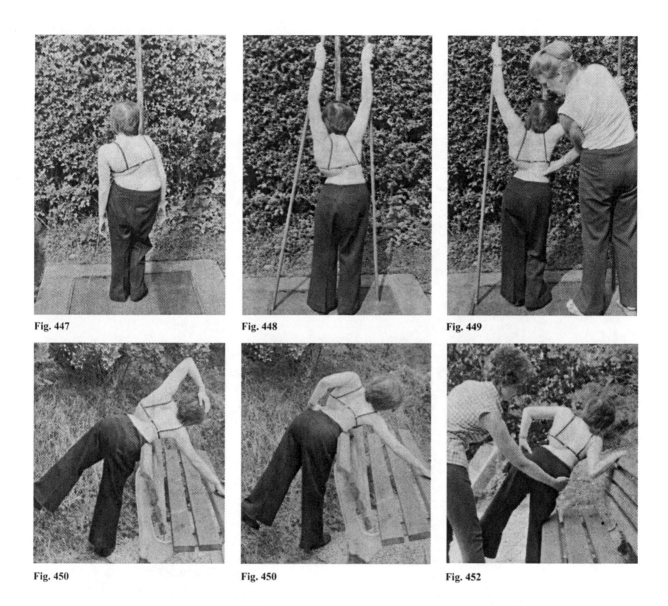

Fig. 447   Fig. 448   Fig. 449

Fig. 450   Fig. 450   Fig. 452

Figs. 447 - 452, Case D: Congenital scoliosis and static decompensation

447: 25-year-old patient with congenital scoliosis and static decompensation. a 4 cm shorter leg on the left, which is compensated by orthopaedic shoes. Nevertheless, she still shows 'scoliotic balance' of the body. During the initial physical examination, it was not clear whether she had left- or a right-sided scoliosis. This could only be determined during exercises.

448: The patient lifts her upper body out of the pelvis using poles firmly pushed against the ground. We now see real thoracic left-sided scoliosis with a prominent hip on the concave side and a clear weak area below the convexity.

449: The weight is shifted to the right leg to correct the faulty balance. The lumbar curvature is derotated manually forwards and inwards while RAB is guided into the left concavity.

450: The newly acquired body awareness produced by the therapist is now being reproduced by the patient on her own. The back of the bench fixes the pelvis. The weight of the upper body is carried by the weak muscles of the lumbar concavity which, as a result, is being stretched and strengthened.

451: Variation: The left hand guides the left hip backwards and downwards. The thumb checks if the correct muscles are being activated.

452: Second variation: Additionally the right arm applies active traction which moves the shoulder diagonally upwards and outwards. Manual aid from the therapist reminds the patient that the protruding hip has to be brought in. At the end of each corrective inhalation, the muscles are tightened firmly during exhalation, an isometric contraction to retain the corrective results.

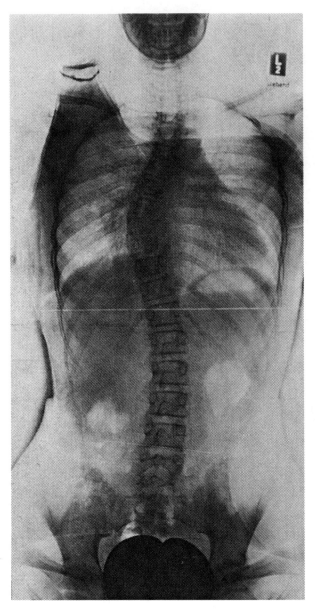

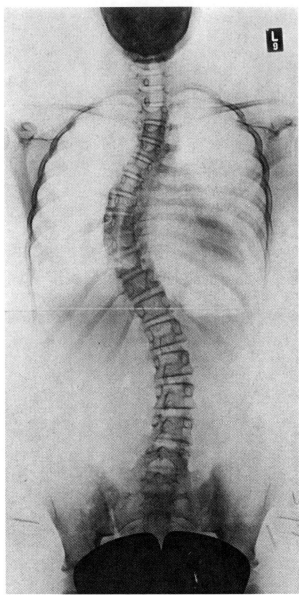

Fig. 453:
12-year-old girl in a plaster cast.

Fig. 454:
5 months later, increase in curvatures:

Cervical	21° to 29°
Thoracic	32° to 52°
Lumbar	18° to 36°
Lumbosacral	7° to 7°

These pictures show the increase in curvature after taking off the plaster brace. It would be most beneficial if the patient performed isometric exercises according to Schroth during the corrective plaster cast treatment. Then, after the plaster has been removed, the patient would have muscles ready to work and there may even be an improvement in results.

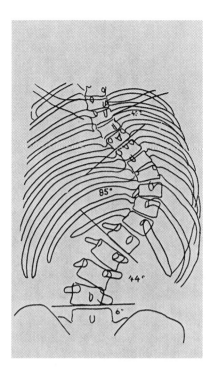

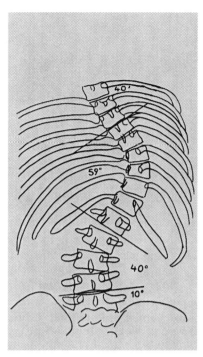

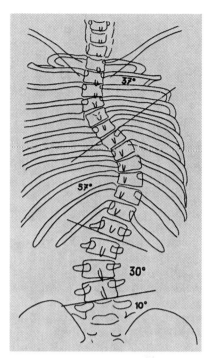

Fig. 455:
Male patient, 20-year-old; 6 months before starting Schroth treatment: 45°, 85°, 44°, 6°.

Fig. 456:
14 months later: 40°, 59°, 40°, 10° following a course of in-patient treatment at our clinic. After this, the patient exercised on his own. The lumbar curvature improved by only 4° and has shifted a little to the left due to the straightening up of the thoracic curve. L4 is now in a minor oblique position of 10°, which puzzled us as well as the patient.

Fig. 457:
Another 5 months later: 37°, 57°, 30°, 10°. The X-ray shows this patient during his third in-patient course of treatment while performing a stretching breathing exercise. The lumbar curvature has been reduced by a further 10°, but the oblique position of L4 remains. A small degree of tilting between L5 and S1 has emerged.

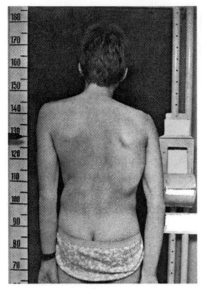 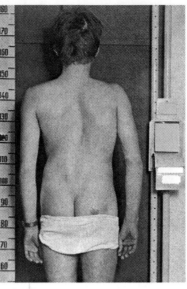 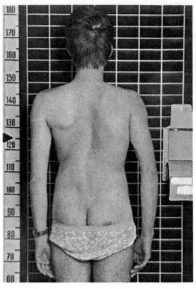

Fig. 458:
Start of a 6 week course of in-patient treatment for the first time; 21 years old.

Fig. 459:
End of a second course of in-patient treatment which lasted 3 weeks, 22 years old.

Fig. 460:
End of the third course of in-patient treatment (3 weeks), age 22 years, 6 months. The shoulders are now level.

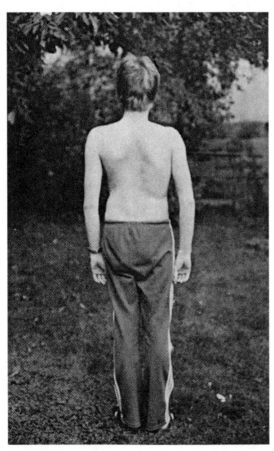 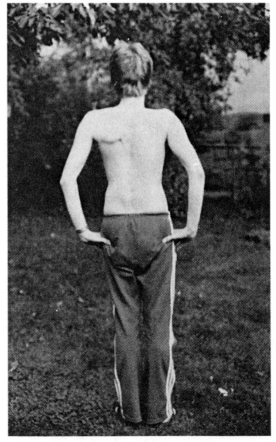

Fig. 461: Normal upright position.

Fig. 462: During a stretching breathing exercise.

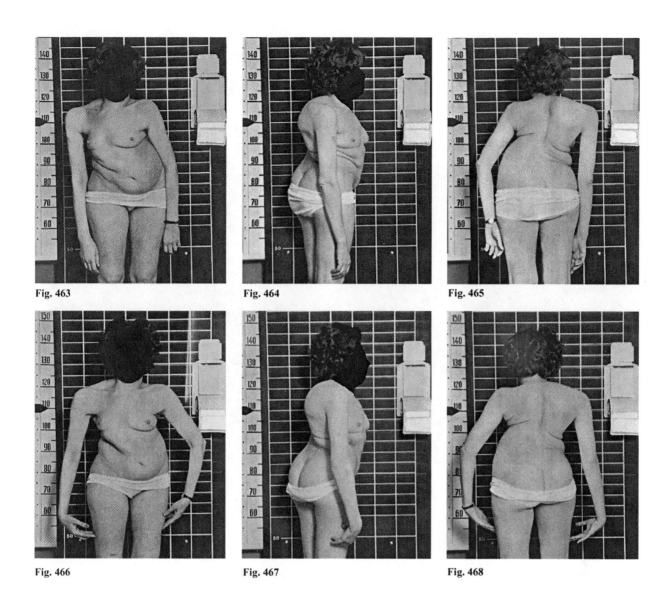

Fig. 463   Fig. 464   Fig. 465

Fig. 466   Fig. 467   Fig. 468

Figs. 463 - 468, Case G, Non-typical distortion of the trunk.

This 41-year-old woman shows non-typical rotation of the upper trunk, i.e. only two twists: the shoulder girdle has rotated together with the rib cage against the pelvic girdle and not, as is usual, against it.

The patient was only able to spend three weeks in the clinic. Nevertheless, it is evident that the lateral shift is starting to improve (see posterior view). You can also see how the frontally depressed ribs are gradually rising (see anterior view). The highest point of the rib hump is linked to these depressed ribs: they have sunk down and have moved backwards. Thus, we have to start here, at the depressed area with guided RAB to lift these ribs and not, as one might expect, to push the dorsal ribs forward. Although the right shoulder is too far backwards in relation to the right hip, we have to start correction in the usual way by derotating the rib cage and pelvic girdle. Under no circumstances may we rotate shoulder girdle against the pelvic girdle – this would enlarge the convexity.

The lateral view shows a stage at which the distorted pelvis had not yet been corrected (see lateral view). Nevertheless, the results were astonishing, considering that the patient had a vital capacity of only 400 cc, which unfortunately she was unable to improve during the 3-week treatment. However, her height increased by 1 cm. In Fig. 463 the shoulder girdle is not aligned; in Fig 466 it is more horizontal.

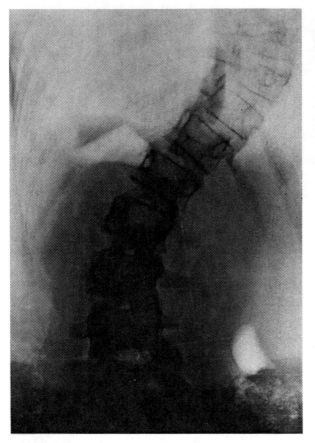

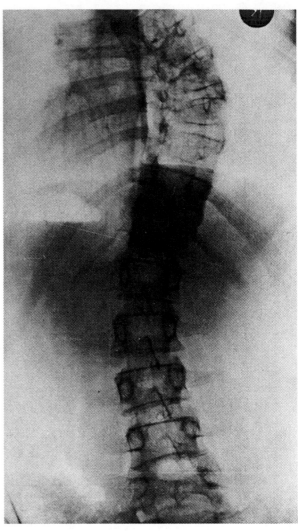

Fig. 469: Unstable scoliosis. Girl, 11 years old.

Fig. 470: The same patient during a rotational breathing exercise against the static decompensation.

Figs. 469 - 470, Case H, Prepubertal unstable scoliosis.

Improvement:
Thoracic: from 74° to 51°
Lumbar: from 48° to 27°
The patient, still before onset of puberty, was able to compensate statically for a very unstable scoliosis.

The degree of straightening achieved by the Schroth exercises was remarkable, but she was to maintain this during everyday life. We recommended a Milwaukee brace which was fitted during the best possible Schroth correction and could be adjusted later on continuously, and we advised wearing it well beyond the end of puberty.
Only with this combination of treatments was it possible to achieve good results.

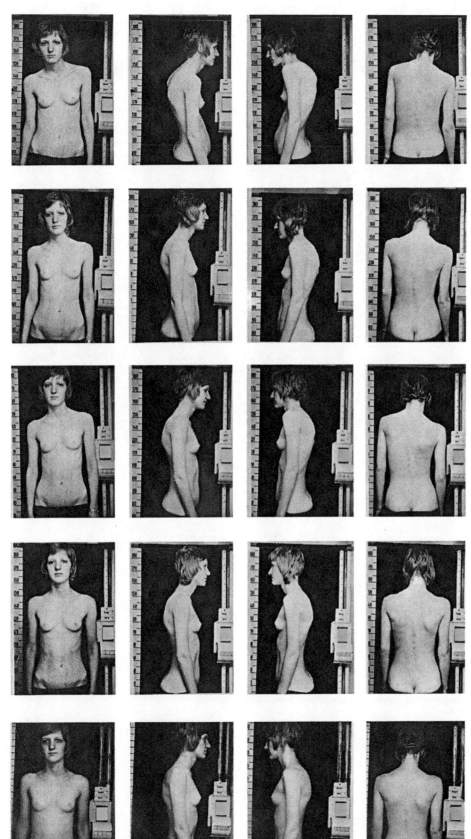

Fig. 471:

In addition to severe Scheuermann's disease with fixed kyphoscoliosis, this 19-year-old patient exhibited a number of psychological problems, was unable to cope, and had to quit her job for some time. Spasms forced her repeatedly into her original malposture.

During the exercises, we constantly encountered psychological obstacles. We extended the usual time of treatment from 6 to 13 weeks because there were promising signs of improvement. During her time at the clinic there were often days when she would lie in bed cold and motionless, needing psychological support.

After 13 weeks she was discharged with a better posture and psychically strengthened.

Shortly afterwards she had new psychological difficulties which compromised her results. Her upper trunk sagged markedly sideways and she underwent several courses of treatment in different clinics. Some positive results were finally achieved with stereotactic surgery, but did not last long.

Years later she was diagnosed with torsion dystonia and was treated successfully, whereupon her physical condition improved again.

163

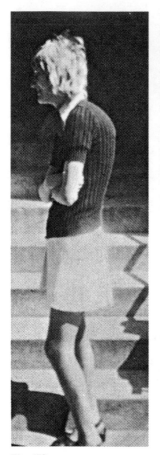 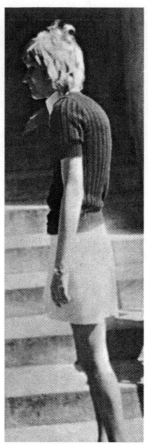 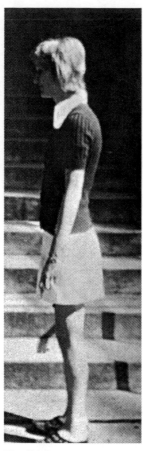 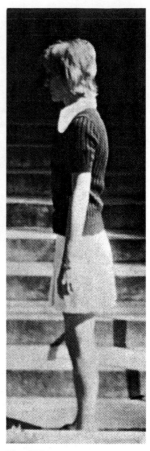

Fig. 472   **Fig. 473**   **Fig. 474**   **Fig. 475**

Fig. 472: Habitual unfavourable posture and rigid deformation before Schroth treatment.

Fig. 473: Best possible posture before treatment.

Fig. 474: Habitual posture after 12 weeks of treatment.

Fig. 475: Best possible posture after 12 weeks of treatment.

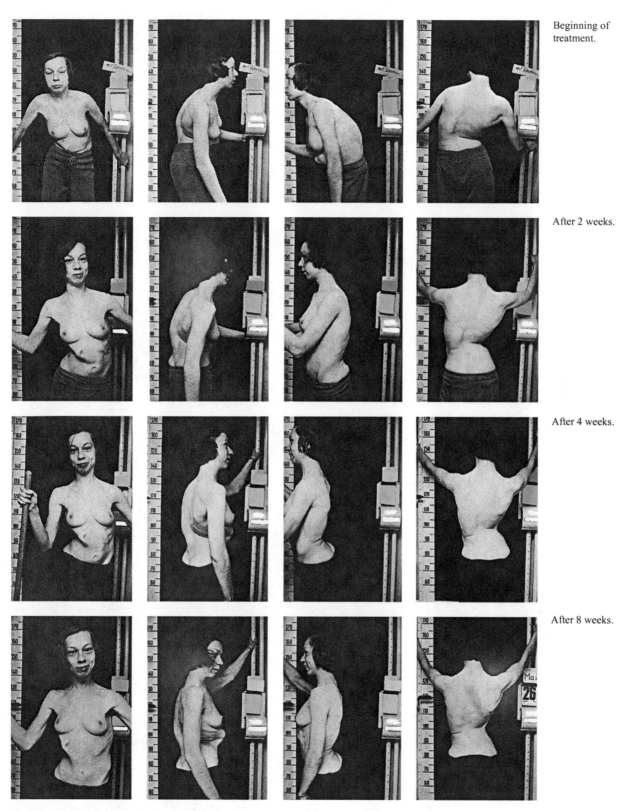

Beginning of treatment.

After 2 weeks.

After 4 weeks.

After 8 weeks.

Fig. 476, Case K, Scoliosis due to cerebral palsy
This 18-year-old patient suffered from cerebral palsy. She was admitted in a wheelchair and could only stand up while holding on to something. Her upper trunk inclined markedly towards the right. In the beginning, she was carried upstairs and downstairs. With much care and effort, it was possible to teach this patient a better posture. Holding on to the arm of a therapist, she was finally able to walk and even climb the stairs. It was not possible to improve her VC because she did not close her lips during breathing. Nevertheless, the respiratory measurements improved from 3 to 7 cm (axilla), 3 to 6 cm (chest) and 1 to 6 cm in the waist.

165

3. Validity of X-ray monitoring during in-patient treatment

The results of the treatment of scoliosis must be evaluated by X-ray. The therapist can work more effectively if there is an X-ray for reference. X-rays are also important for patients, as they enable them to see the scoliotic posture in its full length and better understand how to perform the required exercises. The X-ray can be copied onto tracing paper and the progress can be monitored in this way.

This does not imply that one has to rely solely only on X-rays – it is also important to monitor the cosmetic appearance. This is where photographs are important!

Often, major bone defects are hidden under musculature and not visible at once. In such cases, it may be better for the patient not to see the X-rays to avoid worry.

During her initial professional years – starting in 1921 – Katharina Schroth rarely had X-rays to rely on. In most cases, she had to decide on the basis of the clinical appearance and her experience. It was not until between 1947 and 1951 that she was able to gain experience based on adequate numbers of X-rays that had been taken by authorities of the Saxony Social Security Department. An example is the X-ray of a 36-year-old woman shown in Fig. 477 a 1, about which the following can be said: the ribs on the concave side show breathing in and those on the convex side breathing out. This is

CASE L: THE CLINICAL AND RADIO-LOGICAL PICTURE

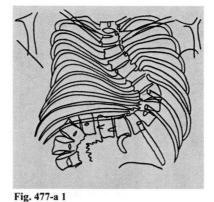

Fig. 477-a 1

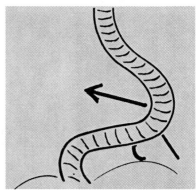

Fig. 477-a 2

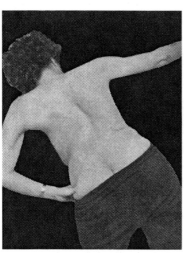

Fig. 477-b 1

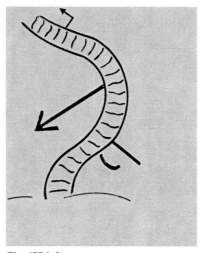

Fig. 477-b 2

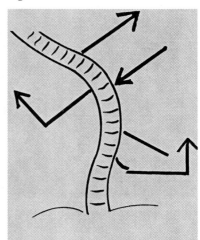

Fig. 477-b 3

Fig. 477:

a 1) X-ray image; 37-year-old patient.

a 2) Course of the spinal column and 11th and 12th ribs, right, in extreme exhalation position. The 12th rib is deformed and rubs on the iliac crest (see b1). The arrow shows the direction of the ribs on the concave side, which are in the maximum inhalation position.

b 1) Schroth exercise: The upper body is elongated actively to the left so the lumbar concavity on the right is relieved and stretched. Now the false ribs can be raised laterally and cranially. The inactive lumbar musculature is forced to hold and thus to strengthen. The lumbar curve is straightened. The concavity on the left is also relieved so that these ribs can be widened laterally and cranially, and moved backwards. The neck has a small certain hump as well, and a concavity because of distortion. This small curve can be corrected easily by performing the occipital push, during which the head is inclined towards the concave side, and the chin turns towards the convex side.

b 2) Visualization of the desired exercise direction: straight positioning of the lumbar spine, maximum anatomically possible stretching of the spine, as well as the concave thoracic areas 'at right angles'. This stops the pain below the rib hump. Shoulder countertraction has to be performed above the rib hump. This exercise involves horizontal traction of the right arm to the outside, combined with derotation on contraction of the dorsally and laterally protruding rib hump.

166

the result of the curvature of the spinal column and the deformation of the costovertebral joints. The body has compensated for this in this way to avoid complete collapse. If it were possible to achieve suppleness in the rigid vertebral joints to allow active elongation of the spine to the left, the ribs on the concave side could be brought to point downwards again (Fig 477 b 2).

The 11th and 12th left ribs are considerably elongated, presumably to give support to the left dorsal part of trunk. The floating ribs on the right, however, have been pushed caudally and ventrally due to the weight of the rib hump pushing down against the pelvic rim, and they are deformed. Often, the floating ribs below the dorsal convexity point vertically into the abdomen and irritate the liver, in particular. A fold is visible on the outside. According to the Schroth method, the floating ribs belong to the pelvic girdle in the case of three-curve sco-

liosis, as they have rotated in the same direction. They have to be derotated together with the pelvic girdle. This is only possible if there is enough space. Space is created by leaning – *not bending* – the trunk to the left. Initially this is an exercise, but after some time it should have become a habit. In such cases, exercises start with the treatment of the lumbar curve for a variety of reasons:

1. The left hip is pulled inwards.
2. The bodyweight rests on left leg or left buttock
3. By shifting the upper body to the left, weight is taken off the right waist region. Only now is it possible to move the right floating ribs outwards. This is realised by an actual and imaginary descending action of the diaphragm on the right side. X-ray films show that this breathing technique moves the intestines and fills the lung base like a cushion. The ribs are pushed

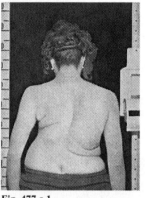

Fig. 477 c 1

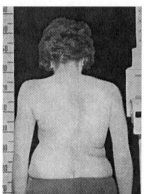

Fig. 477 c 2

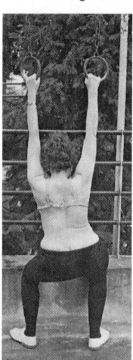

Fig. 477 d 1   Fig. 477 d 2

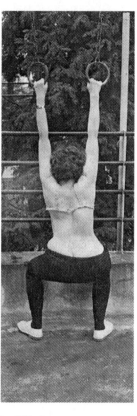

Fig. 477 e 1   Fig. 477 e 2

Fig. 477:

c 1) picture at the beginning of treatment
c 2) results of six weeks of treatment

d 1) Lateral flexing the upper body towards the convex side results in an enlarged lumbar curvature. The lumbar curve is pushed towards the left side. This increases the distortion and will have an effect on the upper curves.

d 2) Lateral flexing the upper body to the concave side will enlarge the thoracic curve. The pelvis is now more aligned. Active correction according to Schroth may now begin. It forces widening 'at right angles' and ventilation of the cranial concavities. This transforms disadvantages into advantages. There should never be lateral flexing in scoliosis. Only leaning towards the concave side, in which no narrowing occurs on the left or the right side, can positively influence deformations of the trunk.

e) 'Hip loop' exercise which contains all five pelvic corrections. Elongating both sides of the trunk, this exercise affects all concavities.

e 1) Imperfect performance: the right hip is still lifted and the lumbar concavity can be neither stretched nor ventilated.

e 2) Diagonal traction with the right side of the pelvis will stretch the left concavity and the lumbar concavity below the rib hump on the right waist to the right. This aligns the lumbar spine. This is the best starting position for RAB. After each exercise, all muscles must be tightened to form a muscle mantle for stabilization during the exhalation phase.

sideways (laterally, cranially and dorsally The only thing that can raise these ribs is breathing.

Although the ribs on the concave side (X-ray on the left) are horizontal, the approved technique must be followed. The ribs have to be spread sideways, upwards and backwards while the diaphragm is depressed. The patient must follow this process mentally and consciously feel it physically.

Costo-diaphragmatic breathing movement is performed with the thorax and pelvis in a corrected or overcorrected position. The result is that the atrophied and weakened lumbar muscles are also activated. This, in turn, causes the lumbar spine to move towards the middle. The waist region seems to be less wedge-shaped. As the trunk is inclined towards the concave side, it forces the lumbar muscles to work or to provide support (Fig. 477 b 1). This means that they become *long and strong*, while previously they were short, contracted and inactive, and consequently atrophied. The fact that pressure has been taken off this area of the thorax forces air into it. At the same time, the ribs on the concave side, being in the inhalation position (as shown by the X-ray), move into a more normal position and derotate the spinal column. This is the reason why it is important to guide breathing to these ribs sideways and upwards. The success of our treatment method depends on knowing these facts and on regular practice. Treatment is a continuous learning process which motivates the patient to keep exercising for weeks, months or even years without external assistance.

The X-ray shows only the bony parts of the skeleton, which often have serious structural changes. The angles can be measured two-dimensionally according to Cobb or others. The extent and depth of the rib hump is not measurable by X-ray. The skin folds, structure of the muscles and blood flow are not visible.

The external appearance is what concerns the patient most. The Schroth method therefore treats the entire scoliotic body with all its varieties of deformities and functional changes. Postural correction starts with the feet. As a rule, we treat the feet and legs as well during an in-patient stay. The ribcage breathing movements created by the RAB technique move the costovertebral joints and are capable of partially derotating the spine and flattening the rib hump. The effects of this can actually be seen.

It is conceivable that by derotation of the thorax against the pelvis on the one hand and against the shoulder girdle on the other, different degrees of pressure are created in the lungs, and the diaphragm, which may also be distorted, takes on a more normal position and thus functions more properly. This explains why the ribcage can achieve a corrected posture (Fig. 606) although the X-ray may not show a significant improvement in the degree of curvature. The result was obtained by the following.

1. Reversal of false body statics ("scoliotic balance") of skeleton and muscles, which is a decisive factor.

2. Overcorrection during exercises, since only in overcorrection are the former atrophied muscles forced to work, and concave areas of the thorax are relieved to allow them to be better ventilated.

3. All this is combined with elongation, i.e., active stretching of the spinal curvatures and the lateral areas of the trunk.

4. And only after this is derotation of the spinal column and the ribs possible.

5. In this corrected position, the isometric-orthopaedic tension (tensing of all the muscles concerned) is at its maximum and all corrections are maintained (otherwise the scoliotic posture would stabilize even further).

There is no other way to normalize the many deformities of idiopathic scoliosis in a conservative manner.

The scoliosis therapist has to be aware of the above facts, to learn them and be able to explain them to the patient. The patient and therapist must be secure in the knowledge that the improvement brought about by these methods, initially in appearance, will also result in a decrease in curvature – measurable by X-ray – and an overall improvement in health. At first, the treatment seems to be very time-consuming, but it is worthwhile, since risks are avoided.

Scoliosis cannot be treated schematically since all cases are different, and this what is so fascinating for the therapist. Treatment is always interesting because each new patient is a new challenge. The visual impression helps to decide where and to what extent overcorrection is needed to reach the goal of optimum correction. Schroth aims for the impossible to achieve the anatomically possible. This forms the basis for the pedagogic principles of the Schroth method.

Our efforts aim to restore muscular and skeletal equilibrium by training the muscles in the range of what is anatomically possible. The skeletal segments have to be aligned in a way that brings the scoliotically deformed parts of the trunk close to the normal position. The important lifting force in the **nuclei pulposi** of the intervertebral disks deviates to the back and sides in scoliosis and has to be redirected to the middle to enable it to work cranially. This is the reason why Schroth primarily corrects incorrect body balance. *Without* the indispensable correction of this equilibrium, patients exercise desperately without achieving any positive results. *Only after* the correction of balance can the ribs be employed as levers which derotate the vertebrae, supporting by breathing. These ribs are blocked before correction. Efficient scoliosis treatment must therefore include rotational breathing therapy. These exercises have to be practised even if derotation of segments of the spine seems hardly possible because the lever arms of the Mm. rotatores and its muscle volume are in a disadvantageous position and can only be used as an aid. It is our opinion that the Mm. rotatores, which form the innermost muscular group, are the last muscles to be used. Fig. 481 shows a hypermobile person whose trunk is bending into a scoliotic posture. Would you say that these shifts were caused only by the Mm. rotatores? Even if the origin of scoliosis stems from such a posture, the rotation of the outer body parts is initiated automatically. The Schroth method visualizes ribs as long lever arms that unwind the distortion of the vertebral bodies. Adding internal pressure from breathing to this creates an improvement in shape that would not be possible without guided breathing. It is necessary to be aware of this, otherwise the theoretically impossible muscle functions are regarded as a problem which cannot be solved in theory and therefore, nor in practice. But it is the *practical* impact that is decisive! May we add the following phrase attached to the wall at the entrance to a French aircraft manufacturing company:

"The weight of the bumblebee in relation to its wings makes it *theoretically* impossible for this bee to fly. But the bumblebee does not know about this, and flies anyway!"

Experience has demonstrated that the rotation of the spine is still possible while scoliosis is developing, otherwise scoliosis would never occur! Schroth declares: What can develop on the one hand must be able to be eradicated by exercise on the other. Theoretically,

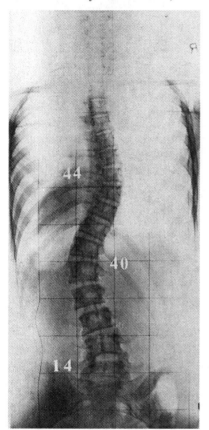

Fig. 478:
15-year-old female patient, before Schroth treatment

Thoracic	44°
Thoracolumbar	40°
Lumbosacral	14°

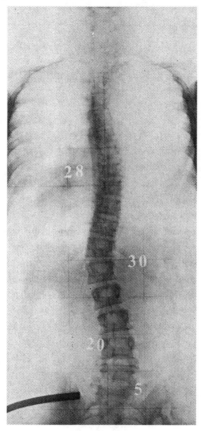

Fig. 479:
15½-year-old female patient

Thoracic	28°
Thoracolumbar	30°
Lumbosacral	20° = + 6°

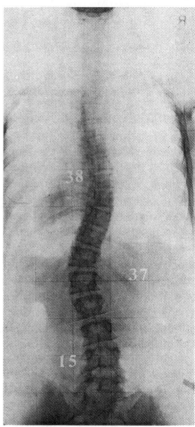

Fig. 480:
16-year-old female patient

Thoracic	38°
Thoracolumbar	37°
Lumbosacral	15°

CASE M: SPINE UPRIGHT BUT DEVELOPING A LUMBOSACRAL CURVE

Fig. 478:
Case M, 15-year-old female patient, idiopathic scoliosis. The lumbosacral curve deviates 14°, swinging to the side of the rib hump. Afterwards the pelvis is horizontal. The patient had a 6-week course of in-patient treatment using all available corrective aids and the five active pelvic corrections.

Fig. 479:
After 6 months, the X-ray shows a marked straightening of the thoracic and lumbar curve. The lumbosacral curve increased due to the 4th and 5th pelvic correction (hip below the rib hump backwards and downwards). Oblique position of the pelvis 5°. Obviously, the pelvic corrections act positively on the lumbar curve. If the caudal curvature is very extreme, as in this case, these two pelvic corrections should be omitted.

Fig. 480:
The patient continued exercises at home for seven months. She did not pay attention to pelvic derotation. The lumbosacral curvature straightened again. However, this had a negative influence on the upper spinal curves. Our question: What is more beneficial: a horizontal pelvis and larger spinal curves or a scoliotic pelvis and smaller spinal curves?

169

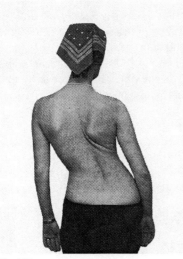
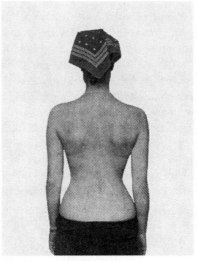
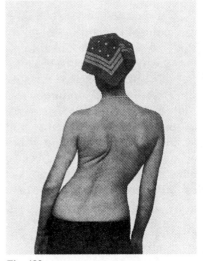

Fig. 481:
Normal, hypermobile body of a 22-year-old female patient with a scoliotic posture to the left.

Fig. 482:
The same patient in a normal, upright position

Fig. 483:
The same patient performing a scoliotic posture to the right.

scoliosis can be reversed. The actual ability to do so lies within every patient who has been taught well and in whom spinal arthrodesis has not yet taken place. The breathing reaches the areas where pressure is taken off the trunk segments and the natural width has been restored. The parts of lungs which had once been restricted are supplied with oxygen again, and consequently, regain strength through recaptured function. We have witnessed patients who have been freed from susceptibility to colds, nervous asthma, abdominal cramps and other complaints. The great advantage is the new lease of health when the wedged parts of the spine and body are mobilized and the function of the diaphragm is normalised. X-rays show how much stronger the spinal structures become.

Training is fundamental for each postural improvement. The way patients think also has to be changed. This results in a more harmonious balance of the skeleton, the musculature and the ligaments which, in turn, creates a better shape and a measurable decrease in curvature. The patient has to be motivated to continue permanently doing the Schroth exercises and to integrate them into all other activities. Awareness and the sensation of a new and straighter posture lead to benefits in other areas of life as well.

Photos taken at intervals also play an important role in motivation. The positive results of a 4- or 6-week in-patient course have not yet been stabilised and will worsen to a certain degree after the patient leaves the clinic. Trained muscles cannot, however, suddenly be reactivated, just as one may not discard a supportive brace without preparing the body. The improvement in curvature and posture come about slowly as in nature, but they do come constantly and thoughts and perceptions have to be directed predominantly in the same positive direction. Nature does not take shortcuts either. When we stand under an apple tree in springtime and blow warm air onto the blossoms, we do not expect ap-

ples to ripen immediately. A patient who guides physical growth in the right direction and shakes off bad habits will get results, and these will show on the photos. We have often seen scoliotic patients with better posture than non-scoliotics.

4. Accessory rotation in lateral flexion of the upper trunk (Fig. 484)

Sketch a) shows the sacrum and lower 3 lumbar vertebrae in the vertical position. The vertebrae may be seen as faces: the spinous process is the nose, the articulations are the eyes, and the transverse processes are the ears.

Sketch b) shows lateral flexion in a person without scoliosis and accessory rotation according to Lewitt (Lewitt 1987). The face looks toward the inner side of the arch and downwards.

Sketch c) shows two inclined lumbar vertebrae (kyphotic), and

Sketch d) shows the same vertebrae reclined (lordotic). The marked points show more flexibility. The areas pressed together have no mobility.

Vertebral bodies in a physiological lumbar lordosis tend to deviate laterally, mainly the apical vertebra.

As the area of the vertebral arch is relatively fixed due to the connecting articulations, and the area of vertebral bodies remains relatively flexible, only the vertebral body can pursue a lateral tendency. This means that the vertebrae rotate. The vertebral bodies turn towards the convex side of the curvature. The same happens in physiological lateral flexion of a healthy person. The effect of these forces is even stronger in real scoliosis since the scoliosis has become evident already and the trunk (including the head) weighs down on the spine and increases the curvature to such an extent that torsion becomes the result.

170

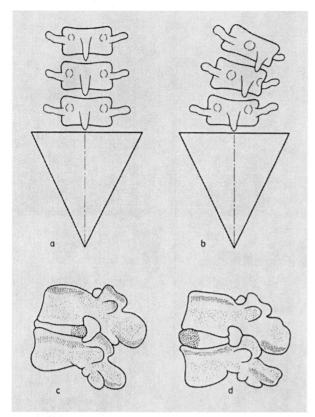

Fig. 484

If we study the 'muscle cylinder' exercise (Fig. 107) we notice that stretching the concave side of the lumbar curve results in derotation which, of course, is supported by muscular activity in this area. This exercise straightens up lateral flexion and reduces the tendency of vertebral bodies to shift to the convex side. We are using rotatory forces and decrease rotation this way.

The *thoracic spine* has a physiological kyphosis of about 30°. The vertebrae are closely connected to the ribs and fixed. The intervertebral disks are slimmer. Here, the vertebral bodies shift again to the convex side in lateral flexion. Vertebral rotation is the result, analogous to the lumbar spine: the spinous processes turn towards the concave side of the curvature.

According to Dickson and Tomaschewski, lordosis presents itself in the thoracic spine. This is only visible when a X-ray shows a lateral view of the vertebrae of the main curvature. However, the body of the vertebra has to be in oblique rotation. Simply taking an X-ray from the side does not show this. Our derotational correction of breathing – moving the narrow front forwards and upwards and then contracting the lateral intercostal musculature during exhalation – has to be performed nevertheless, independent of an existing lordosis of the thoracic spine. The 'forwards' is not to be understood as movement in the sagittal plane, but rather rotation in the transverse plane.

Theoretically we may think of the cervical spine as a cranial continuation of the thoracic spine, similar to the lumbar spine and described as 'lordotic'. The spinous processes also rotate to the concave side. This is countered by the Schroth corrective head pose: the head is inclined towards the concave side while the chin points towards the convex side. The neutral vertebra, transition from one spinal curvature to the next, is not affected. This vertebra shows only an oblique position and is not rotated.

5. Puberty

Children pose a special problem at the time of puberty; girls especially, before the time of menarche. At this time, many cases of scoliosis worsen tremendously, even if there had been a fairly good corrective result before. Physiological changes lead to weaknesses in some girls. In combination with the stress of school and growing up, they may not be able to exercise as much as needed and therefore not be able to maintain corrections. A number of mothers have reported that they observed the scoliosis worsening daily, even though their daughters exercised for an hour a day. These young patients are overstressed physically and emotionally. They need mental as much as physical support. In such cases, a well-fitted brace aiming at overcorrection seemed appropriate. These braces can be adapted to changing states of the body. There are also patients who are not worried about their condition, and do nothing for their back and do not exercise at all. We cannot offer such patients much help (Fig. 485). By the time they change their attitude it is usually too late. These young patients need our help, especially during puberty. We came to the conclusion that a 14- to 16-year-old girl who is not menstruating yet and shows angles of 30-40° has to have a brace. Otherwise the scoliosis worsens without a support.

It is generally known that scoliosis above 50° represents an indication for surgery. There are, however, patients who do not want this or may not undergo surgery. They may be helped conservatively, provided they work hard and continuously for years. This is illustrated by the figures in this book. Training only the body does not help in these cases. The patients have to 'work' mentally as well, using visualization and imagery, feeding their mind with desire and an unbreakable will to change their body. They have to be very consistent and develop a strong will.

6. Correction of the shifted sternum

The sternum forms the middle of the anterior rib cage. In scoliosis it may shift to the side. In a strongly decompensated three-curve scoliosis with a protruding hip on the concave side, the sternum has often shifted towards the convex side (Fig. 53). In the case of scoliosis with an aligned pelvis or a protruding hip on the convex side (four-curve scoliosis), the sternum shifts to the concave

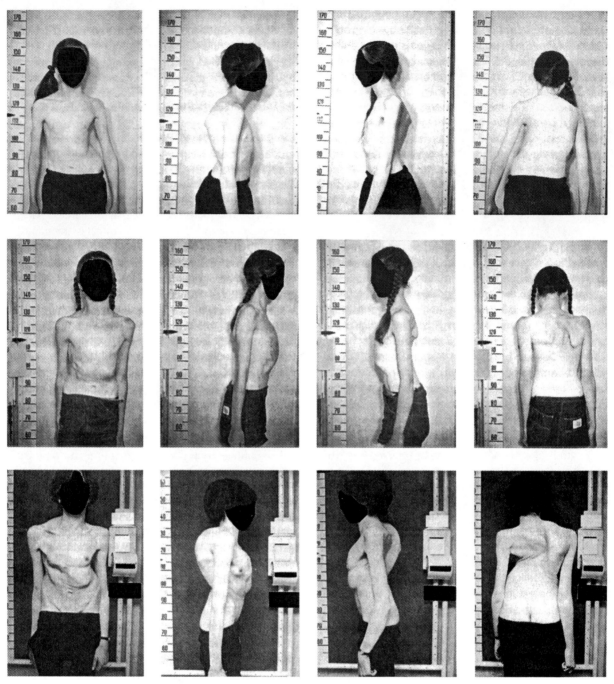

Fig. 485:

Upper row: 13-year-old girl at the beginning of treatment. Faulty balance of skeleton and musculature; scoliotic pelvis. Very prominent rib hump. Multiple broken line of the trunk. Oblique shoulder girdle.

Middle row: Same patient after a 6-week course of in-patient treatment. Corrected balance of the skeleton. The body is aligned vertically. The shoulders are levelled.

Bottom row: The same patient after nine years. As she was indifferent about her disorder, she neither practised at home nor did she come back for in-patient treatment. There was no motivation at all. The deformities worsened until she showed ribs in the front which overlapped and created a large dorsal rib hump. At this point it was obviously much harder and more laborious to correct.

side (Fig. 52). This requires a different method of treatment. The patient checks the position of the sternum with the fingertips and observes in the mirror. Now they move the rib cage in a way that aligns the sternum, and keeps a close watch while correcting. The movement of the rib cage forwards and upwards is continued with the aim of moving the rib hump from dorsal to ventral. This breathing rib cage movement has to be performed vigorously to move the narrow area of the chest forward so that it covers the other side of the chest when observed from the side. The shoulder and pelvic girdles have to counterhold, of course. The direction 'inwards' is changed to 'obliquely to the outside and upwards' (in the case of Fig. 52, this meant diagonally to the right and upwards). The inward movement is performed only by contraction of the lateral intercostal muscles. This pushes and shifts the spine to the middle, while RAB on the concave side pulls the spine to the middle and derotates it.

The RAB movements described have to start precisely dorsally since the concavity is located dorsally and only the posterior rib portions can pull and have a lever effect on the spine. Using the hands and eyes to observe, the patient can practice a certain oblique breathing technique. Once the sideways and upwards phase has been successfully managed, the concavity arches backwards and upwards, and the ribs spread. The patient can feel this sensation of 'bursting' of the muscles very well. The shoulder girdle and pelvic girdle are counterheld, and the lumbar hump is derotated strongly at the same time. Powerful shoulder countertraction on the right completes the result.

7. Correction of the shoulder on the concave side

When moving the shoulder on the concave side forwards, one has to pay attention that the entire shoulder with the scapula is moved, not only the side of the top. If only the latter were done, this might result in a shoulder hump above the dorsal concavity. The corrective cushion has to be placed so that it elevates the entire scapula forwards. Placing this cushion higher could result in tilting of the shoulder girdle and not the desired derotation. Very important: avoid pulling with the arm on the concave side alone to lift the shoulder off the ribs. This would enlarge the cervical curvature in most cases. Refer to the exercise 'Shoulder countertraction'. See Figs. 107 and 108.

8. Correction of the anterior rib hump

The anterior rib hump must not simply be pressed manually backwards or inwards in order to make it disappear. Manual pressure on these ribs would provoke an oblique pushing movement to the posterior rib hump and thus enlarge it. The anterior rib hump aligns itself once the same ribs on the concavity in the back have been breathed and rotated backwards and upwards. Manual assistance on the front (as in Figs. 92 and 93) often has to be omitted, and other exercises to spread the dorsal concavity have to be performed.

9. Correction of flatback in combination with scoliosis (Figs. 487–499)

According to Tomaschewski, some segments of the thoracic spine are characterized by restricted anteflexion in case of flatback syndrome. The erector trunci muscles are shortened. The symmetrical contraction of the erector trunci muscles may, with decreasing stability, change into asymmetrical contraction which leads to pathological rotation (scoliosis). This may be triggered by a blockage.

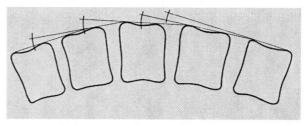

Fig. 486:
Radiological measurements: Functional X-ray of the spine in anteflexion. The cervical spine also in anteflexion. Measurements were taken of the tangents at the dorsal rims of two neighbouring vertebrae. They form angle A as a measure for the anteflexion that a vertebral body is able to perform in relation to its neighbour.

Tomaschewski measures flatback in the so-called 'package-position' and takes lateral X-rays. Thoracic lordosis is often not detectable in the standing position. The vertebrae imaged on an X-ray in this position are measured in a special way (Fig. 486). The larger these angles, the greater the physiological rounding of the back. The smaller these angles, the less physiological the thoracic spine. Tomaschewski examined students of different grades and selected children with restricted anteflexion. Follow-up showed that in most cases these children also developed scoliosis. A flat back is as abnormal as kyphosis. Most of our scoliotic patients also have a flat back. Sometimes flatback is combined with lumbar or cervical kyphosis.

The sagittal diameter is low in flatback, and thus breathing is restricted. The rib cage is deformed anteriorly and the rib hump is hardly visible. When dressed, these patients have an 'extraordinary upright posture'. In later life flatback may lead to back and low back pain symptoms.

Observing the scoliotic back from the concave side at the level of the thoracic curvature, it is obvious that lordosis exists here, and not kyphosis, as was suggested earlier. The kyphosis is simulated by the rib hump.

In case of flatback, RAB is even more important, because it has the effect of mobilizing the anteflexion, especially in the thoracic region. RAB aims at increasing the sagittal diameter of the thorax.

This breathing technique is a very advantageous instrument in the treatment of major scoliosis. Katharina Schroth recognized this fact in her early years, although kyphoscoliosis was dominant at the time.

173

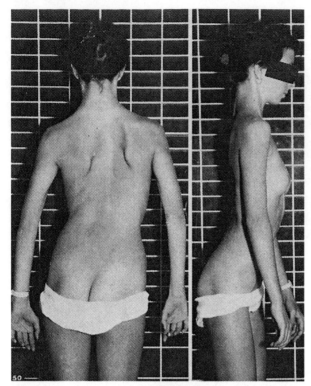

Fig. 487: **Flatback in connection with scoliosis.**

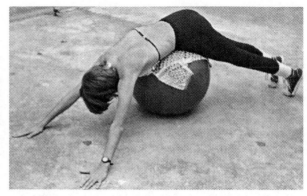

Fig. 489:
Exercise for thoracic lordosis, hyperlordosis in the lumbar spine, flatback and a severely twisted trunk.

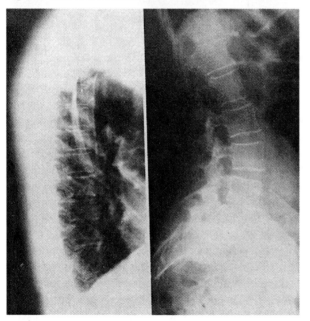

Fig. 488:
Lateral view of flatback. Left: thoracic spine; right: lumbar spine.

She put great emphasis on exercises like the 'Great arch' (Figs. 201–203). These exercises have an excellent effect on the derotation of vertebrae. She named this phase of the RAB 'vertebral derotational breathing'. Special attention should be paid to movements which 'fill' and widen the dorsal concavity when treating scoliosis in combination with flatback.

Exercises which are directed forwards should be done with great care and the back should be kept in a good middle position while performing the concluding corrective contraction.

There is no corrective cushion under the dorsal rib hump in case of flatback. In flatback without scoliosis, the cushions are placed laterally under the scapulae and the lowest part of the buttocks. You may also do the latter in case of hyperlordosis of the lumbar spine. All elements that contribute to creating kyphosis are very important. The ball exercise (Fig. 489) is also very advantageous. The patient's abdomen and pelvis are across the ball and the chest adopts the shape of it. This position makes dorsal breathing especially effective. The extended arms create a good starting position to build up muscle tension between the scapulae. The therapist may place the fingertips on the spinous processes of each segment with restricted anteflexion. The patient reacts by breathing and extending intensively. The therapist may also use circular stroking movements to enhance breathing. These are performed from the inside of the main curvature in the intercostal spaces and lead to the sides. The patient breathes against these stimuli. The same technique should be used in all other exercises.

Performing the exercise with the trunk hanging forward (Figs. 490, 491, 492) is also very good. The weight of the head results in elongation of the spine, during which derotation of the vertebrae is very successful when applying RAB.

The exercises already described (Figs. 201, 203, 240 and 253) can also be used to treat flatback.

174

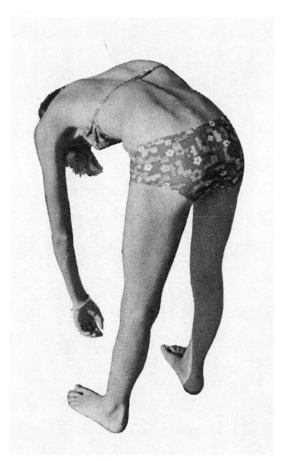

Fig. 490: Suitable starting position to ventilate the dorsal concavity.

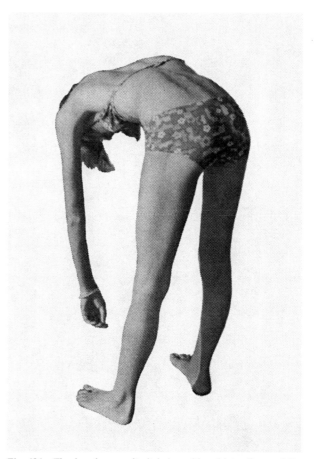

Fig. 491: The dorsal concavity is being widened laterally, cranially and dorsally by RAB.

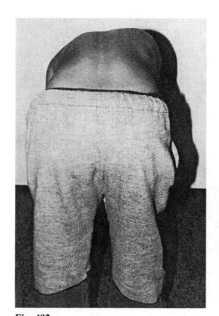

Fig. 492:
Inclining the body forward.

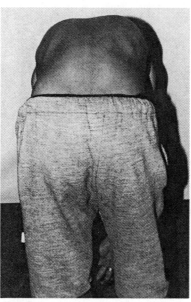

Fig. 493:
RAB while inclining the body forward.

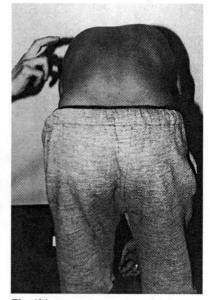

Fig. 494:
Using tactile stimulation.

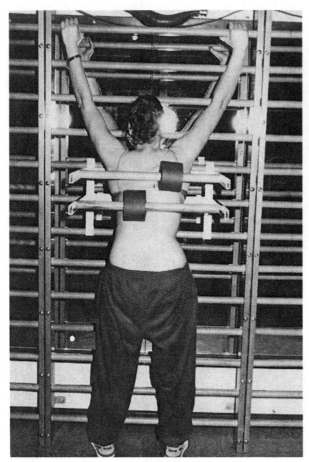
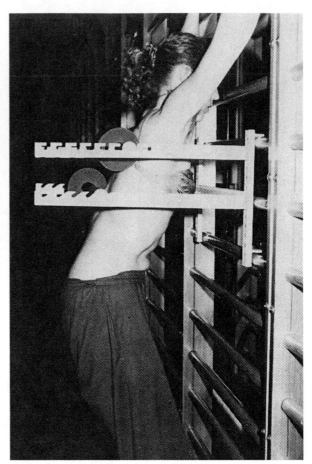

Fig. 495 a and b:
Exercises with the Flexomat. The protruding areas of the back are being fixed. The concave areas are being widened by RAB.

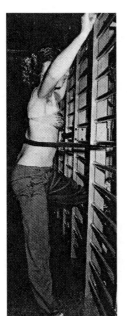
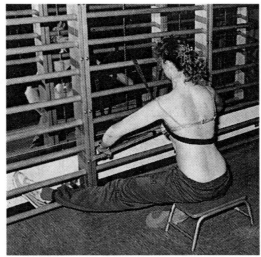
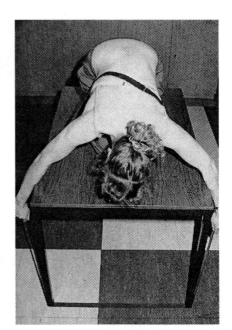

Fig. 497 (above)

Fig. 496 (left)   Fig. 498 (right)

Fig. 496: Ventilation of the lumbar concavity by using a resistance band as a counterhold..
Fig. 497: The resistance band is pulled tighter on the left to derotate the lumbar hump.
Fig. 498: The resistance band is positioned diagonally across the dorsal concavities and fixed with the legs of the table. The patient pulls the band sideways and upwards.

176

Flatback exercises using the 'Flexomat' (Fig. 495)

The device is attached to the wall bars at rib hump or lumbar hump level. Corrective cushions are placed under the rib hump and the lumbar hump. The patient performs the 'Great arch' exercise so that both the concavity below the rib hump and the concave side come into contact with the posterior pole during RAB. The number of corrective breathing movements is increased steadily until a rotatory movement between the rib cage and the lumbar area can be felt. The corrective result is then stabilized by contraction of the abdominal muscles or tension of all muscles to form a muscle mantle. For three-curve scoliosis, the patient may place the leg of the convex side about 5 cm further back to derotate the pelvis. Then the concave side is counter-moved by RAB towards the posterior holding position.

Pressing the back against the derotational spacers and forming kyphosis at the same time makes possible passive mobilization into anteflexion as well.

Flatback exercises at the wall bars using a resistance band (Figs. 496-498)

The band is either stretched across the concavities so that it can be breathed against when performing RAB, or it is placed behind the convexities to hold these forward while they are filled against the resistance.

Exercise with two resistance bands and the 'Bandscho' at the wall bars (Figs. 499 and 583)

One band is attached to the wall bars and is placed around the lumbar hump or the weak area below the

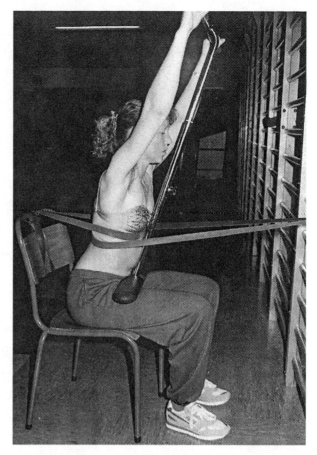

Fig. 499: Exercise with a resistance band and the 'Bandscho'.

rib hump. Slightly more tension is placed on the lumbar hump, so that it turns passively forwards. The other band is attached to the back of a chair and is placed over the protruding rib humps from in front, to pull them back-

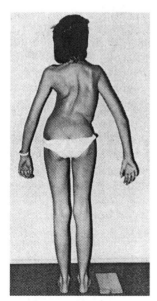

Fig. 500
12-year-old patient with idiopathic scoliosis and a severe static defect of the pelvis which increases the curvatures cranially.

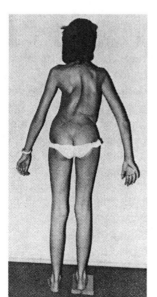

Fig. 501
Leg-length compensation on the right to straighten the thoracic convexity – increased lumbar curvature.

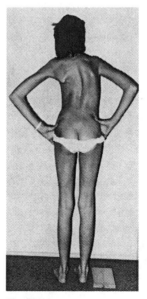

Fig. 502
The patient tries to tuck in the left hip with manual help. The lumbar curvature straightens.

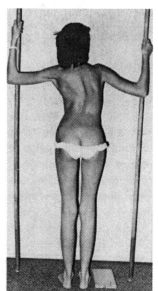

Fig. 503
Alignment of the pelvis happens actively. The straightening of the trunk is stabilized by the isometric push of the poles.

177

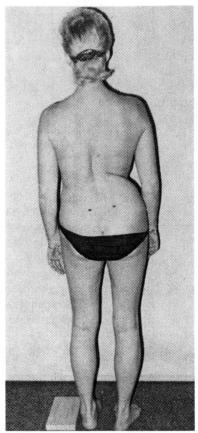

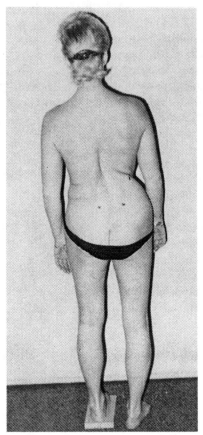

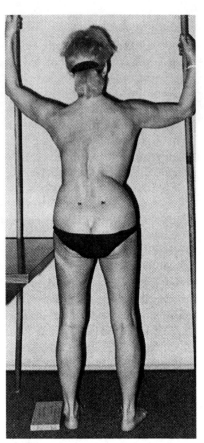

Fig. 504
40-year-old patient with a very prominent lumbar hump on the left and a lumbosacral curvature of 26°. Oblique pelvis of 1.7 cm.

Fig. 505
An LLC of 1.7 cm; the pelvis does not become completely horizontal. The right hip still shifts laterally. This increases the lumbosacral curvature.

Fig. 506
During exercise. Aligning the pelvis above the middle corrects the functional oblique pelvis as well.

wards. The 'Bandscho' is positioned very high. The patient now leans the extended trunk slightly forwards, and in doing so, stretches the back so that the dorsal concavities can be extended and filled with air. In the exhalation phase, the position achieved on inhalation is maintained and the entire front is tensed or pulled together.

10. Correction of the scoliotic pelvis (Fig. 500)

Heels or shoes should only be elevated if the legs have anatomically different lengths. Compensation for leg length (LLC) difference may result in an increase in the lumbosacral curvature (among other things) if lateral shifting, rotation and distortion of the pelvis are not corrected.

It is almost impossible to straighten up a laterally sagging upper trunk by increasing heel height, because the lumbar spine shifts to the opposite side in such cases. This enlarges the fold below the rib hump (Fig. 501).

It is our opinion that leg-length compensation should not be used in such cases and that it is preferable to reach a certain length below the rib hump and to move the lumbar spine to the middle by exercises (Figs. 502 and 503). The unilateral hip elevation often disappears as soon as the lateral shift has been corrected. If LLC is necessary, shoes with adjusted height should be worn permanently, also during exercises as well. Otherwise each step

includes movements which are disadvantageous to the spine. We found that after roughly one year it was no longer necessary in some cases to adjust the height of shoes. The shorter leg seemed to have been stimulated by correction and to have grown.

The usefulness of compensation has to be considered very carefully in the presence of a lumbosacral curve. Improvement of the lumbar curve may worsen the lumbosacral curve, and vice versa. In case of doubt apply the rule: no compensation, even moreso if it can be expected that the protruding hip will shift to the middle with exercise. In such cases, the oblique position of the leg changes as well and makes compensation unnecessary, because the pelvis and the iliosacral joints are realigned (Figs. 500-506). In almost all cases, the laterally shifted hip has turned backwards as well. The X-ray shows a seemingly wider wing of the ilium: in three-curve scoliosis on the left (Fig. 507); in four-curve scoliosis on the right (Fig. 508).

During brace treatment, an LLC is sometimes prescribed 'to make the brace fit better'. This results in an artificial pelvic obliqueness, as Fig. 510 shows. It is our opinion that the patient has to learn the specific pelvic corrections before the plaster cast for the brace is made (Figs. 506 and 513). This may certainly lead to a more effective brace treatment.

178

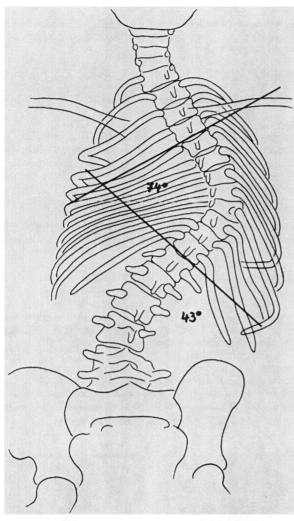

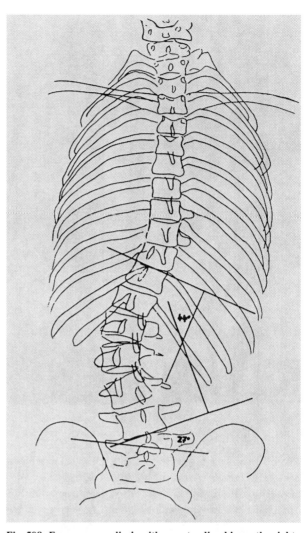

Fig. 507: Three-curve scoliosis with a protruding hip on the left.

Fig. 508: Four-curve scoliosis with a protruding hip on the right.

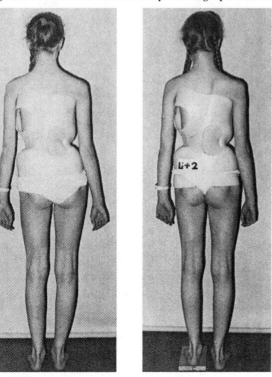

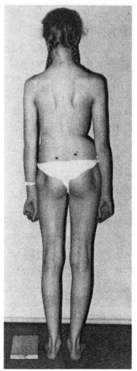

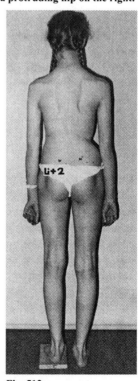

Fig. 509

Fig. 510

Fig. 511

Fig. 512

179

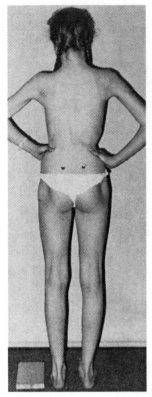 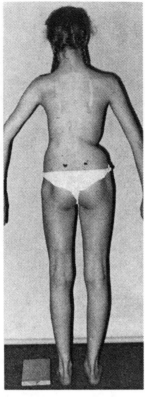

Fig. 513   **Fig. 514**

Fig. 509:
12-year-old girl; Chéneau brace. Without an LLC, the upper body sinks to the left. The bodyweight rests on the left leg and the right hip shifts to the right.

Fig. 510:
Due to the LLC of 2 cm the body is in a more vertical position. But now the two gluteal folds are at different heights.

Fig. 511:
The same patient without brace. The wings of the ilium are positioned obliquely, as are the gluteal folds, higher on the right. The 'waist-tri-angle' on the left has become less visible. The right hip is prominent. The pelvis seems distorted: on the right upwards and backwards, on the left forwards and downwards.

Fig. 512:
An LLC of 2 cm on the left does not align the pelvis completely. But the right hip is not quite as prominent. The waist-triangle' is develop-ing again.

Fig. 513:
The same patient exercises 'taking in' the hip and breathes the ribs on the right side sideways and upwards and backwards and upwards. She stabilizes the correction result with an isometric push against the pelvis. The gluteal folds are horizontal. The hips are more even. And thus without leg-length compensation.

Fig. 514:
The patient tries to reach correction without manual support, only with body awareness and mirror control. The functionally scoliotic pelvis has not been resolved. But with consistent exercises the pelvis will be aligned, and this without leg-length compensation.

The difference in hip height can clearly be seen when a person is dressed. Most of the time it is due to a func-tionally scoliotic pelvis. Very often, the prominent hip is higher. The belt 'hangs' obliquely, and one leg of the trousers seems shorter. This is the reason why we urge the patients to look into a mirror as often as possible to correct the faulty posture. Fig. 515 shows the 'oblique' pelvis. Fig. 516 shows the same patient after 15 min. of exercising the pelvic corrections. The belt is almost hor-izontal and her trouser legs are almost the same length.

11. Multiple-curve scoliosis (Figs. 517 and 518)

Smaller and shorter curvatures are most often present in multiple-curve scoliosis. This makes it harder to ap-ply the RAB which was developed to open several seg-ments.
At first, we try to resolve spinal inflexibility with small wriggling movements of the spine. We try to obtain maximum elongation of the spine. This is, of course, supported by special breathing as well. The result is then stabilized as described above. The most appropriate way is by holding two poles and pushing them against the ground using isometric tension of the upright spinae muscles in the elongated state.
In six-curve scoliosis, as shown in Fig. 517, the exer-cises developed for the lumbosacral curvature also have to be applied.

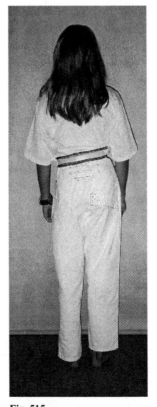 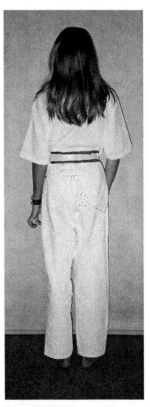

Fig. 515
The belt is oblique, the right leg of the trousers is too short; the right hip protrudes.

Fig. 516
The belt is almost even and the trousers are almost even; the hips are almost even. Both pictures were taken within 15 minutes of each other.

180

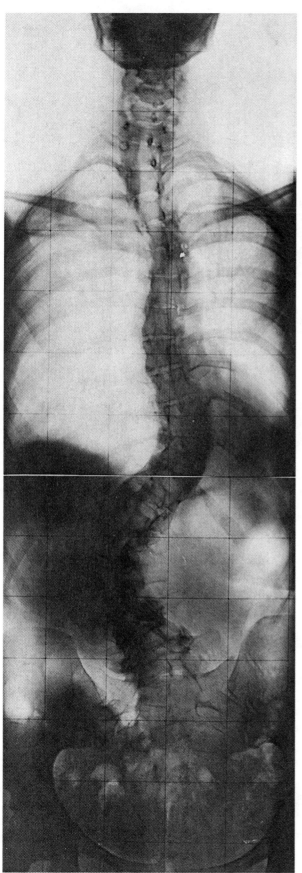

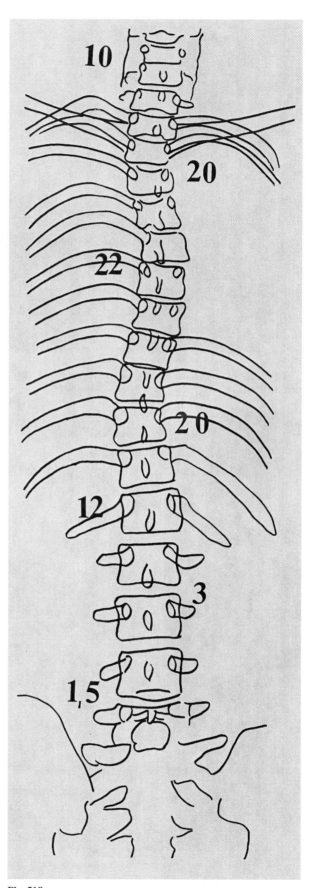

Fig. 517:
Six-curve scoliosis in a 27-year-old woman. The direction for exercise has to be more straight and upwards, as is the case with five- or four-curve scoliosis. The lumbosacral curvature has to be treated as well.

Fig. 518:
Exercise direction is straight upwards in this multiple-curve scoliosis.

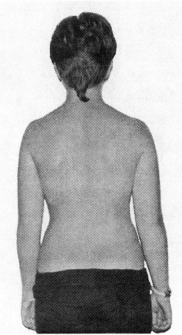

Fig. 519:
Atypical scoliosis: hardly visible in an upright position.

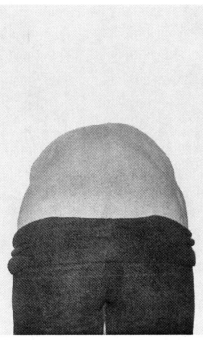

Fig. 520:
In anteflexion, the right side of the back is more prominent.

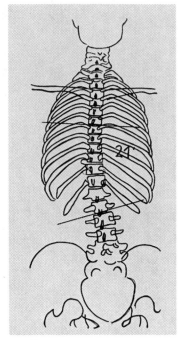

Fig. 521:
Thoracic left scoliosis. The spinous processes also point to the left.

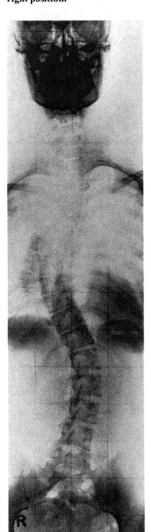

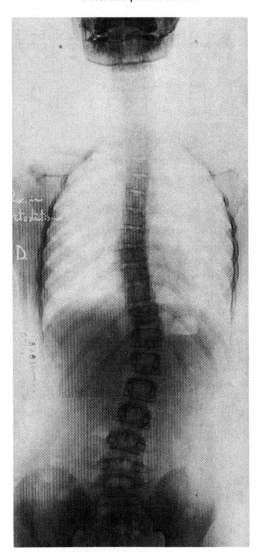

Fig. 522 (left):
16-year-old girl, four-curve scoliosis, pelvis aligned.

Fig. 523 (right):
12-year-old girl with four-curve scoliosis; protruding hip below the thoracic convexity; cervical 10°, thoracic 19°, lumbar 25°, lumbosacral 14°. The laterally shifted pelvis is obvious. The pelvis has to be aligned first before the upper spine can be corrected.

12. Atypical scoliosis (Fig. 519, 567)

Cases of atypical scoliosis are mostly minor, hardly ever exceeding lateral deviations of the spine by more than 20°. There are three categories.

Usually, the spinous processes of the vertebrae turn to the inside of the curve. The transverse processes turn dorsally on the convex side and ventrally on the concave side. They cause the ribs to move in these directions as well. The bigger the distortion, the more severe the thoracic deformity, because the rib hump turns further backwards.

Cases of atypical scoliosis act differently:

1. The spinous processes often point dorsally within the scoliotic curve, i.e., the vertebral bodies have not rotated but have shifted sideways. The scoliosis is not obvious at clinical examination. There is no difference in level when the patient bends forwards. We then exercise straight forward and upwards. Corrective cushions are placed the same way as they would be in the case of kyphosis (right and left lower scapula angles). If the X-ray shows a minor curvature, breathing is directed sideways and upwards as would be the case in a 'normal' scoliosis, but without the backwards component. On the convex side, it may only be necessary to contract the lateral intercostal muscles.

2. If the X-ray shows that the spinous processes point to the convex side at the vertex of the curvature in the thoracic area (Fig. 521), there is usually a rib hump on the concave side. This phenomenon is quite confusing for the therapist. Clinical examination might show a deviation of the trunk to the left which should then be accompanied by a rib hump to the left. But it is usually right-sided (Fig. 520). In such cases, we change the breathing direction and corrective cushions. The cushions can be very flat since there is only a slight rotation: on the concave side, place a cushion transversely under the lower scapula angle. Theoretically, the patient should direct exercises backwards on the convex side. We omit this, since we do not want to cause a more pronounced rounding of the back. It is, however, necessary to contract the lateral intercostal muscles. The concave side is widened laterally and turned ventrally, if visual examination allows this. We advise additional exercises recommended by Niederhöffer in such cases. They involve superficial back muscles and pull only laterally. By doing so, they turn the spinous processes towards the concavity. If there is any doubt, the exercises should only be done straight upwards and without derotation.

3. In many cases the clinical picture shows a quite 'normal' scoliosis with a lateral and dorsal rib hump on the convex side, a kind of scoliosis which only emerges as atypical on X-rays. In such cases, breathing and corrective cushions are as in 'normal' scoliosis.

Correction of false statics has to be done according to clinical findings in any case.

We observed the phenomenon of atypical rotations for the first time in 1982 in X-rays in 1.4% of our patients. In 1983, we observed the same in 3.1%, and in 1984 in 6.8%.

The following table shows the subdivision of the site of the typical vertebral body rotation.

Table 6:

Year	thoracic	lumbar	thoracic + lumbar	lumbo sacral	lumbar + lumbo sacral	number of patients
1982	15	2	-	-	-	17
1983	22	14	-	-	-	36
1984	51	21	3	1	2	78
Total	88	37	3	1	2	131

13. Correction of faulty body statics

People with postural disturbances have lost the normal balance of the body. Those with a symmetrical postural disturbance (Scheuermann's disease, for example) have a so-called "kyphotic equilibrium", whereas patients with scoliosis and kyphoscoliosis have a 'scoliotic balance'. They are no longer statically balanced, but rather falsely adjusted, or decompensated. Their natural static structure is disturbed (Part A). The three trunk segments deviate from the vertical against each other, partially in the sagittal plane and partially in a lateral direction. This may result in complete postural collapse (Figs. 16 and 17) with all the attendant psychological and physical stress.

Some patients with severe scoliosis are not aware of its development and did not recognize the postural destruction that was taking place in their body. This was the case for the patient in Fig. 485. Patients usually consult their physician because of breathing disorders and then the physician diagnoses a scoliosis. The extent of ignorance and indifference among relatives and friends is alarming. With the help of the photos, the patient realizes for the first time how far the body segments deviate. It is only possible to change what has been recognized. This means that an essential part of the Schroth method is to point out and correct even the slightest postural deficiency, because patients must be able to continue helping themselves alone at home.

If the static deviations are due to a difference in leg length, this has to be corrected first with a leg length compensation (LLC). Only after the pelvis has been moved into a horizontal position can the higher body segments be corrected. This causes the lumbar spine to move more to the midline and starts off the straightening of other spinal curvatures. To achieve vertical alignment, we aim for 'overcorrection'. This means that the

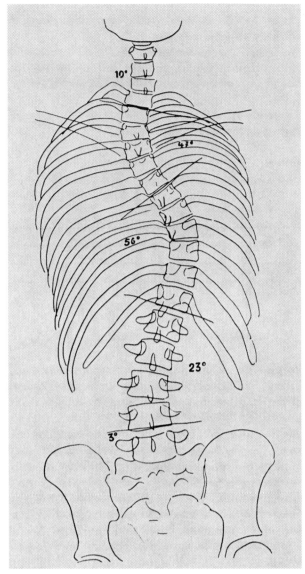

Fig. 524:
Static scoliosis in a 26-year-old woman. The left leg is 1 cm. shorter. The right hip is 1 cm. higher. The spine balances vertically.

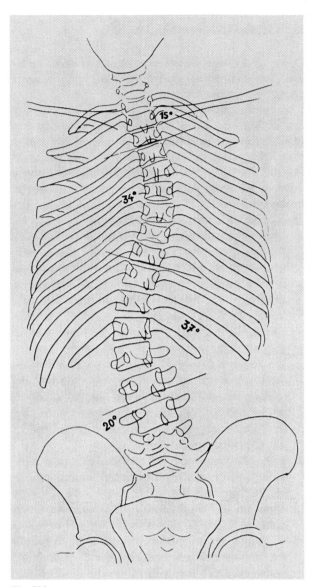

Fig. 525:
Idiopathic scoliosis; 17-year-old boy; the right hip protrudes. Deviation of the trunk is about 4 cm. from the middle towards the left.

concave segments of the trunk should become convex and that the convex segments should become concave during exercise. The trunk segments which protrude too far forwards must be moved backwards and segments that protrude backwards must be moved forwards.

'Overcorrection' changes postural disorders into the opposite, i.e., we create contrary conditions that result in a change in body awareness to what is correct.

The movements necessary to perform overcorrection are really only possible in minor scoliosis. Some of the effects are lost to a certain extent, however, after exercise. Nevertheless, the exercise leaves a special awareness for posture and straightness in the patient's mind; such that the patient subconsciously assumes an upright posture after a certain period of practice. In the case of severe scoliosis, the patient's mind has to be trained and visualisation and imagination lead in very small steps towards the goal. Mobilization and strong motivation

are the best support. The body can then align, even with scoliosis.

Correction of wrongly compensated statics is the concept that runs through the whole of the Three-Dimensional Treatment Method and therefore also through this book.

We must stress again here that each breathing movement of the rib cage has to be followed by forceful isometric tightening of the entire trunk musculature, starting at the anterior upper thighs, passing the groin right up to the costal arches, and from there across the sides to the back, in order to stabilize the corrective results. Exercises alone are not enough because they do not lead to a permanent correction. Only 'orthopaedic-isometric corrective tension' can lead to a stable result which in turn will become the final shape.

Each forceful muscle contraction results in the growth

of new muscle. Attention therefore has to be paid to ensuring that muscle toning not only takes place on the rib hump side (aiming at contraction of the convexity) which would increase the latter visually. The toning has to take place on both sides with the concavity in a stretched state and the convex side in a contracted state after the de-rotational breathing phase.

14. Lumbar kyphosis (Fig. 526)

Kyphosis of this type is most often present in patients without scoliosis. The physiological lordosis of the lumbar spine has disappeared and the spinal segment has moved backwards. It can be observed especially in the sitting position. In most cases, kyphosis of the lumbar spine merges cranially into a compensatory lordosis of the thoracic spine.

Therapists must check very carefully whether an additional minor lordosis exists below L4 or L5. Treatment is complicated in this case because whatever we do may be wrong and therefore it is aimed at elongation only. The aim is to move the spinal column to the middle position and stabilize it by muscle strengthening. Additional movements are not desired.

When the lumbar kyphosis does *not* lead into a lumbosacral lordosis, exercises may be done in the supine position with extended legs. A corrective cushion may be placed under the lumbar spine. If, in addition, flatback is present, the pelvis is kept in middle position.

Exercises performed with the strap and belt need two belts fastened on the right and left to avoid unwanted kyphosis of the lumbar spine.

The starting position for the 'Great arch' exercise includes a pronounced upright position of the pelvis. We have to change this into a "great angle", where the lumbar spine can be brought to midline position with a very slight lordosis.

Exercises for lumbar kyphosis

The following exercises teach the patient to become **aware of pelvic movements** and to control them.
Sitting on a chair. Feet parallel on the floor.

1. One hand is placed on the lower abdomen, one on the lumbar spine. Tilt the pelvis down and up again. Feel while tilting how the spinous processes of the vertebrae move forwards and how the stomach arches forwards. Raise the pelvis to a middle position and feel how the positioning of the pelvis changes the position of the spine. The stomach tightens. Feel how the thoracic spine reacts: if the pelvis is tilted, it is elongated, and if the pelvis is straightened, it makes it "shorter", because the lumbar spine is rounding out again.

2. Fold the hands behind the neck. The neck pushes slightly against the hands. The head pulls upwards. Sit firmly on the ischial tuberosities. Move the

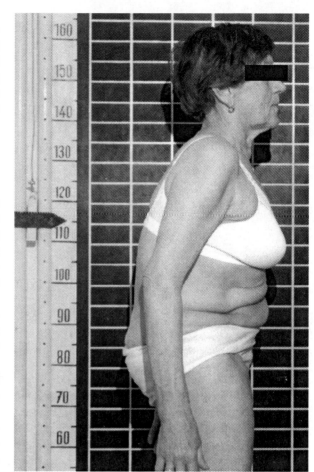

Fig. 526:
Female patient with lumbar kyphosis and idiopathic scoliosis

whole upper body forwards while inhaling and push the feet firmly onto the ground. Move backwards to the starting position while exhaling. Be careful not to form a flatback.

3. The same exercise. Come upwards with oscillatory movements of the spine. Inhale (RAB). Push the elbows wide apart. Exhaling, lift off the chair with hands a little while forming a lumbar lordosis and bringing the flat back backwards.

4. Move the pelvis as far as possible backwards, as if you want to slide under the back of the chair. Maintain an upright position, with your back against the chair. Relax the shoulder girdle and exhale.

5. Sit on the edge of the chair. Feet parallel. Hands on the inside of the thighs; elbows directed sideways. Wriggle with the spine upwards, perform corrective inhalation; then pushing the hands against the thighs while exhaling. Feet stay in position; the soles of the feet pull backwards. This moves the lumbar spine upwards into elongation.

6. Sitting cross-legged on a footstool; back against the wall bars. The ischial tuberosities rest on cushions. The patient sits on a wedge-shaped pillow, the wide part of it in the back, as at the beginning: the pelvis is tilting forwards; RAB. The lumbar spine loses contact with the wall bars. Exhale and let the spine

185

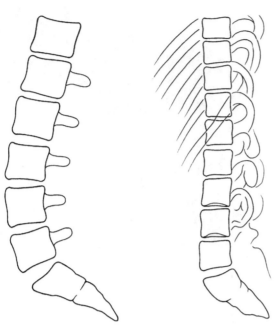 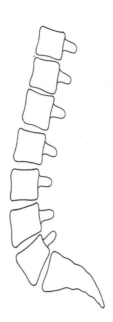 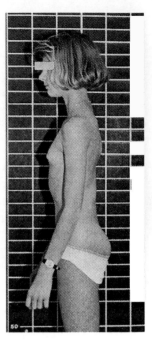

Fig. 527: Normal lumbar spine, lateral view.   **Fig. 528:** Straight lumbar spine   **Fig. 529:** Hyperlordosis   **Fig. 530:** Straight lumbar spine

move backwards. The sternum moves upwards, the shoulders stay backwards and downwards. The head pushes upwards.

7. Relax! Use your hands on the iliac crest to control and feel the movements.
8. Hands folded against the back of the neck. The hands and neck stabilize each other. The head pushes upwards. Stretch while inhaling, tilting the pelvis forwards. Exhale while moving the upper body forwards with small dipping movements. The elbows are pulled apart. Be aware of the region of the lumbar spine. Keep the pelvis tilted.
9. Keep the lumbar spine in a slight lordotic position while sitting anywhere at a table or at work.
10. Prone position. Do swimming movements with both arms.
11. Prone position without corrective cushion or footstool. RAB. While exhaling, stretch and lift arms and legs from the ground.
12. When performing the 'Great arch' exercise at the wall bars, it is better not to straighten the legs, as this rounds the lumbar region, but to bend the knees and perform a 'Great angle'.

The following exercises can be performed supine (also in bed). Slightly pad your lumbar spine. Cover the lower half of your body with a blanket to provide slight resistance during the exercises. Breathe in when going into the movement, which is very small. Breathe out when tensing the muscles, to avoid straining. During the ensuing rest phase, breathe in and out strongly. Always keep your pelvis tilted, i.e., lower the anterior edge of the pelvis so that your coccyx can feel the padded exercise mat underneath you. Your back should lie on the padded exercise mat.

13. Stretch your legs. Push your feet outwards against the slight resistance. Tense all the muscles in your legs and pelvis up to your lumbar spine.
14. Flex your knees and place your feet flat on the floor. Now push both knees outwards against the slight resistance, raising your lumbar spine slightly from the padded exercise mat.
15. As above, but put a resistance band behind your knees and take hold of the ends with both hands. Push both knees outwards against this resistance.
16. With your feet flat on the floor, press your hands against the sides of your thighs. With your lumbar spine in lordosis, push your thighs outwards.
17. With your legs stretched out, raise one leg forwards against the slight resistance. Your back should remain on the padded exercise mat, only your lumbar spine may lift a little.

In any event the pelvis must be pushed backwards during the exercises, i.e., it must remain in the perpendicular axis. A lumbar hump as well as a rib hump starts below with backwards displacement and goes forwards again above the curvature. Therefore there is no point in trying to treat lumbar kyphosis with trunk back bending exercises (section C.VIII) because this causes the 'body axis to be interrupted at multiple points' (section B. II). Therapy must ensure that the region that has deviated backwards is moved again into the perpendicular, while the pelvis remains pushed backwards, no matter how low the lumbar kyphosis. The lower part of the curvature is always forwards and must be displaced backwards without causing the thoracic spine to go into lordosis as a result. Picture how a bow under tension (as in archery,

186

for example) points in the same direction at both ends, while only the central section goes in the opposite direction. Otherwise it is not a bow.

If lumbar kyphosis is coupled with scoliosis, there will be a pronounced lumbar hump on the thoracic concave side (which could be wrongly interpreted as 'lumbar kyphosis'), whereas the lower ribs ('the waist' below the thoracic rib hump) are directed forwards.

In this case it is wrong to speak about lumbar kyphosis. This should be treated as a four curve scoliosis (section C.VII).

15. Spondylolisthesis (Fig. 531)

This is most often caused by the 5th lumbar vertebra slipping forward against the sacrum. Externally, this is evident in hyperlordosis of the lumbar spine. The patient very often suffers from back pain. We have to focus on exercises that counteract this: in the supine position, we place two corrective cushions under the lowest parts of the buttocks to allow the lumbar spine to sink towards the floor. In the prone position, we omit the first pelvic correction (footstool under the pelvis). Instead we put a flat cushion under the abdomen.

The patient sits on a wedge-shaped pillow, the wide part of it to the front.

Schroth exercises and all strengthening exercises for the abdominal musculature are of great importance. Also, additional leg strengthening exercises (hamstrings) and stabilizing exercises for the pelvis are necessary.

Exercises for painful spondylolisthesis (also lumbar hyperlordosis), Fig. 531

Treatment has to concentrate on the shifting vertebrae and a mental image of the X-ray has to be borne in mind to locate where to exercise, since the movements required are diminutive and delicate. They require a special body awareness. To begin, patients stand between two mirrors and perform small circular movements with the fingertips on the hollow area of the lumbar spine, to feel the area. Through this tactile stimulation, they gain a sense for the area which has to be exercised. The following exercises are done in the supine position (in bed). A blanket is folded and put under the legs. Additionally, the buttocks should rest on a wedge shaped pillow whose broad side points towards the legs. This widens the narrow lumbar region. The abdomen relaxes and sinks down. This position itself may already relieve pain. The lower trunk and legs are now wrapped in a blanket to give resistance during exercising. Starting the exercises is accompanied by inhalation. Contracting and tightening is done during exhalation. Avoid any undue force. Take resting periods and breathe calmly.

1. Using very small sideways wriggling movements,

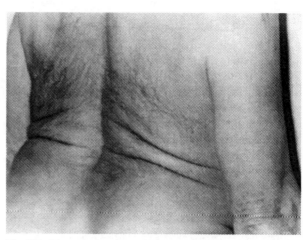

Fig. 531: 46-year-old patient with spondylolisthesis. The slippage of L5 is obvious because of the depression in this area.

the patient 'paints' patterns on the bed while concentrating on the most lordotic area. Patients should try to visualize the disappearance of the lordosis.

2. Knees are carefully pulled up to the stomach. The hands are folded in front of the knees and they pull the knees in this direction while the lumbar spine presses gently against the bed. The coccyx is lifted off the bed a little. Breathing is calm. Avoid undue force (this might happen because of pain).

3. Pull the knees to the chest. They now push against the hands and upwards. The buttocks tighten and the patient tries to lift the lower part slightly off the bed. This may be done on one side or both. There should be resting periods during which the legs are straightened and breathing is calm and natural. Relax!

4. Knees bent; feet on the bed. Wrap a resistance band

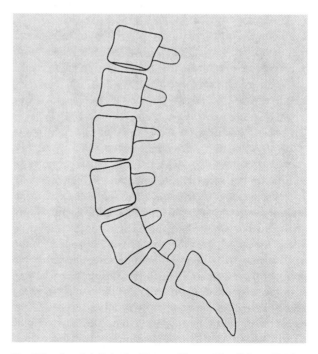

Fig. 532: Spondylolisthesis, 45-year-old man. The sliding of L5 is obvious clinically because of the depression in the lumbar area.

187

around the knees (crossed around the hollows of the knees), and hold both ends tightly. Now push the knees against the resistance while the coccyx is lifted a little off the bed, and the lumbar spine presses against the mattress. Exhale during this procedure while counting to eight. Then relax.

5. Extend the legs carefully. The right foot flexed, the left heel pressing against it. The buttocks are tight, the lumbar spine presses against the bed. Increase the contraction while counting (count to 4, then 8, then 12…). Relax and breathe evenly. Change legs.

6. Extend the legs. Both heels move slowly upwards along the padding, the lumbar spine presses down, and the buttocks and abdomen are tightened. The pelvic muscles are contracted to such an extent that the coccyx lifts off the bed (as far as the pain allows it). Relax. Close the eyes, become aware of the movement; breathe normally.

7. The knees are bent; feet on the bed. Hands are placed on the outside of the thighs. Try to press against this resistance. The coccyx moves upwards again, the lumbar spine against the bed, the stomach tightens. Relax!

8. The legs are bent and slightly lifted. The hands are on the inside of the knees. Apply isometric tension again. The coccyx lifts and the lumbar spine presses against the bed. Then relax.

9. Both legs are extended carefully. The lumbar spine presses against the padding. Lift one leg slightly against imaginary resistance (or against the blanket). Exhale. Switch legs.

10. Legs extended; the outside of the feet press against the bed; the coccyx lifts and the pelvic muscles tighten. Count to eight, lower coccyx. Exhale during contractions. May be repeated.

11. Extended legs, feet flexed. Overstretch the legs and lift up the heels slightly. The feet push away from the body or against resistance. The pelvis tightens. Relax and breathe evenly afterwards.

12. Do exercise 11 on one side and try to relax the other side.

13. Knees bent; feet on the bed. Count to eight while contracting the pelvic musculature and lifting the pelvis a little. Count again to eight while pushing the lumbar spine down. Imagine that the knees are pressing against resistance on the outside. During another count to eight, lower the lumbar spine slowly. Then relax the body slowly.

These are small exercises and do not involve a great deal of movement. They should become important and large in the imagination, however. Doing these exercises in the morning or in the evening before going to sleep will affect the posture positively and take away pain, because the lumbar region is being stabilised and straightened. The stomach flattens and the overall appearance improves. You may verify this in front of a mirror.

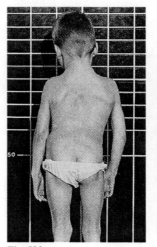
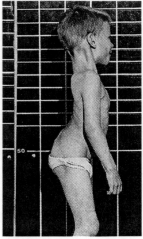

Fig. 533
5 year old boy with a hollow back and congenital scoliosis.

Fig. 534
Hollow back; lateral view; see text for description.

16. The hollow back (lordosis) (Figs. 533 and 534)

In lordosis, the physiological signs are the opposite. Usually patients have lumbar and cervical kyphosis. Sometimes the thoracic lordosis extends all the way to the lumbar spine. In such cases, the sacrum has moved excessively backwards. This leads to a flexion contracture in the hip and knee joints. This calls for stretching the M. iliopsoas, quadriceps and knee joints, and also needs exercises to create kyphosis. In the supine position, the patient puts corrective cushions under the

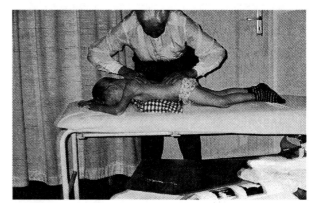

Fig. 535

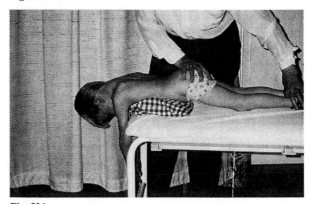

Fig. 536

188

lowest end of the sacrum.

We add the following to the exercises for flatback:

Exercises in the prone position

a) Corrective cushion under the trunk. To guide the breathing towards the back, the therapist gives tactile stimulation by stroking the back along the spine and by softly pulling the shoulder girdle and pelvic girdle apart (Fig. 535).

b) Head, arms and shoulder girdle hang down from the table. The shifted ribs rest on a corrective cushion. The legs are straightened and the therapist fixes the pelvis against the table. The patient ventilates the

widened dorsal area while the therapist gives tactile stimulation (Fig. 536).

Exercises at the wall bars

Standing or kneeling

c) Back to the wall bars. A resistance band is placed around the frontal ribs. The patient tries to put the hands onto the ground while ventilating the hollow region in the back (Fig. 537).

d) Sitting cross legged. The resistance band is pressed forwards; arms extended. This makes room for dorsal breathing (Fig. 538).

e) Standing position, facing the wall bars. The resis-

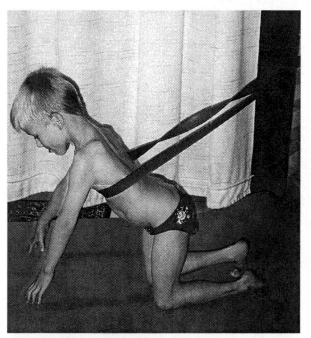

Fig. 537

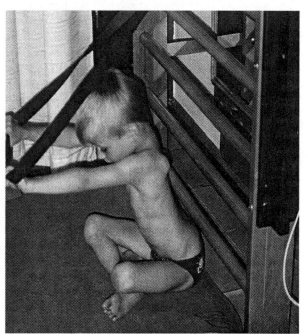

Fig. 538

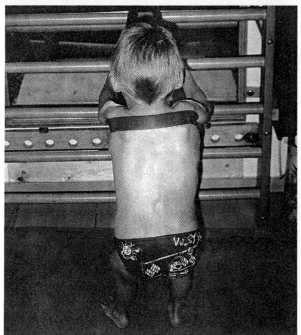

Fig. 539

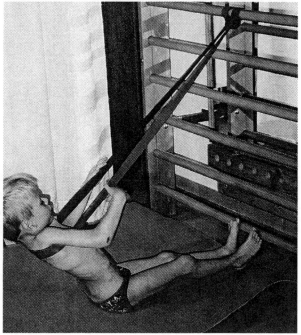

Fig. 540

189

tance band is placed above the dorsal concavity. The patient tries to widen the concavity by breathing. During breathing out, the stomach muscles are tightened and the ribs are drawn in (Fig. 539).

f) Sitting in front of the wall bars. Legs extended. The resistance band as in e). The feet push strongly against the lowest bar. The hands try to reach the wall bars (Fig. 540).

17. Rotational slippage of vertebrae (Figs. 541–546)

The clinical picture is characterised by a weakness of the connective tissue. This usually does not become apparent until adulthood, although young people may be afflicted as well (Fig. 543). In most cases, symptoms appear in the lumbar region, sometimes also in the thoracic spine (Fig. 546). Patients complain of extreme back pain due to the strain on ligaments and muscles, and especially nerves. This usually calls for a surgical solution. Fig. 545 shows that even minor scoliosis of 25° may involve slippage of vertebral bodies combined with rotation between L3 and L4.

When a patient complains of increased back pain while doing the muscle cylinder exercise in kneeling or standing position, the therapist should be very cautious. The pain may be due to rotational vertebral slippage, and treatment must be adapted accordingly. We know from experience that it is impossible to stop this rotatory displacement by manual countermanipulation. Slippage continues, as we have observed on X-rays (see Case A, p. 153). It is necessary to perform the important muscle cylinder exercise only in lateral position, the lumbar hump

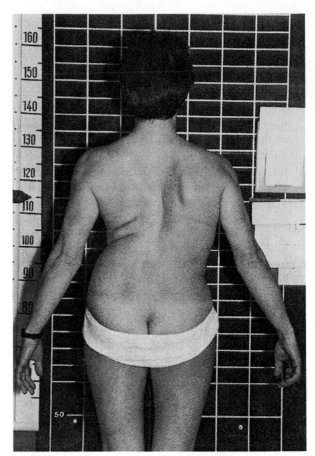

Fig. 541

having first been derotated manually. This applies even if the slippage has been diagnosed by X-ray and the patient has not yet developed pain.

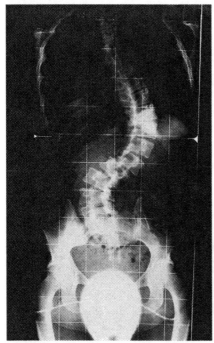

Fig. 542:
40-year-old woman suffering from a painful rotational vertebral slippage between L1 and L3.

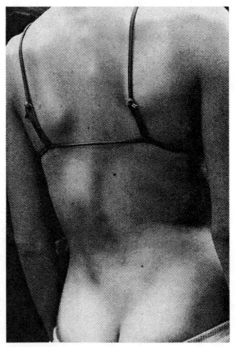

Fig. 543:
15-year-old patient; rotational vertebral slippage in the lumbar region.

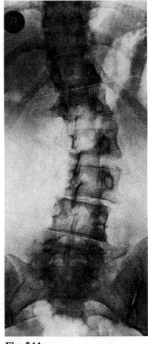

Fig. 544:
X-ray of a 38-year-old patient. Rotational vertebral slippage L3/L4

190

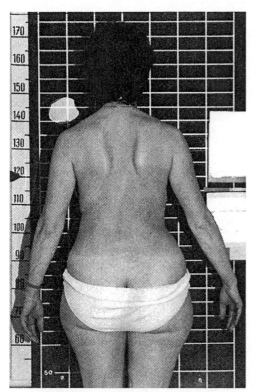

Fig. 545 (left): The same patient as in Fig. 544. Rotational vertebral slippage of L3/L4

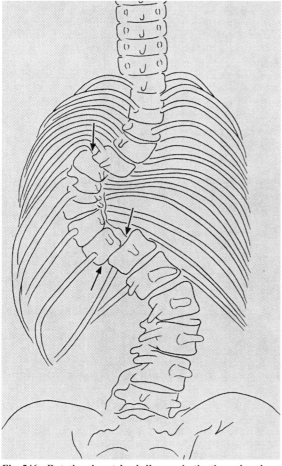

Fig. 546 : Rotational vertebral slippage in the thoracic spine, which is uncommon. T5/6/7 and T 11/12

18. Thoracolumbar scoliosis (Fig. 547)

This type of scoliosis poses a problem since the therapist must decide whether to treat as a three-curve or a four-curve scoliosis with a lumbosacral curvature. One has to experiment with several different approaches: which method achieves the better appearance?

If the curvature extends very high into the thoracic region, to about T9, four pairs of ribs are affected. We then treat as we would a three-curve scoliosis. The patient lies on the concave side and the corrective cushions are placed under the hip and shoulder girdle.

If the curvature extends only up to about T11, we treat it as a curvature of the lumbar region. The patient rests on the lumbar convexity, but only after it has been derotated forward manually (Fig. 369).

Below are positionings and exercise positions in the case of a thoracolumbar scoliosis, here left-convex (Fig. 547). To simplify the explanations, we assume a left-convex case and refer to left and right side rather than convex or concave.

Supine position
a) Cushion under right shoulder along its length.
b) Cushion under left convexity starting at lower angle of scapula.
c) Cushion under right hip to rotate it forwards.
d) Left leg bent and dropping towards the floor – or leg extended and rotated outwards. Omit push of heel (stretching must not extend into the rib hump part).

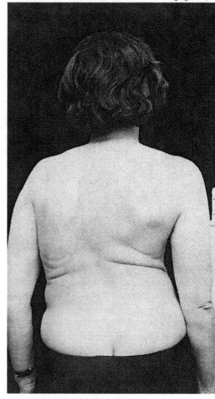

Fig. 547: Thoracolumbar scoliosis with convexity on the left.

Lateral position

a) On the right side, lower leg bent 90°, upper leg on a footstool.
b) Cushion under hip and shoulder girdle.
c) In case of a low thoracolumbar part: patient rests on the left side and treats the curvature as if it were a lumbar hump (cushion underneath); upper leg on a footstool; no active lifting, no pushing with the heel.

Prone position

a) Footstool under the pelvis.
b) A roll under frontal rib arch if necessary.
c) Cushion under left shoulder when hands are under the forehead or on poles.
d) Cushion under right anterior rib hump.
e) Cushion under left hip to rotate it backwards.
f) Both legs straight; left leg may be rotated backwards to bring medial border of foot to the floor.

Sitting cross-legged

a) Both buttocks carry equal weight; when visual evaluation requires it, move weight slightly to the right. No cushion under either side.
b) Left leg bent first to turn the hip backwards.
c) Check knees to see if pelvis is horizontal.
d) Exercise at the wall bars requires visual evaluation. Does it look better if the left leg has a cushion in front? Otherwise omit.

Head position

Lean head to the right; chin points to the left if the cervical curve is large and distorted. If this segment of the spine appears straight, it is usually not distorted. Leave the head in the middle position.

Standing

Weight is on the right leg with simultaneous contraction of right hip towards middle. Trunk leans over to the right without narrowing ribs. Shoulder countertraction on the left.

Exercises to activate the M. iliopsoas to achieve derotation

The following four figures show a person with a high lumbar convexity on the left and a rib hump on the right side. The exercises derotate the lumbar convexity and flatten it (Figs. 548–551).

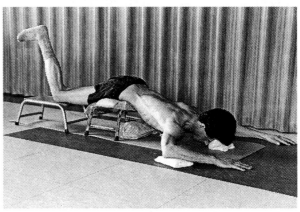

Fig. 550:
Prone position; pelvis on a footstool; corrective cushions. After RAB, the right knee pushes forward against a second footstool. Occipital push.

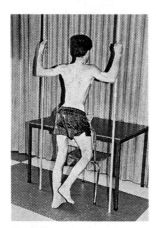

Fig. 548:
Standing in front of a table under which a chair is positioned. Pushing the poles into the ground lifts the trunk out of the pelvis. RAB into the concavities and maintaining the results by pushing the right thigh against the chair forwards and inwards during exhalation. The right hip is kept in by muscle contraction.

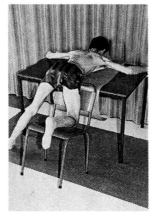

Fig. 549:
The upper body is across a table. The right knee pushes against the back of the chair. RAB into all the sunken trunk segments. During exhalation, the result is stabilized and the hands pull the side of the table towards the body.

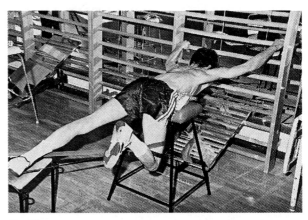

Fig. 551:
Patient lies across a high chair which is kept at a certain distance from the wall bars. The right hand grasps one bar higher (shoulder girdle derotation). The right hip has a cushion underneath. The left foot is extended and rotated outwards and holds the resistance band, which runs around the right knee and thigh. After corrective inhalation, the patient pulls the bar towards himself and at the same time pushes the right knee forwards and inwards.

192

Exercises with a resistance band for thoracolumbar scoliosis or a high lumbar convexity

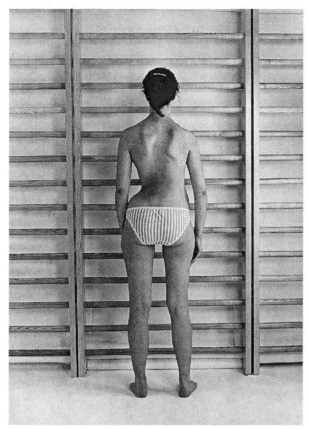

Fig. 552:
The patient shown had Wilms tumour surgery followed by radiation treatment. The left kidney was removed. The scar tissue was very rigid. The left hip is prominent. This appears even more so as the tissue above it is very atrophied. There is also a fourth curve, a lumbosacral curvature to the left. The lumbar hump is very rotated. The patient also has flatback.

The countercurvature in the thoracic region deviates to the left. Schroth calls this a thoracic left scoliosis (rib hump) with a strong thoracolumbar convexity to the right and a lumbosacral fourth curve to the left.

Fig. 553:
The left leg is bent 90°/90°, the knee resting on the third bar. The right leg is straddled and rotated outwards on a bar. The pelvis is horizontal and is derotated and pulled in on the left.
Exercise: The lumbar hump is turned forwards, upwards and inwards. The left concavity is being widened by RAB to the outside and backwards. During exhalation, the bar is pulled down forcefully.

Fig. 554:
Muscle cylinder position. The rubber ball applies counterpressure for the thoracolumbar curvature.
Exercise: After pelvic corrections, the lumbar hump is derotated forwards, upwards and inwards. At the same time, the patient guides breathing into the left concavity. The shoulders are pulled laterally. During exhalation, the entire body musculature is contracted isometrically. The weight of the trunk activates the muscles in the left waist area. We might further stimulate this musculature by moving forwards in small movements.

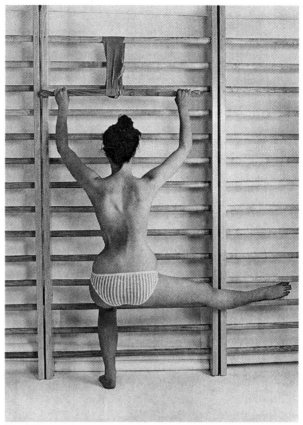

Fig. 553

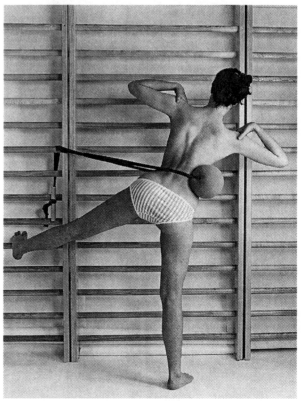

Fig. 554

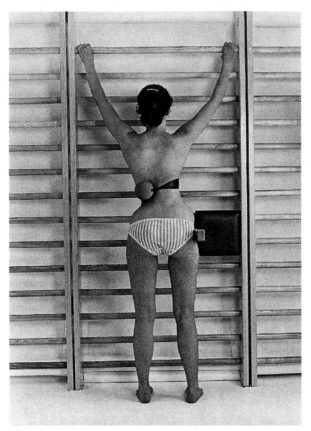

Fig. 555

Fig. 555:
Standing position. Hip bar on the right to support taking in the prominent left hip. The resistance band is fastened to the wall bars and guided around the lumbar hump. The rubber ball is in the concavity to help guide RAB.

Exercise: The fixed point is the right thigh, which has been rotated outwards. The moving point is the pelvis, which is rotated inwards. The left hip is turned backwards to realign the pelvis. This leads to a marked thoracolumbar derotation. The right hip then pushes against the hip bar and the left heel pushes into the ground for horizontal alignment of the pelvis. During exhalation, the patient pulls the upper bar down to activate the lateral erecting musculature.

Fig. 556:
a) A resistance band around the right hip; this acts in the same manner as the hip bar in Fig. 555. Pelvic corrections are the same.
b) A second band is wrapped around the waist with the ball in the concavity. RAB aims to push it away. The band derotates the lumbar hump forwards, upwards and inwards.
c) A third band, fixed above, is pulled outwards and down during exhalation. The elbows pull outwards and upwards. This strengthens the neck-shoulder musculature. Attention! Do not work into the flat back. The thoracic spine should rather become somewhat kyphotic. During the entire exercise the patient should try to overcome the pressure on the right hip, to facilitate awareness of the new postural sensations.

Fig. 557:
A resistance band around the left thigh. Exercise: The left thigh contracts in flexion and adduction after pelvic alignment (activation of the M. psoas). RAB starts at the left concavity. During exhalation, both arms pull the bands outwards and down. The head pushes upwards.

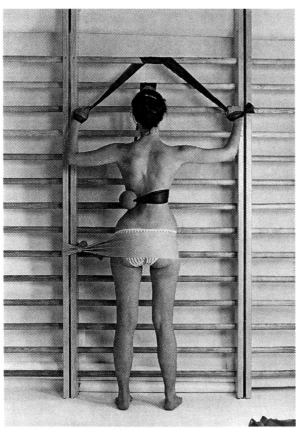

Fig. 556

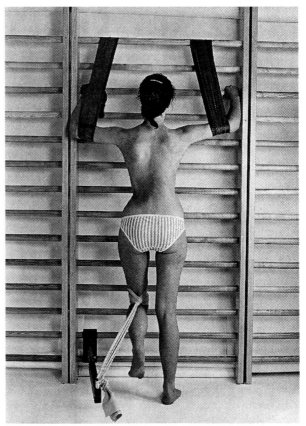

Fig. 557

Fig. 558:
In a sitting position, the right leg is rotated outwards, slightly abducted, flexed 90° at the hip, and placed on a bar. This leads to a movement of the right hip dorsally and cranially. The entire pelvis must be pulled towards the right side. The left hip is corrected backwards, either by a cushion (passively) or actively. Ensure that the pelvis is horizontal. The bodyweight may be shifted towards the left buttock. The band is placed around the lumbar hump and fastened to the wall bars to make it pull towards the left.
Exercise: RAB into the left concavity against the band. Push the poles against the floor while exhaling.

Fig. 559:
Sitting on a chair; both feet against each other on the lowest bar.
a) A band around the right knee. Tense the right knee while abducting and rotating outwards).
b) The second band fixed around the left knee. The knee in flexion and adduction; the knee now pulls in the direction of the right shoulder (activates M. psoas).
c) The third band around the lumbar hump. The ball offers resistance to the left concavity, which should be overcome by RAB. During exhalation, the upper bar is 'pushed together' and pulled down at the same time.

Fig. 560:
Sitting on a ball; hip bar on the right; band around the left knee.
Exercise: The left knee pulls inwards and upwards. At the same time, the upper bar is 'pushed together' and pulled down.
Remark: This patient did not pay attention to the left rib overhang, which has shifted outwards towards the side. It is important to bring the entire segment above the lumbar hump towards the right side. Shoulder countertraction should also be applied on the right.

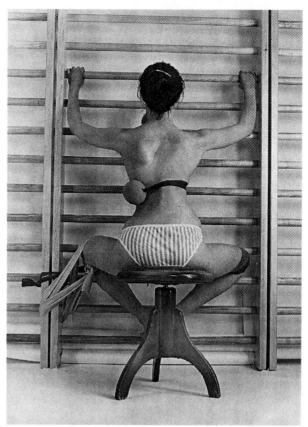

Fig. 559

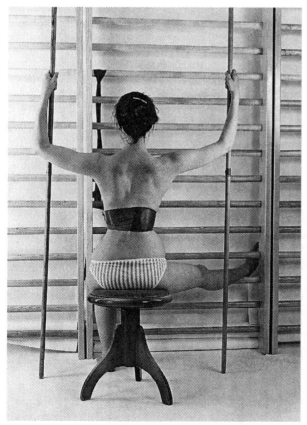

Fig. 558

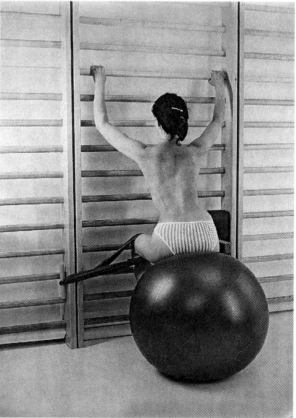

Fig. 560

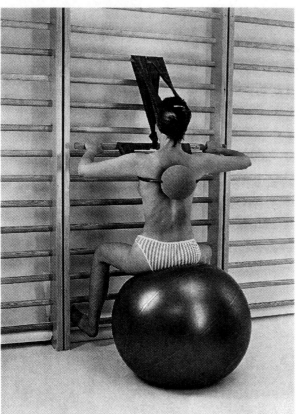

Fig. 561

Fig. 561:
Sitting on a ball; legs spread. A band is placed around the upper trunk and fastened to a pole and the wall bars. The ball is placed in the area of the flat back – here it is between the scapulae. The patient breathes against it. The second band is placed around the back of the head which should push upwards. During exhalation, the horizontal pole is 'pushed together' and pulled down.

Fig. 562:
Lateral position on the side of the lumbar convexity. Cushions are placed under the convexity to align the lumbar spine almost straight in the middle. The patient has derotated the lumbar hump manually beforehand. The upper leg is on a footstool, the lower leg is straight. The heel of the lower leg holds the band, which is placed around the knee of the upper leg. A second band is held by the right hand after it has been placed around the lower part of the upper left arm.
Exercise: RAB and pulling of the right arm. During exhalation, the lower leg pushes against the floor. The right hip should pull behind the corrective cushions. The left knee pushes against the band and the footstool, flexed and adducted. The patient should not move either backwards or forwards. To compensate, the right hip has to pull a little backwards. Derotation of the pelvis around the fronto-transverse axis after maximum derotation of the lumbar spine and pelvis. The goal is the physiological position of the lumbar spine.

Fig. 562

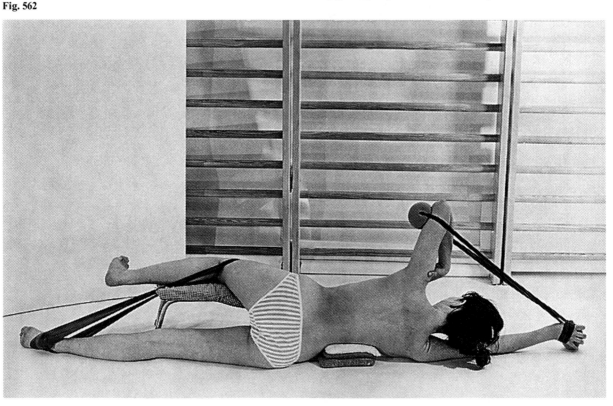

Fig. 563:
Prone position parallel to wall bars; right side towards wall bars; pelvis placed on a roll; left knee on a cushion; knee bent 90°; frontal rib hump (left) corrected backwards by a cushion; band around the left concavity and fastened at the wall bars.

Exercise: Head pushes upwards; RAB against resistance of the band. During breathing out, the corrections are maintained, felt, sensed. Additional push of the left knee (activates M. psoas) to deflex and derotate the thoracolumbar spine. Shoulder countertraction should be applied if necessary. The patient in the picture is performing shoulder countertraction on the left and the right. On the right, the lumbar hump has to derotate forward, upward, and inward against the countertraction. On the left the thoracic curvature also has to be contracted against it, forward, upward, and inward.

Important: The patient has to work against the band during the entire exercise. Afterwards, the band has to be removed immediately.

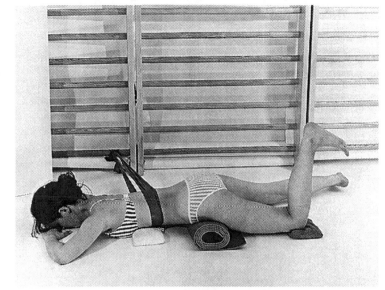

Fig. 564:
Upper trunk and pelvis lie across a table. The pelvis rests on a roll. The left frontal rib hump is corrected by cushions. The hands hold on to a bar. The right foot is on a chair. The right heel holds the band, which has been placed around the left knee.

Exercise: The left knee pulls the band forwards. The left hip is kept back. RAB. During breathing out, the patient pulls the bar towards the body. Elbows are far apart.

Variation: The patient may instead lie on a ball, which can then serve as an additional resistance for the left thigh. Keep the left hip back.

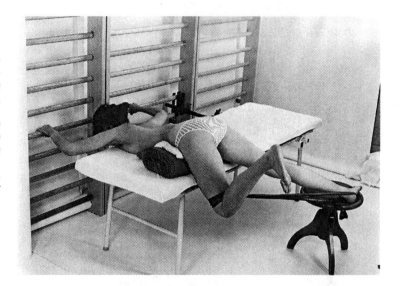

Fig. 565:
A special high chair has been fixed to the wall bars with a spacer. The upper body rests on the chair. A resistance band has been fastened around the stretchers at the base of the chair. This serves as a resistance for the left knee and the ventral thigh. A second band is placed around the lumbar hump on the front of the chair, and is tied to it. There are corrective cushions under the ventral rib hump. The hands hold the bar. The right foot is placed on another chair, straddled, and is rotated outwards.

Exercise: RAB into the left concavity. During breathing out, the instep of the right foot pushes against the chair and the left ventral thigh against the horizontal resistance band. The arms pull the wall bar towards the body.

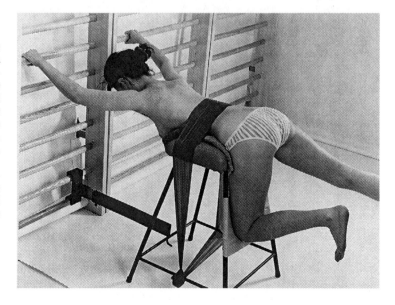

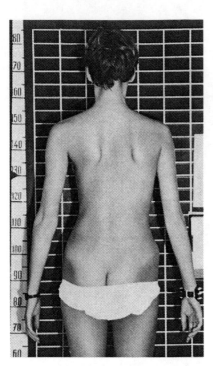

Fig. 566

19. Double curvatures of the lumbar spine (Figs. 566 and 567)

Sometimes the lumbar spine shows two curves. They are very small since they include only 5 or 6 vertebrae, i.e., each of these curves affects only 2 or 3 vertebrae. Clinical observation shows one larger lumbar area. Nevertheless, we have to omit the muscle cylinder exercise because one of the curvatures would be enlarged. Exercises have to be symmetrical in such cases.

20. Cervical kyphosis (Fig. 568)

The cervical spine usually presents only mild lordosis. This is physiological. However, sometimes we do see a cervical spine with a dorsal curvature. It is seldom visible. It does, however, become obvious in X-rays taken in the lateral view.

Patients suffer from headaches of unclear origin. They may be due to the deviation of the cervical spine in the sagittal plane. In such cases, we omit the exercise phase 'neck backwards and upwards' and the occipital push. Instead, we use pushing of the crown of the head. We also omit the head and neck extension exercise (Figs. 282–284, 295) and the 'hanging from the back of the neck' exercise (Figs. 183 and 184).

If headaches develop during neck elongation exercises, this is a warning sign that may indicate cervical kyphosis or a straight cervical spine, or possibly blockage of the neck joints. Treatment must then be altered accordingly. Cervical kyphosis and steep thoracic spine sometimes occur together.

Exercises for cervical kyphosis

Sitting position (on ischial tuberosities)
- Circulating movements with the top of head pointing to the ceiling; upper body upright; switch direction.
- Nose performs "figure-eights"; small at first, then larger. Do not cross the pain threshold.
- Both hands push against forehead while the chin is lifted slightly. Hands give resistance and vice-versa; neck shows a slight lordosis.
- Right ear is pulled upwards while right shoulder pulls down; change sides.
- Semi-circular movements with the forehead; chin slightly upwards; nose pointing to the front. Do not exceed the pain threshold!

Supine position with a small roll under neck
- Both fists next to the shoulders; stretch right arm above head – eyes follow the movement; fist back to starting position. Alternate sides!
- Same movement, but more forceful. Inhalation while straightening the arm; exhalation while pulling it back.

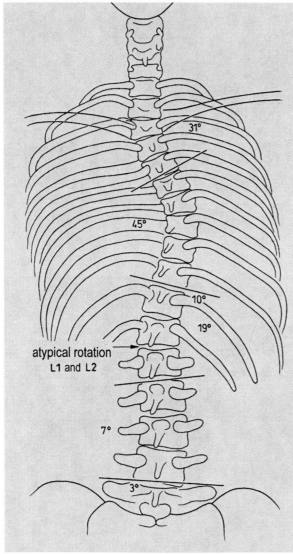

Fig. 567: Atypical rotation of the spinous processes of L1 and L2.

198

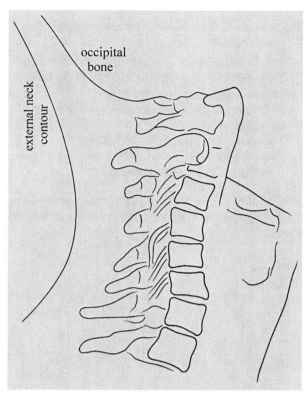

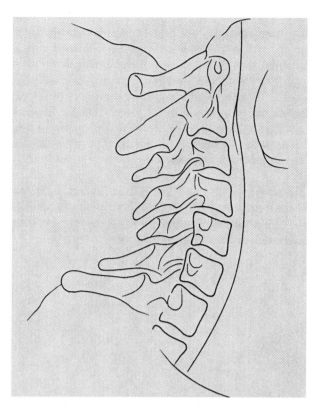

Fig. 568: Cervical kyphosis, lateral view. Labeled curves at top left represent the external contour of the neck and the occipital bone.

Fig. 569: Normal cervical spine. Lateral view.

– Hands folded above forehead; elbows stay on the floor; chin slightly lifted; hands offer resistance to the push of the head.
– The same without resistance; hands folded above the head on the floor; crown of head tries to reach the hands.
– Nose makes small "figure-eights", then larger ones. Do not cross pain threshold.
– One ear pushes upwards, shoulder on the same side downwards; alternate sides. This may also be done intermittently. Sides of neck are stretched.
– Chin lifted slightly; back of head performs circles against the floor. Change directions.
– Chin lifted a little; place fists under the chin. Fists press against chin resistance and vice-versa. Variation: chin presses once against left fist, then against the right one.
– Fingers left and right of cervical spine; massage softly by pushing forwards and upwards; massage each vertebra.

21. Final tensing of the muscle mantle

It is not always true to say that "the journey is the destination". Without starting out on the journey, people will never reach the destination. That's why it is so important to practise the relevant exercises with the correct breathing and to monitor the results in the mirror. Only in this way is it possible to reinforce the **exercise outcome**. Without reinforcement, the exercise remains an unfin-

ished work. That's why it is rounded off with what we call 'Tensing in 12s' or 'Twelve-Count-Tensings'. As they breathe in, patients assume the best possible corrected posture They then hold this result by counting to 4 while breathing out and tensing all the surrounding muscles firmly and hard (lengthening the concave ones, and shortening the convex ones). When they next inhale, they try to improve further on the result. in the following exhalation phase, they again count to 4 (think "re-in-force-ment" = make as hard as rock).
Inhaling for the third time, patients again correct everything, and during the exhalation phase they again tense all surrounding muscles (the Muscle mantle) as they count to 4. After that, the patients should rest and allow the exercise to run through their mind again like a film. Only in this way does the good exercise outcome lead to improved body shape.

Katharina Schroth even went so far as to make her patients tremble with the effort during this exhalatory tension phase.
If the work is done in this manner, success is bound to follow. Patients who are very strong can extend the exercise up to a count of 16 or 20. Those who are less strong may find it enough to stop after the first or second corrective tension step.
However, some patients think, "I've just made such an effort, so now during my leisure time (at mealtimes or watching TV) I'll sit or stand as I please." Those with this attitude are certain to slip back into

their former malposture. And this means that they thereby perform an incorrect exercise that will sadly negate the good corrective outcome. The end result is then just as if they hadn't exercised at all, and the time has been wasted. But in the end of our exercises it should become part of the very fibre of their being, so that the patients aren't even tempted to think about letting themselves slouch again deliberately. If they are tired, it's better for them to lie down and relax.

To investigate whether this method of exercising might be too strenuous, patients' pulse rates were measured in our Clinic before and after these exercises. In every case the result was beneficial (see Section D.II.8).

22. Diagnosis of cases of externally invisible minimal scoliosis

a) Patient in supine position, legs bent, feet on the floor. Therapist holds patient's knees. The patient pushes the knees sideways or inwards isometrically. If it is easier to press inwards, the thoracic curve runs in the opposite direction.
b) The same, but both knees are pulled towards the chest. If it is easier to press inwards, the thoracic curve runs in the opposite direction.

The therapist can choose the appropriate exercise and variation for patients from the various exercises offered above.

IX. Therapy aids to support corrections

(See Figures 570 - 597)

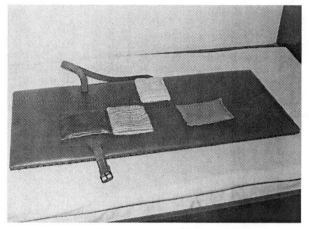

Fig. 570:
Board for resting with corrective cushions. 50 x 100 cm. A belt is attached at the height of the pelvis to fixate the latter. This prevents it from turning during sleep. Arrangement for three curves.

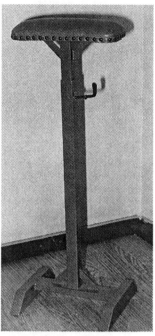

Fig. 572:
Support for the forearm for patients with a severely depressed concave side. To be used during meals, while watching TV, etc.

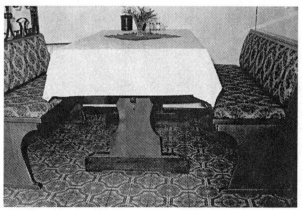

Fig. 571:
Wooden blocks to raise tables. They are easy to put on and take off, and assist in sitting upright during meals.

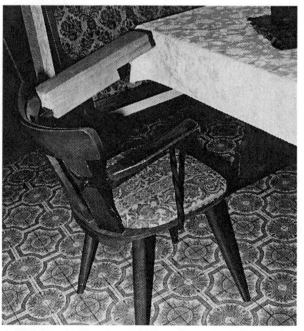

Fig. 573:
Supportive device for the forearm to be slipped on the arm of the chair.

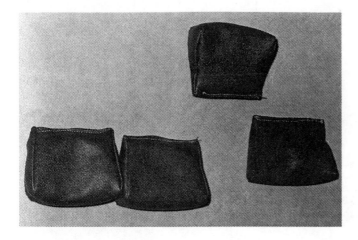

Figs. 574 and 575:
Corrective cushions to be used as passive aids. Some of them are small bags filled with 200 g of rice. Some are wedge-shaped cushions to be used on the board, mat or in bed to derotate the hip or lumbar hump. Arrangement for three curves.

Fig. 575: Sewing directions for a wedge-shaped cushion.
Make a paper pattern first!
Material: The lining is cotton and the cover is coloured material that can be washed easily.
Filling: Rice or grain

1. Cut the cotton lining as shown in the picture.
2. Cut the cover 1 cm larger.
3. Draw the broken lines onto the material.
4. Use zigzag on the edges.
5. Sew the broken lines (about 2 or 3 cm from the fold).
6. Close the sides.
7. Leave an opening on the inside. Turn inside out.
8. Take a piece of paper and form a funnel to fill the inner cushion.
9. Close the opening well.
10. The outside case is made in the same way, but leave a wide side open and use any way of closing (buttons etc).

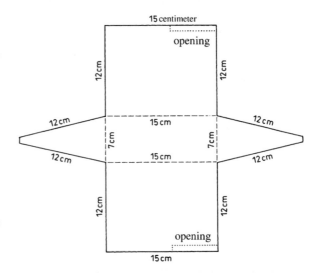

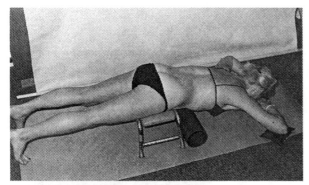

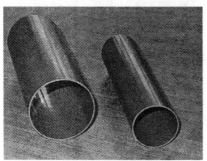

Fig. 576

Fig. 577

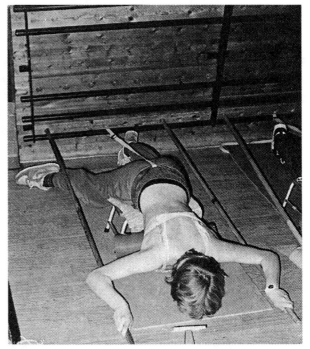

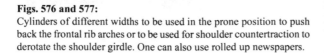

Figs. 576 and 577:
Cylinders of different widths to be used in the prone position to push back the frontal rib arches or to be used for shoulder countertraction to derotate the shoulder girdle. One can also use rolled up newspapers.

Fig. 578:
Belt and strap to fix the pelvis at a certain length to the wall bars. The poles are about 2 meters long. They are helpful to 'lift' the upper trunk from the pelvis and to stabilize exercises when all muscles are tensed at the end to form a muscle mantle.

Fig. 579 (a and b):
Door-bar as a substitute for the wall bars. It can be fixed by a guide rope (gag) under the door.

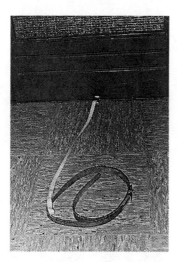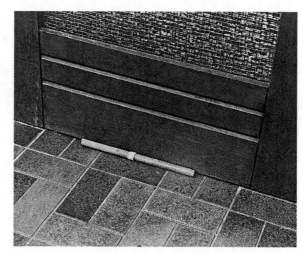

Figs. 580 and 581 (below left and right):
A device to broaden the back of the chair. It is needed in exercises which are supposed to broaden the upper trunk. The pole across the seat widens the seat. The footstool gives support for the first and second pelvic correction.

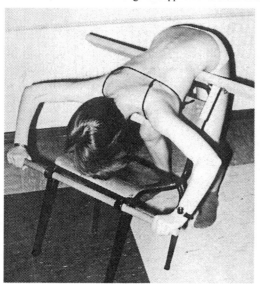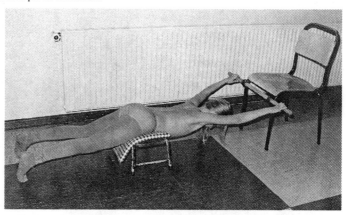

Fig. 580 :
The back of the chair holds a device to broaden it. There are two iron rings through which a pole can be threaded and then held by the patient.

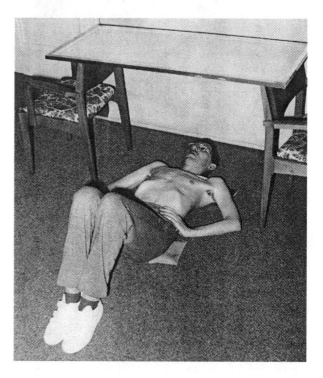

Fig. 582:
A light mirror is placed across two chairs. The patient can observe the corrections. This special mirror can be used everywhere in almost any position.

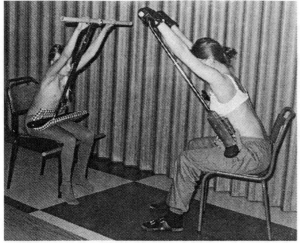

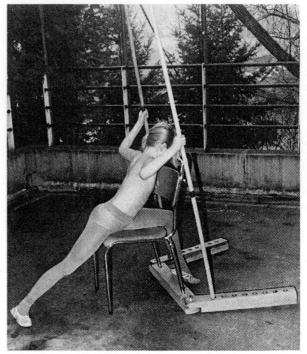

Fig. 583:
"Bandscho", a device to exercise against flatback. Place a thick cushion between the device and the patient's frontal rib arches. A bar on top allows a wider grip. The hollow part of the back is arched backward through RAB.

Fig. 584:
Wooden board with holes. The legs of the chair and the poles are fixed so they do not slip during exercise (here the 'rotational sitting' exercise).

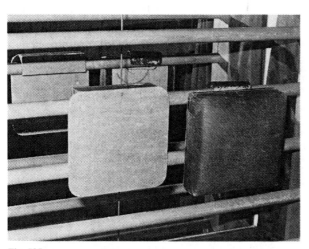

Fig. 585:
This small board is used at the wall bars behind the head to keep it from being pushed against the wall bars (see Figs.212 and 337). These boards may also be used as an aid in the hip bar exercise and – if padded – as a derotational device for the hips and shoulder girdle.

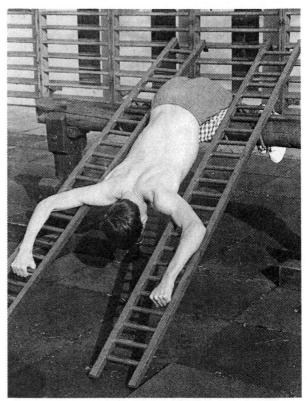

Fig. 586:
The mini double wall bars are put in an oblique position. These are used to elongate the sides of the trunk and the spine. The patient has the chest between the wall bars and the head downwards. He pushes the elbows out sideways and pulls while breathing out. Complete tension of all muscles involved at the end to from a muscle mantle. RAB.

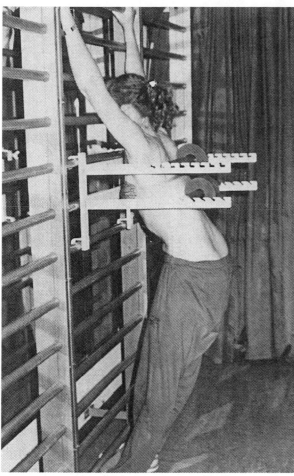

Fig. 587:
The 'Flexomat' is used during exercises against lordosis or flatback. The patient guides RAB against the cushions in the concavities. It may also be used at the convexities to induce contraction.

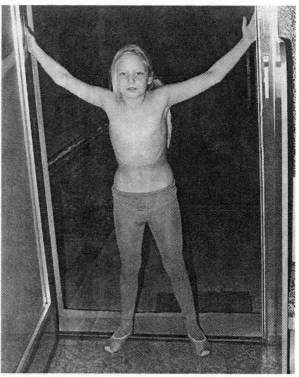

Fig. 590:
The door frame may be used as an exercise aid: to stretch the pectoral musculature during RAB with closing isometric tightening of the arms against the frame.

Figs. 588 and 589 (below and right):
Spacer to be used against stiff kyphotic backs and to stretch the pectoral musculature. The patient has to lift the pelvic rim. Do not use for flatback or lumbar kyphosis.

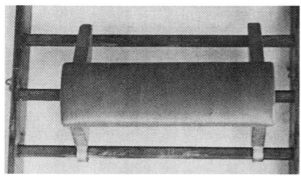

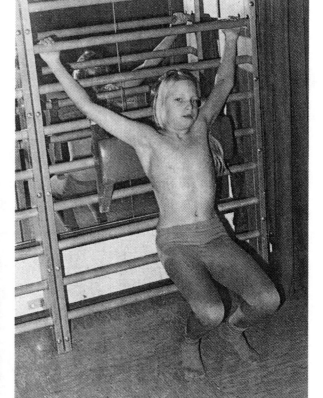

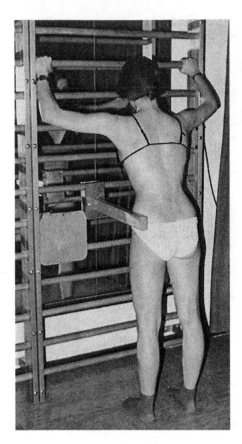

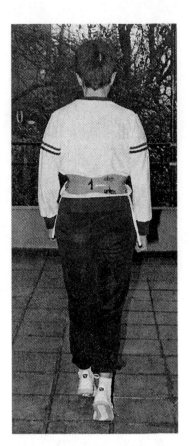

Fig. 591 (left):
"Hip bar", to be adjusted at the wall bars. A counterhold used to correct the protruding hip in four-curve scoliosis. The small board stops the device from sliding. Also for exercises where the head needs to be pushed against the wall bars.

Fig. 592 (right):
"Trunk lifter", the patient walks with this belt in front of a mirror, the hands pushing downwards, and becoming aware of the lifting and elongation of the trunk.

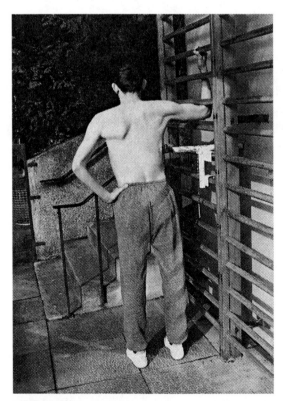

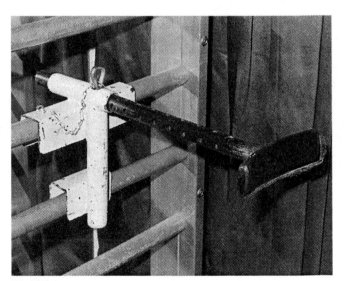

Fig. 594

Figs. 593 and 594:
Spacer to maintain a certain distance from the wall bars during strengthening exercises. Using it prevents the rib hump from shifting laterally.

Fig. 593:
This picture shows clearly that the shoulder on the thoracic concave side has to be moved forwards – otherwise the concavity cannot be filled out.

Fig. 595:
The bench may be used to stretch the pectoral muscles and to contract the convexity. Omit this exercise for flatback or lumbar kyphosis.

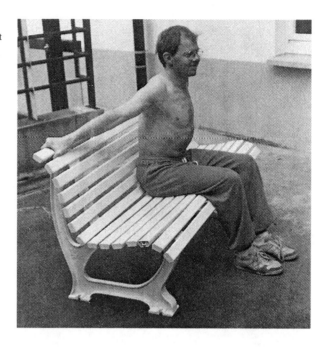

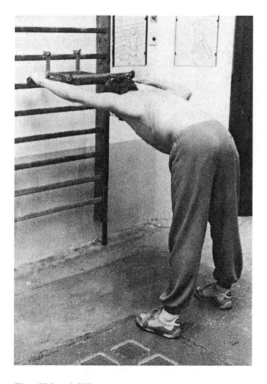

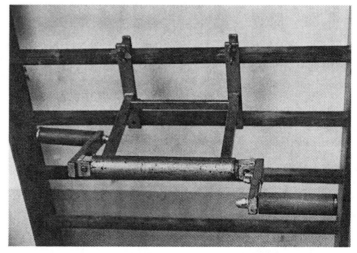

Figs. 596 and 597:
The crank is used in case of a very stiff back (Scheuermann's disease) to mobilize the upper spine and the shoulder girdle. Direction of movement: backwards to bring the scapulae against the rib cage.

PART D
Documentation

The "Island" (Figs. 598–600)

In postural collapse and Scheuermann's disease with the tendency for scoliotic deviations of the spinal column, besides the endangered section of the spine, we often find a depression of M. erector trunci near the spine, caused by muscular insufficiency. The short row of spinous processes in the middle of the spine appears like an island between two rivers. A spinal column can have more than one of these 'islands'. We see this as a sign of the body developing an abnormal posture. We do, however, sometimes see such islands during exercises to treat scoliosis and this is a sign for us that this scoliosis is retrogressive. All three photos show the 'island'.

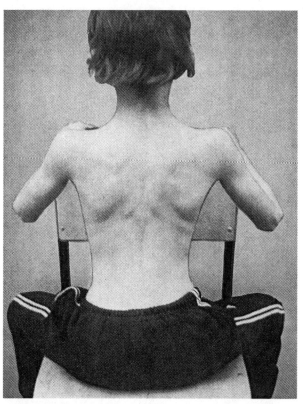

Fig. 599: 10-year-old patient.

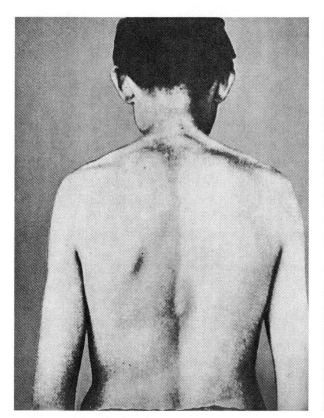

Fig. 598: 16-year-old patient.

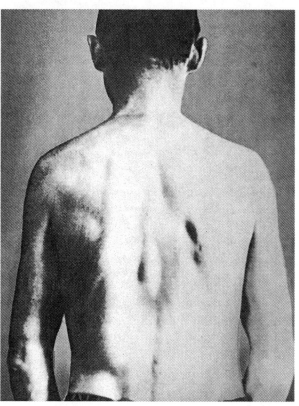

Fig. 600: 57-year-old man.

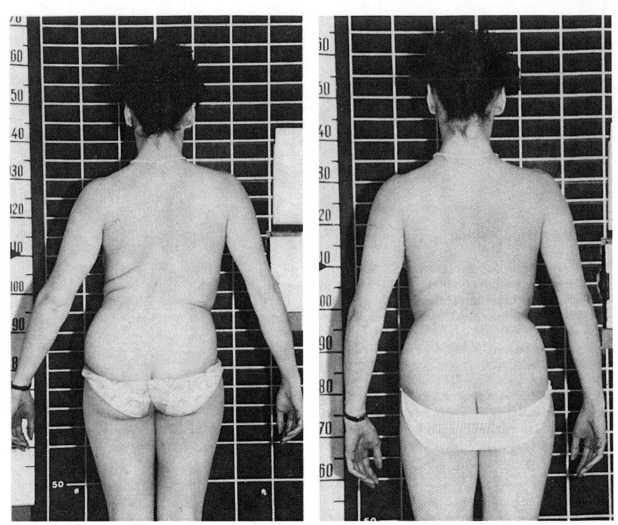

Fig. 601

Fig. 602

Figs. 601 and 602:
29-year-old patient with idiopathic scoliosis at the beginning (Fig. 601) and end of a 4 week course of in-patient treatment (Fig. 602).

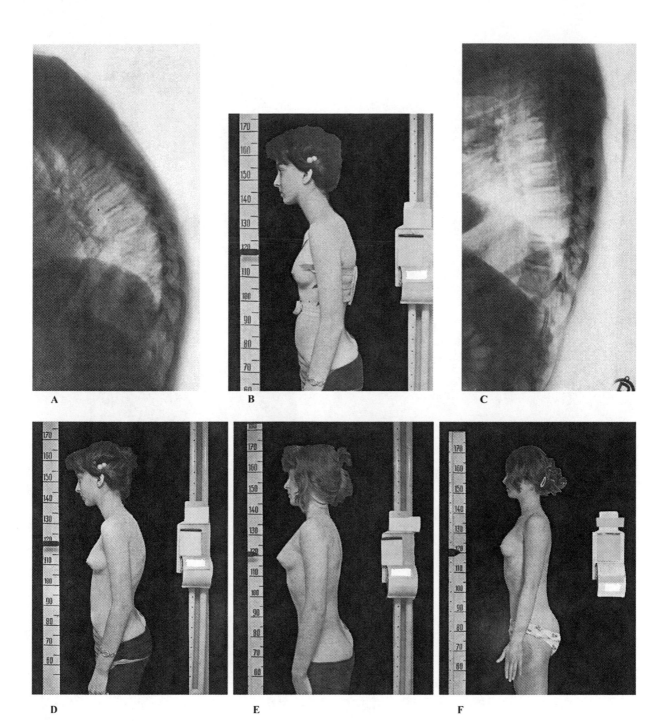

Fig. 603 (A-F):

Fig. 603 A: X-ray of a 13-year-old girl with Scheuermann's disease.
Fig. 603 B and D: The same girl with a brace at the beginning of in-patient treatment; age 13 years, 1 month.
Fig. 603 C and E: The same girl 4 months later following 6 weeks of in-patient treatment.
Fig. 603 F: The same girl, 16 years and 4 months old, after two more courses of treatment of 4 and 3 weeks duration.

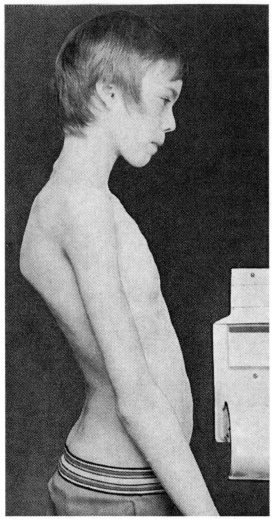 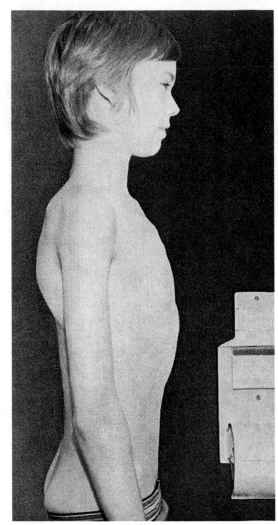

Fig. 604:
12-year-old girl with Scheuermann's disease.

Fig. 605:
After 5 weeks of Schroth treatment.

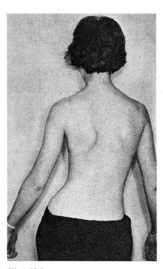 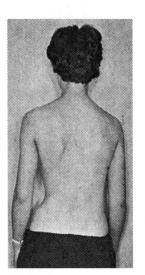 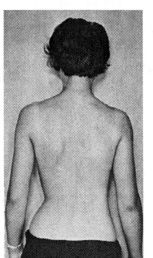 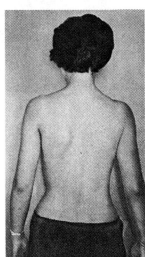

Fig. 606 a   **Fig. 606 b**   **Fig. 606 c**   **Fig. 606 d**

Fig. 606 (a-g): A 14-year-old girl with idiopathic scoliosis.

Figs. 606 b, c and d: The girl during her first 2-month course of in-patient treatment. The X-ray does not clearly show the straightening of the spine. Reduction from 30° to 15°.

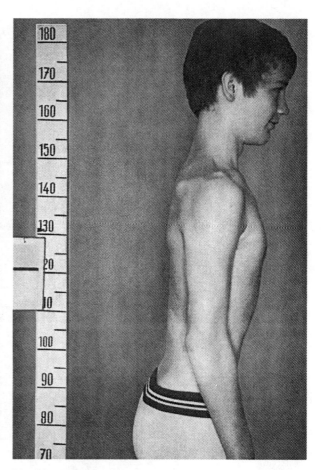

Fig. 607:
17-year-old patient with Scheuermann's disease and asymmetry of the chest.

Fig. 608:
After 5 weeks of Schroth treatment: the chest has evened out.

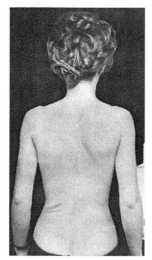

Fig. 606 e

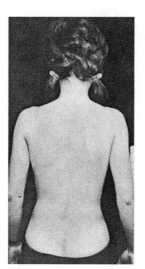

Fig. 606 f

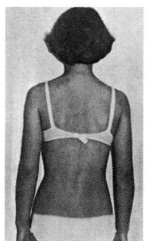

Fig. 606 g

Fig. 606 (continued):

e) The same girl, two years later after another two months of treatment.

f) Seven years later, the same girl, 23 years old.

g) A picture sent from home. She did not need any further in-patient treatment, since she kept on exercising at home while at the university.

215

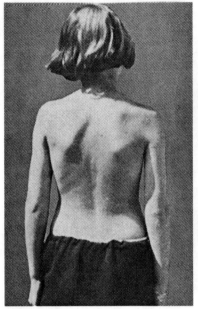

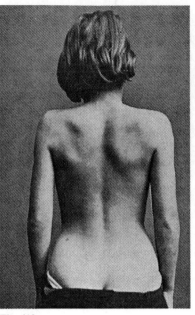

Fig. 609
10-year-old girl with at onset of left dorsal scoliosis.

Fig. 609

Fig. 610

Fig. 610
After eight weeks of Schroth treatment. It is obvious that it is very important to treat incipient scoliosis, i.e., a scoliotic malposture, immediately, before there are structural changes. Early treatment may make further in-patient courses of treatment unnecessary. It is never too early for treatment. This girl did not have to come back to the clinic. We saw the patient again at the age of 18 years, and she had maintained her normal, straight posture.

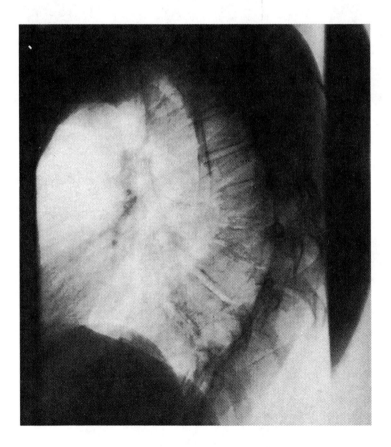

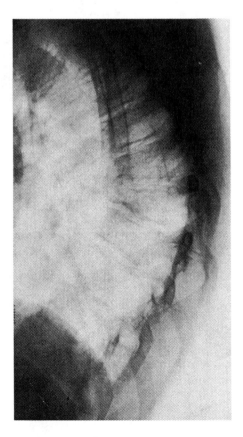

Fig. 611:
X-ray of a 17-year-old boy with Scheuermann's disease. The 7th thoracic vertebral body is severely deformed due to a fall from a tree as a child. The adjacent intervertebral discs are compressed.

Fig. 612:
Same patient, almost 20 years old, after 6 weeks of intensive in-patient treatment. The injured area is straightening slowly. The intervertebral discs have filled out. The deformed vertebra is starting to normalize. The kyphosis seems to have straightened. Improved upper and lower surfaces. This appears to verify the theory that a bone adapts to every change in pressure and traction applied to it. The Schroth method applies muscular pressure and traction differently.

216

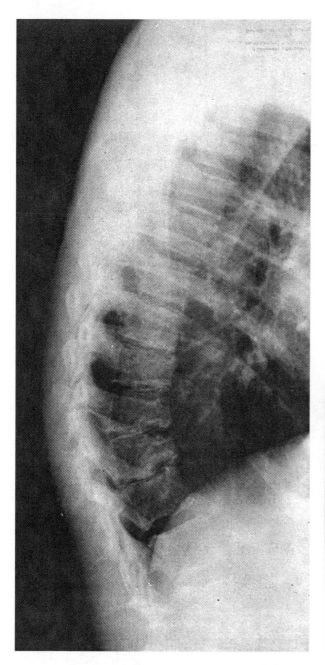

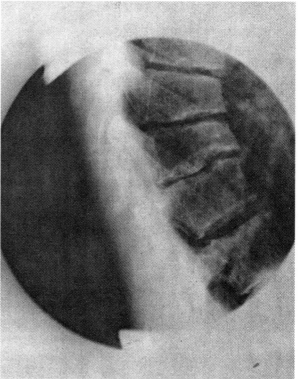

Fig. 613
17½-year-old patient with extremely severe Scheuermann's disease with fixed kyphosis. Very irregular base and surfaces on the vertebral bodies.

Fig. 614
The same patient 1½ years later after a 6-week course of Schroth inpatient treatment and continued exercise by himself at home. The X-ray shows a clearer baseline and surfaces and that the vertebrae on the ventral side are starting to rebuild.

217

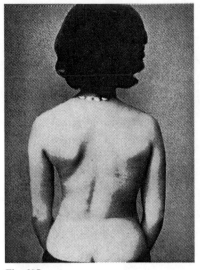 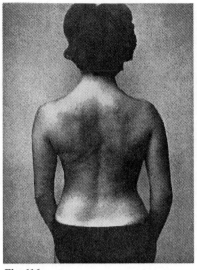 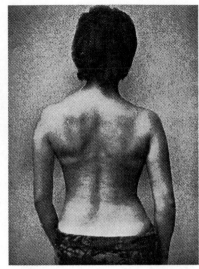

Fig. 615:
16-year-old girl with idiopathic scoliosis.

Fig. 616:
After 3 months of Schroth treatment.

Fig. 617:
After 5 months of Schroth treatment.

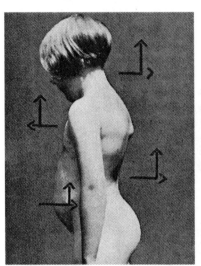 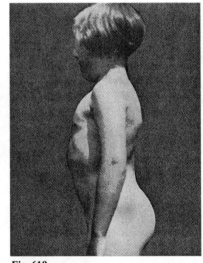 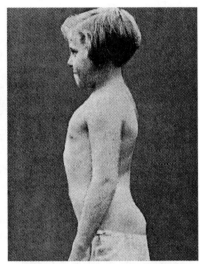

Fig. 618

Fig. 619

Fig. 620

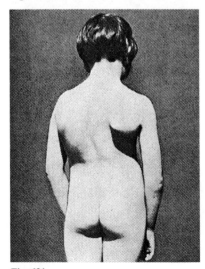 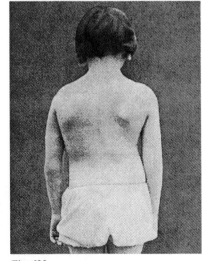 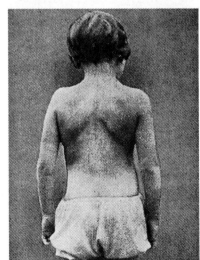

Fig. 621

Fig. 622

Fig. 623

Figs. 618 and 621:
9-year-old girl with left convex scoliosis.

Figs. 619 and 622:
After 6 weeks of Schroth treatment.

Figs. 620 and 623:
After 13 weeks of Schroth treatment.

218

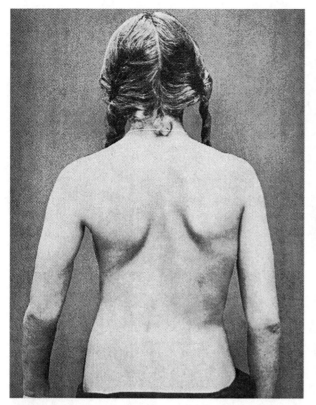

Fig. 624

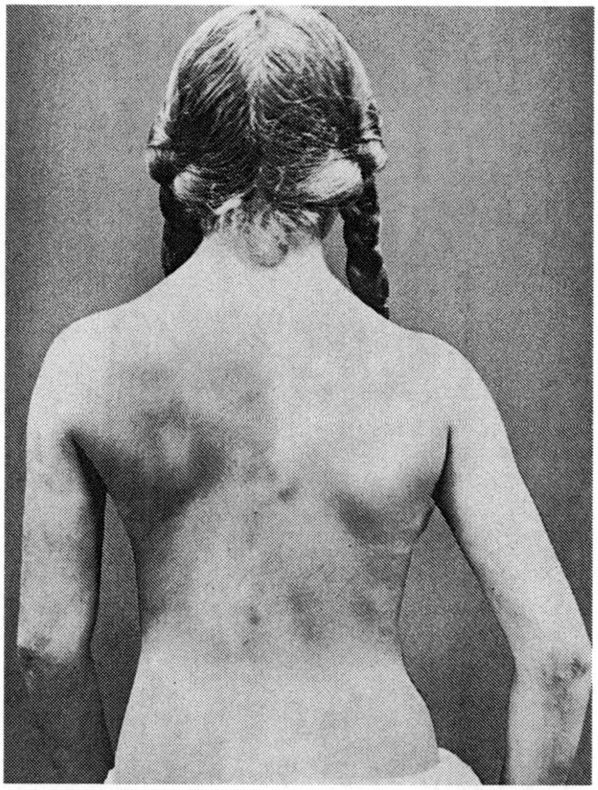

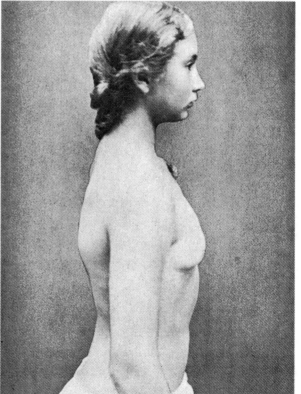

Fig. 625

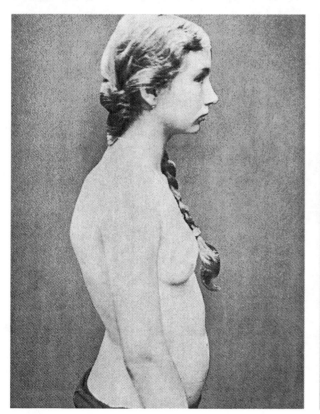

Fig. 626

Fig. 627

Figs. 624 and 626:
17-year-old girl with idiopathic scoliosis

Figs. 625 and 627:
The same girl after 8 weeks of Schroth treatment.

219

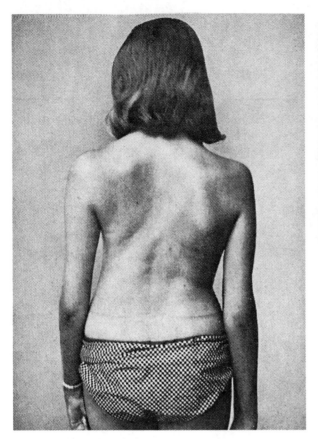

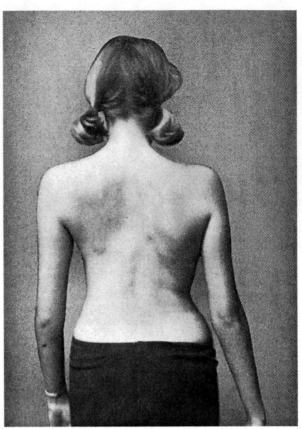

Fig. 628: Idiopathic scoliosis.   **Fig. 629: The same girl after 8 weeks of Schroth treatment.**

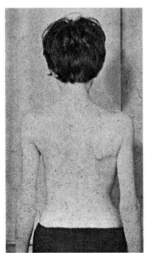 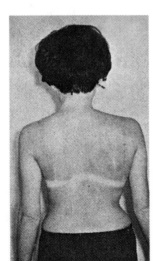 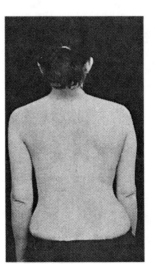 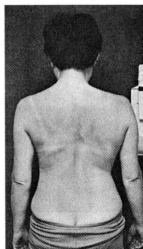

Fig. 630 a   **Fig. 630 b**   **Fig. 630 c**   **Fig. 630 d**

Fig. 630

630 a: 19 years, 4 months old with idiopathic scoliosis, at start of treatment.
630 b: 21 years, 10 months old, after two courses of in-patient treatment of 3½ weeks each.
630 c: 23 years, 5 months old. Patient had two weeks of in-patient treatment and continued exercising on her own.
630 d: 29 years, 7 months old. Exercises at home and a 6-week in-patient course of treatment.

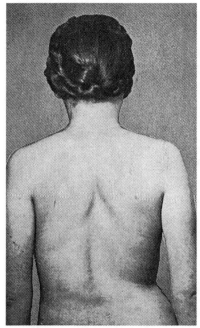
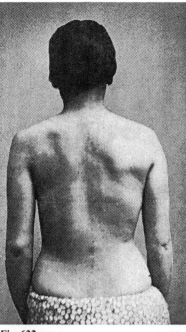
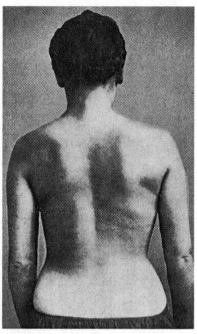

Fig. 631:
16-year-old girl with thoracolumbar scolio-sis, left. Protruding hip on the right.

Fig. 632:
The same girl after 6 weeks of Schroth treatment.

Fig. 633:
The same girl, the following year at the beginning of a course of in-patient treat-ment. She had been able to maintain the corrected posture.

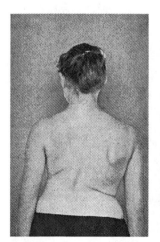
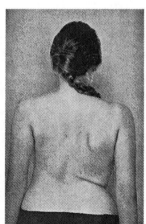
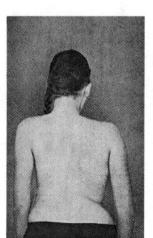
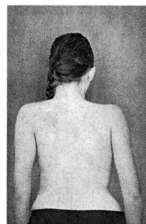

Fig. 634 a **Fig. 634 b** **Fig. 634 c** **Fig. 634 d**

Fig. 634

634 a: 14-year-old girl with idiopathic scoliosis.
634 b: The same girl after 3 weeks of Schroth treatment.
634 c: After another four-week course of in-patient treatment the following year.
634 d: After yet another-four week course of in-patient treatment the year after that.

221

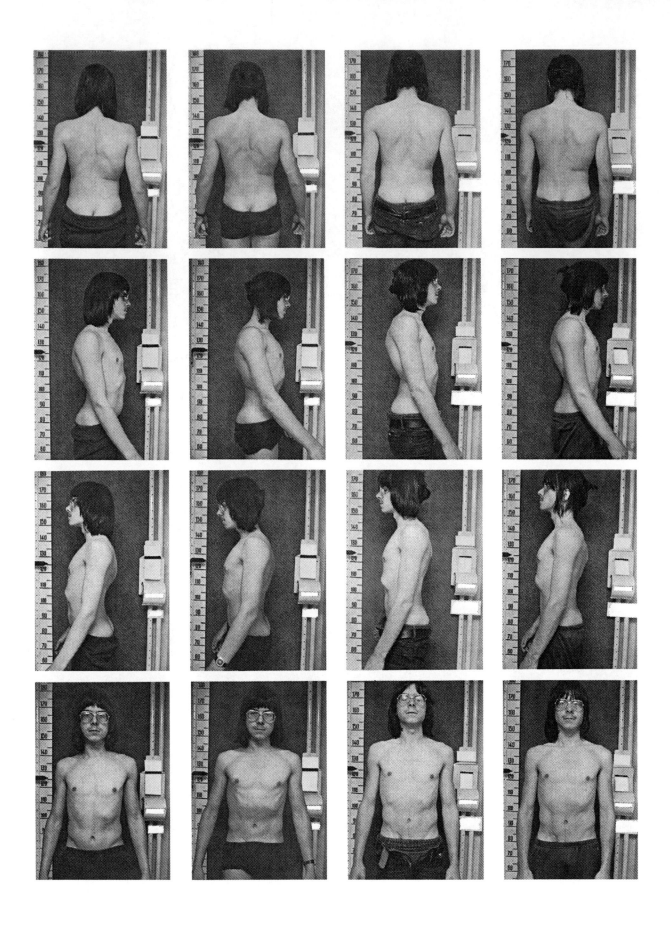

Fig. 635, Set A **Fig. 635, Set B** **Fig. 635, Set C** **Fig. 635, Set D**

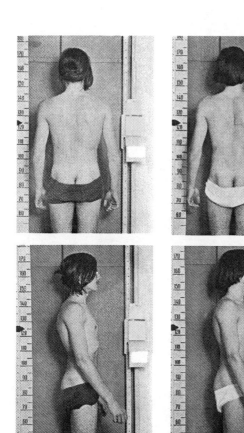
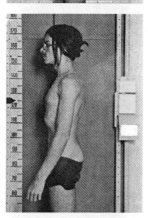
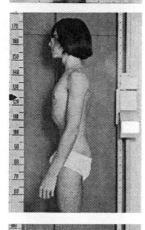
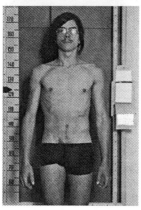
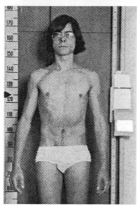

Fig. 635

Set A: 16-year-old patient at the beginning of a course of treatment. Marked postural collapse. Scoliosis. 1.67 m tall. VC of 3700 cc.

Set B: After three weeks of intensive Schroth treatment, correction has begun. 1.68 m tall. VC 4200 cc.

Set C: One year later. Beginning of the second course of in-patient treatment. He had continued the same exercises at home. 1.68.5 m tall. VC 4100 cc.

Set D: After 4 weeks of treatment, a slight improvement in posture is visible. 1.69.5 m tall. VC 4600 cc.

Set E: One year later. This intelligent patient knew that he had to be individually responsible and continue exercises at home. The result was a further improvement at home. The back seems slimmer; the body contours more normal. 1.69 m tall; VC 4400 cc.

Set F: After 3½ weeks intensive in-patient treatment, he further improved in shape and posture. The rib arches are better aligned, the lordosis has mostly evened out. Compared to set A, the rib hump has flattened significantly. 1.69.5 m tall; VC 4600 cc.

During their stay at the clinic, patients are motivated to continue the exercises at home as correctly as possible. This patient was so encouraged by the Schroth method that in addition to the first in-patient course of treatment financed by insurance, he returned for two more self-paid follow-up treatments, In all, he came for three courses in two years, which of course had a decisive effect on his improvement.

Fig. 635, Set E   **Fig. 635, Set F**

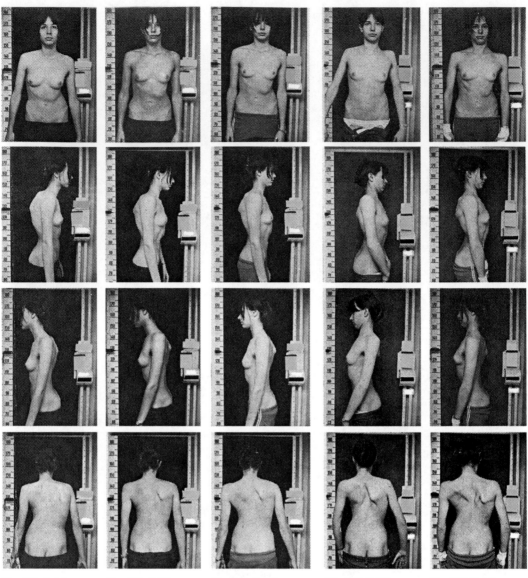

Fig. 636, Set A   **Fig. 636, Set B**   **Fig. 636, Set C**   **Fig. 636, Set D**   **Fig. 636, Set E**

Fig. 636

Set A: 15-year-old girl with severe idiopathic scoliosis and postural collapse. There are no X-rays.

Set B and C: 4 weeks of intensive Schroth treatment as an alternative to surgery. During this time, the anterior rib cage widened and was lifted from the pelvis, which made the uneven rib arches more obvious. The bodyweight rested on the right leg but was shifted over. Thus, the horizontal pelvic correction led to a correction of her postural collapse. Her shoulders were not yet properly aligned.

Set D: Second course of treatment, one year later, 15½ years old. Unassisted exercising at home resulted in a partial loss of the pelvic correction, but an improvement in shoulder alignment.

Set E: After 3 weeks of intensive in-patient treatment, muscle packets are now clearly visible on the concave-side (left) ribs. The faulty balance has been corrected again.

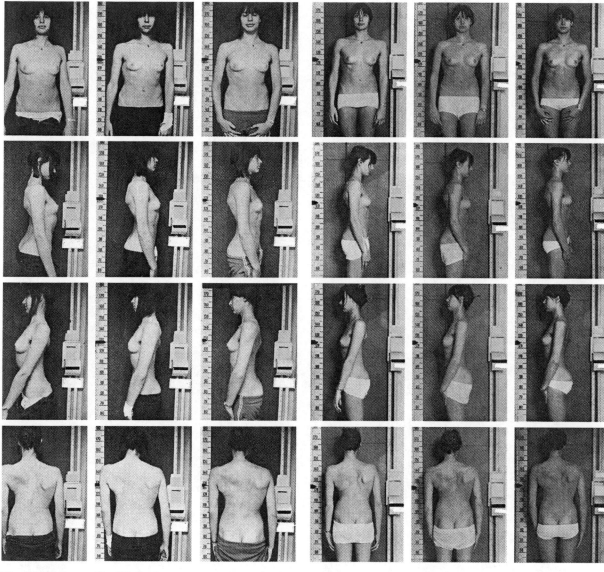

| Fig. 636, Set F | Fig. 636, Set G | Fig. 636, Set H | Fig. 636, Set I | Fig. 636, Set K | Fig. 636, Set L |

Fig. 636 (continued)

Set F: Third course, 16½ years old. Once again, exercising on her own resulted in pelvic distortion, but the shoulders are horizontal.

Set G: After two weeks, there was a marked widening on the concave side. The patient had also gained more postural awareness. The pelvis has been derotated again.

Set H: After the 4th week, the forward rib hump is aligned and upright posture is stabilised.

Set I: Fourth course of in-patient treatment, 17½ years old. Exercising at home brought very good results: upright posture and marked flattening of the dorsal convexity.

Set K: After two weeks, a further improvement: shoulders aligned; a strong M. trapezius.

Set L: After 4 weeks, stabilization of a more appealing frontal view (90° Cobb). Retrospectively, the patient was happy about her decision not to have surgery, since she would have been hospitalised for more than a year. She was proud of her success. She had four courses of in-patient treatment and exercised for one hour daily and was satisfied with the Schroth method. She felt that her efforts had been rewarded, and recognised the overall improvement in her body and appearance, even though the curvature stagnated (still 90°).

This patient's case shows clearly the success and importance of Schroth treatment for scoliosis, especially during the growth period and up to the end of growth. Naturally, for treatment to be efficient, the patient has to show a great deal of self control. Precisely this self control is essential, both for the physical as well as the patient's psychological aspect.

225

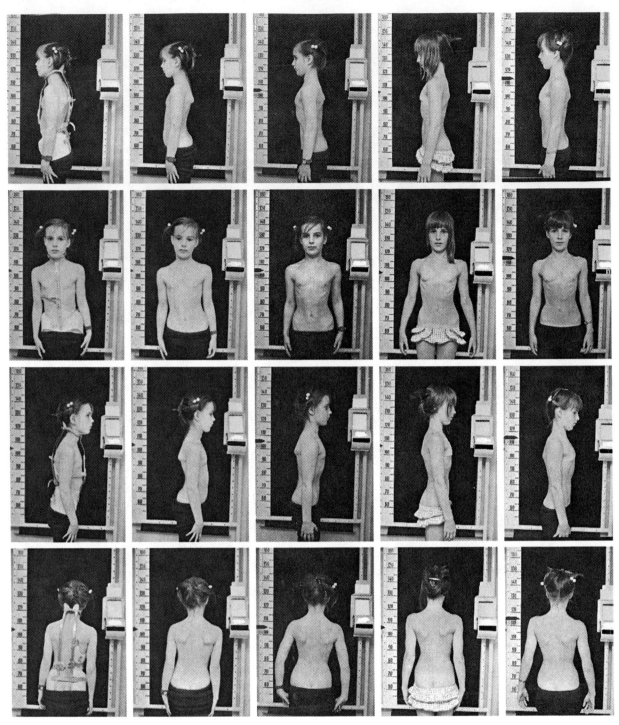

Fig. 637, Set A   Fig. 637, Set B   Fig. 637, Set C   Fig. 637, Set D   Fig. 637, Set E

Fig. 637

Set A: Patient 10 years, 4 months old, wearing a Milwaukee brace.

Set B: Start of treatment.

Set C: End of the first four-week course of in-patient treatment. Improvement in posture. Correction of body statics.

Set D: 11 years, 9 months old, beginning of the 2nd course of in-patient treatment. The results of the first treatment had been maintained.

Set E: After the 3-week course of Schroth treatment. Strengthening of the erecting muscle groups.

226

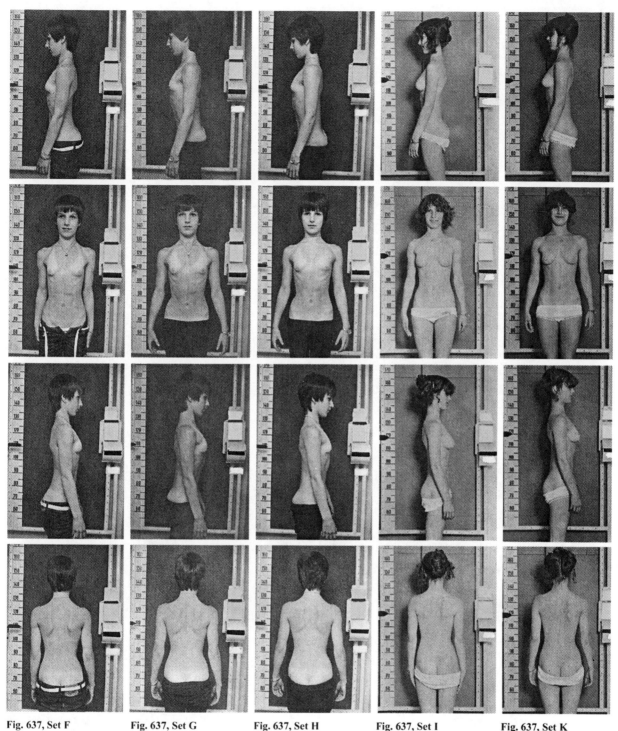

Fig. 637, Set F   **Fig. 637, Set G**   **Fig. 637, Set H**   **Fig. 637, Set I**   **Fig. 637, Set K**

Fig. 637 (continued)

Set F: 12 years, 8 months old. Start of the third course of in-patient treatment (6 weeks).

Set G: Corrected posture after 4 weeks.

Set H: End of this course of in-patient treatment. Corrections are stabilized.

Set I: 14 years, 7 months old. After an interval of 2 years, a slight loss of correction.

Set K: After 6 weeks of intensive treatment, the correction has been restored.

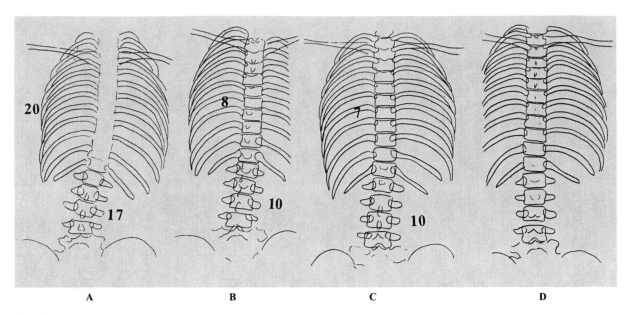

A   B   C   D

Fig. 638

A: The 10-year-old girl from Fig. 637; 6 months before treatment. Milwaukee brace. 20° and 17° curves.

B: 10 years, 5 months old, after a 4-week course of intensive treatment. 8° and 10° curves.

C: 11 years, 10 months old, after a further 3-week course; 7° and 10° curves. She is still wearing the Milwaukee brace.

D: 12 years, 10 months old. After a further 6-week course of treatment. See the previous series of pictures of this patient (Fig. 637). The original X-rays were indistinct and thus could not be reproduced.

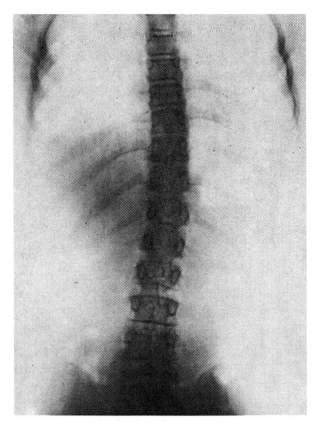

Fig. 639:
Girl, 15 years, with idiopathic scoliosis.

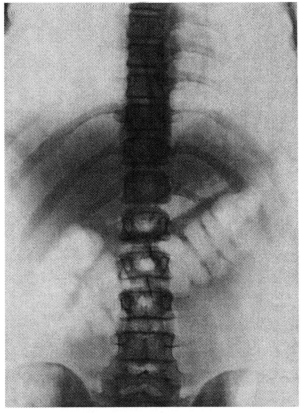

Fig. 640:
After 1 year of out-patient Schroth exercises with the help of a physical therapist..

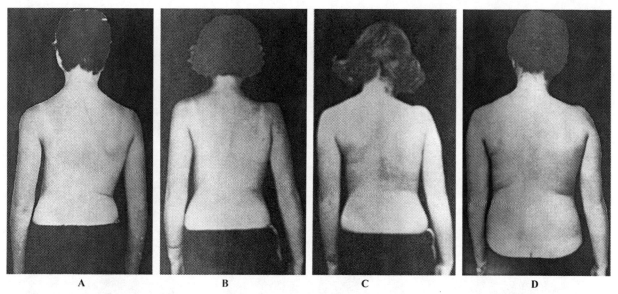

A   B   C   D

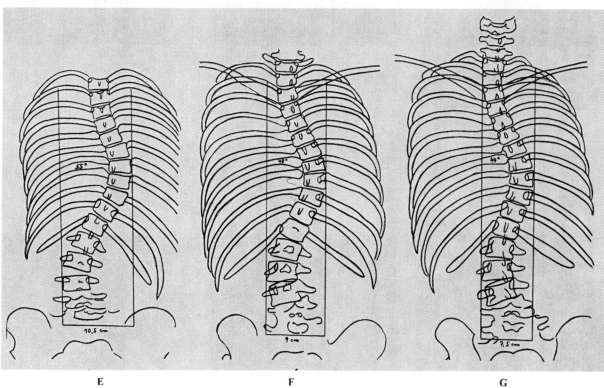

E   F   G

Fig. 641

A: Start of treatment, 12 years, 9 months old. VC 2150 cc, 2.5 cm respirational excursion.

B: 13 years, 11 months old. VC 2600 cc, 4.5 cm respirational excursion, 9 weeks of treatment.

C: 15 years, 4 months old. VC 2800 cc, 11 cm respirational excursion, another 7 weeks of treatment.

D: 18 years,10 months old. VC 2990 cc, 12 cm breathing excursion, another 11 weeks of treatment.

The patient performed Schroth exercised on her own between in-patient sessions.

E: 13 years, 3 months old, 2½ months after the first 6-week course of treatment. 55°, curvature width 10.5 cm.

F: 17 years, 3 months old, after 23 weeks of treatment (altogether). 48°, curvature width 9 cm, thus 1.5 cm smaller.

G: X-ray taken on the same day as f) while exercising and using RAB. 44°, curvature width 7.5 cm, another 1.5 cm smaller.

The original X-Rays were too indistinct to be reproduced.

229

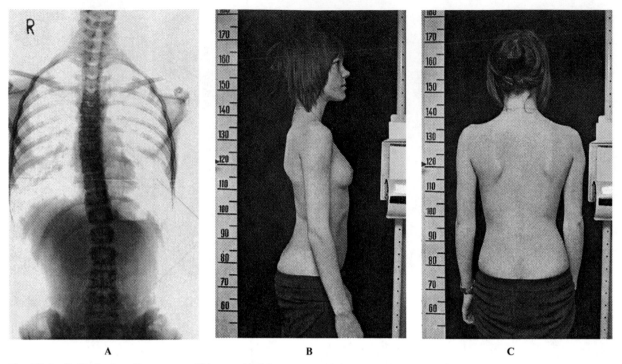

A   B   C

Fig. 642 A - C: Beginning of treatment; 13½-year-old girl.

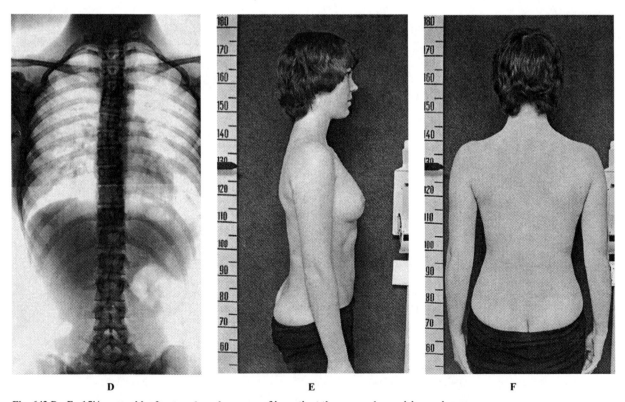

D   E   F

Fig. 642 D - F: 15½ years old, after two 6-week courses of in-patient therapy and exercising on her own.

230

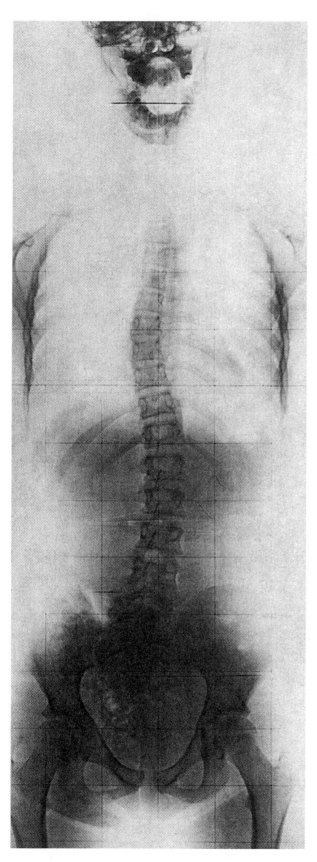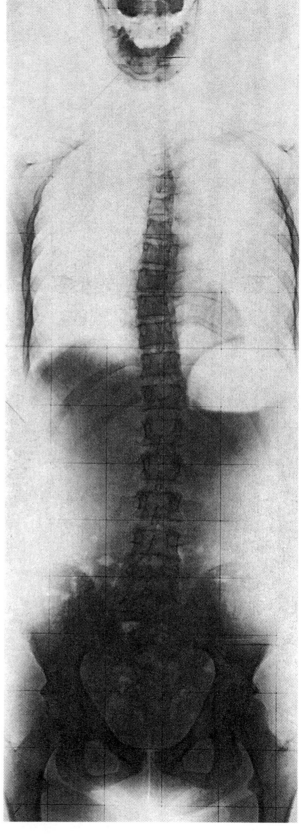

Fig. 643 A:
Girl, 13 years, 4 months old; idiopathic scoliosis.

Fig. 643 B:
14 years, 1 month old, after two courses of Schroth in-patient treatment (3 and 6 weeks).
Improvements: thoracic 22° reduced to 10°
                    lumbar 22° reduced to 11°

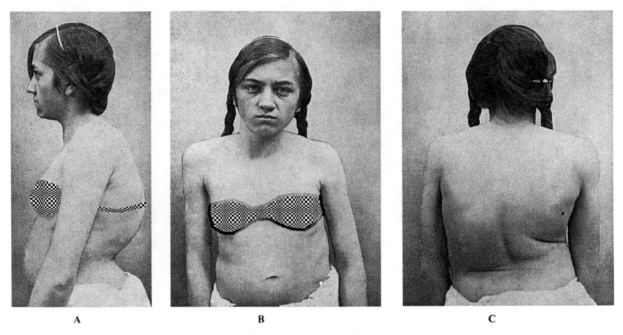

A   B   C

Fig. 644, A-C: 18-year-old girl who had suffered from poliomyelitis. Depressed facial expression.

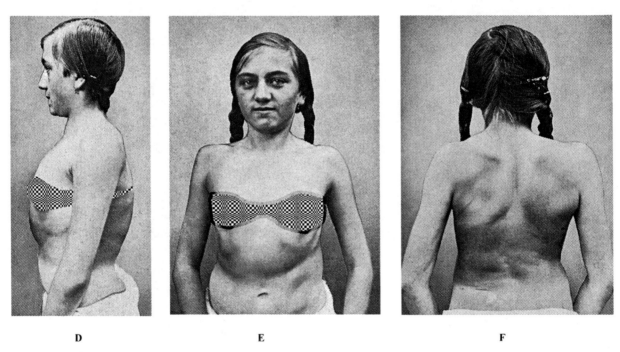

D   E   F

Fig. 644, D-F: After 4 months of Schroth treatment; much straighter posture and more hopeful facial expression.

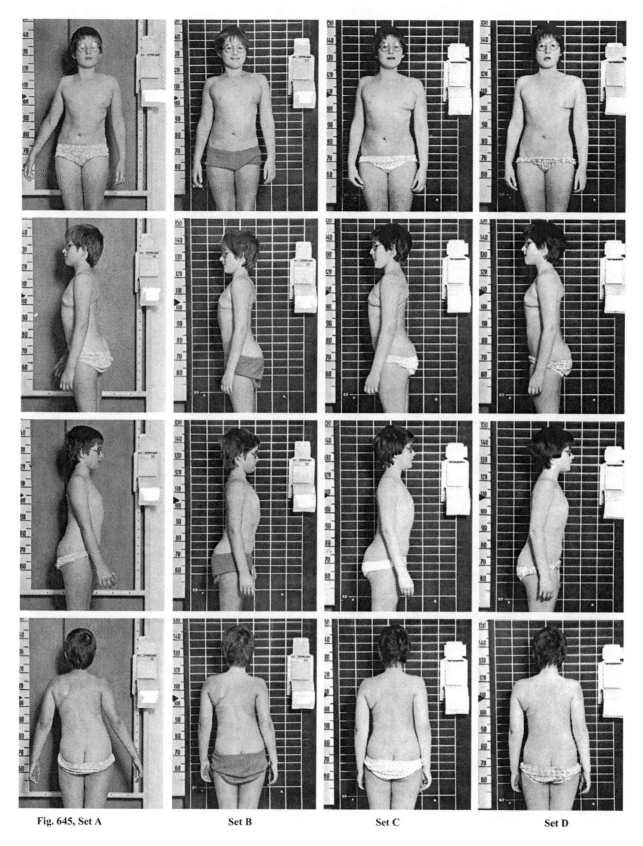

Fig. 645, Set A   Set B   Set C   Set D

Fig. 645

Set A: 10-year-old girl; start of treatment; scoliosis due to the development of wedge vertebrae, surgically fused at the age of 6. During her growth, a steel cable in the instrumentation broke.

Set B: At the end of a 6-week course of Schroth treatment.

Set C: 8 months later; start of the second course of in-patient treatment. Her physical condition was well maintained by her home exercises.

Set D: At the end of a 3-week repeat course of treatment.

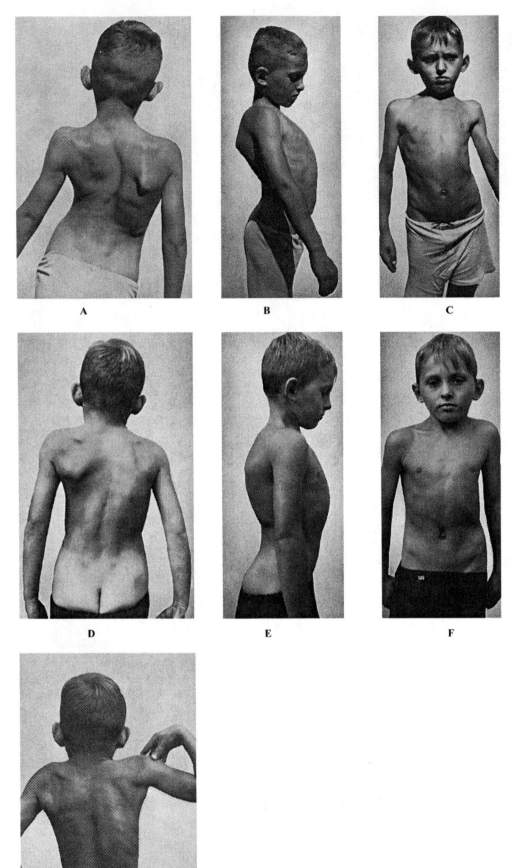

Fig. 646 A - C: 9-year-old boy: condition after poliomyelitis.

Fig. 646 D - F: After 12 weeks of Schroth treatment.

Fig. 646 G: The same boy during an exercise.

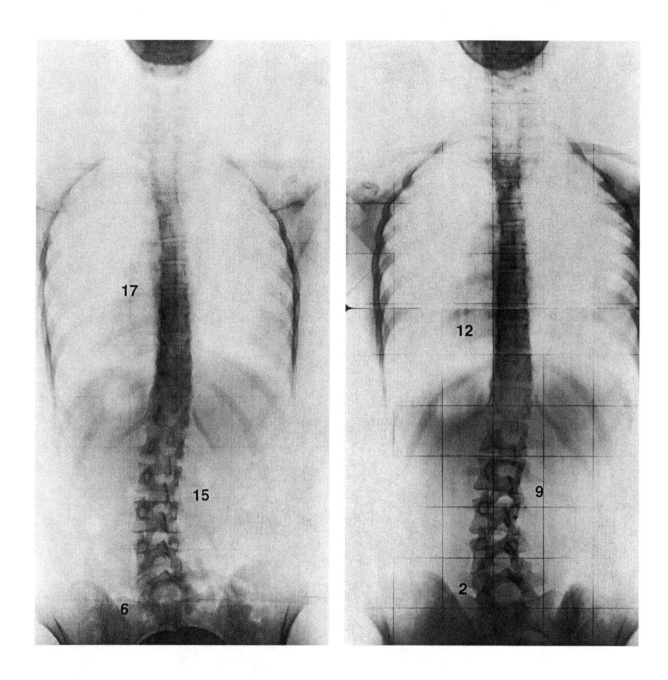

Fig. 647 A:
16-year-old girl with idiopathic scoliosis. Her younger sister had scoliosis as well.

Fig. 647 B:
The same girl at age 17, after three courses of in-patient therapy (twice for 3 weeks and once 2 weeks). Between courses she continued performing the exercises herself. The thoracic curvature improved from 17° to 12°; lumbar curvature from 15° to 9°; lumbosacral curve from 6° to 2°. This improvement was achieved during the difficult time of puberty.

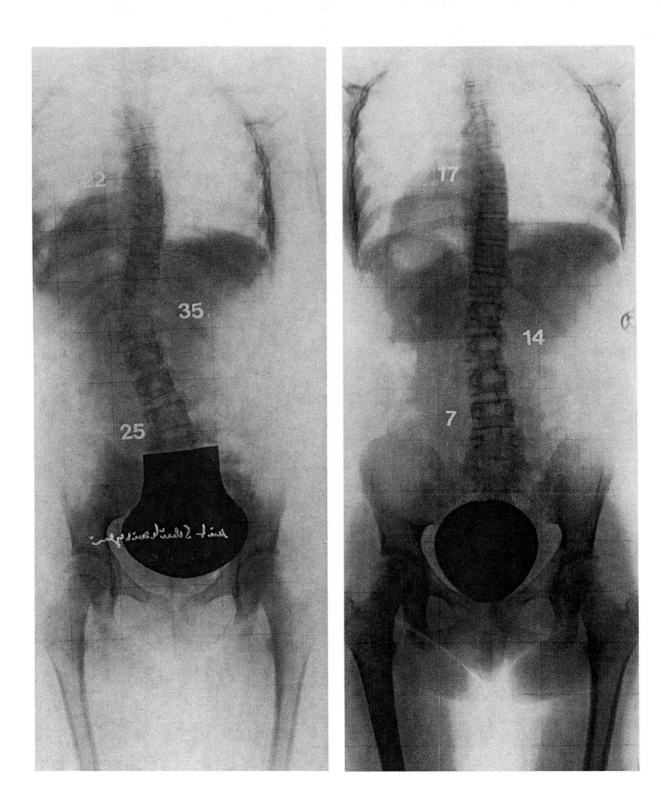

Fig. 648 and 649:

15-year-old girl; slight right thoracic curvature; the left lumbar curvature is much more pronounced;
she also has a lumbosacral curvature to the right.

Improvement after 6-week course of Schroth therapy:
Thoracic curve from   22° to 17°
Lumbar   35° to 14°
Lumbosacral   25° to 7°

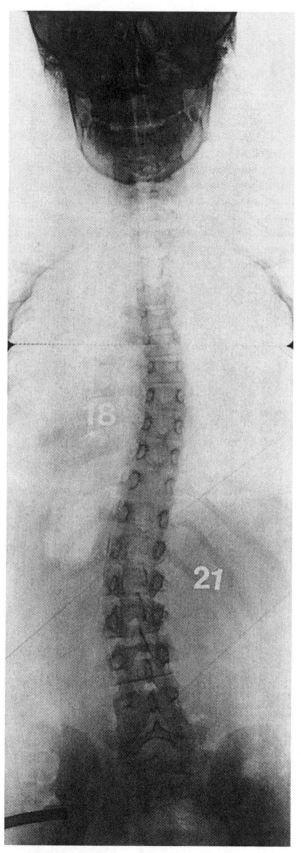

Fig. 650 A:

10-year-old girl before Schroth treatment. She first had 20 Schroth treatment sessions with an outpatient physical therapist, then 4 weeks of in-patient treatment.

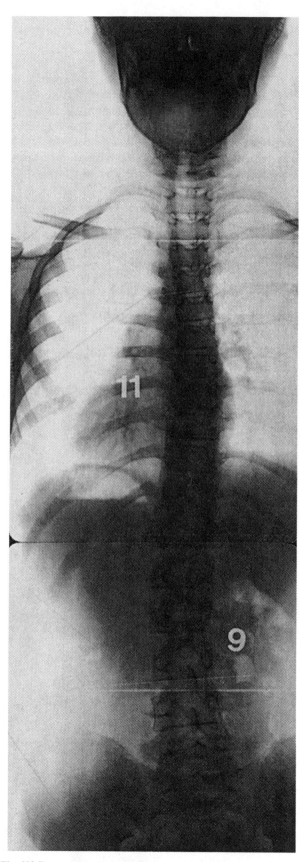

Fig. 650 B:

Improvement after 4 weeks:
Thoracic	18° to 11°
Lumbar	21° to 9°
Lumbosacral	12° to 4°

237

II. Statistical evaluation of treatment results

In every case at the Katharina Schroth Klinik, documented findings were recorded before and after treatment. Patients were questioned about their subjective judgment as far as well-being was concerned. The overall assessment was positive. Now that several studies have been completed on Schroth three-dimensional treatment, we would like to report here on the findings.

1. Changes in vital capacity

One study focused on 2,013 scoliotic patients who had come to the Schroth clinic for initial treatment over a period of two years. 93 % of these patients experienced an increase in vital capacity, with an average baseline of 400–600 cc. (Fig. 651).

A retrospective long-term study (Weiss 1989a) of 10- to 13-year-old patients showed a highly significant increase in VC. After an initial course of treatment for 6 weeks, there was an increase of 20.85 % (p < 0.001). After repeated treatments, there was an average increase in VC of 10.7 % (p < 0.001) (Fig. 652a).

In another study, the increase in VC in teenagers and adults was compared (Weiss 1989b). The young patients showed a highly significant increase in VC (n = 278). The increase was 18.94 % over baseline (p < 0.001). This corresponded to an average gain of 445 cc (base-

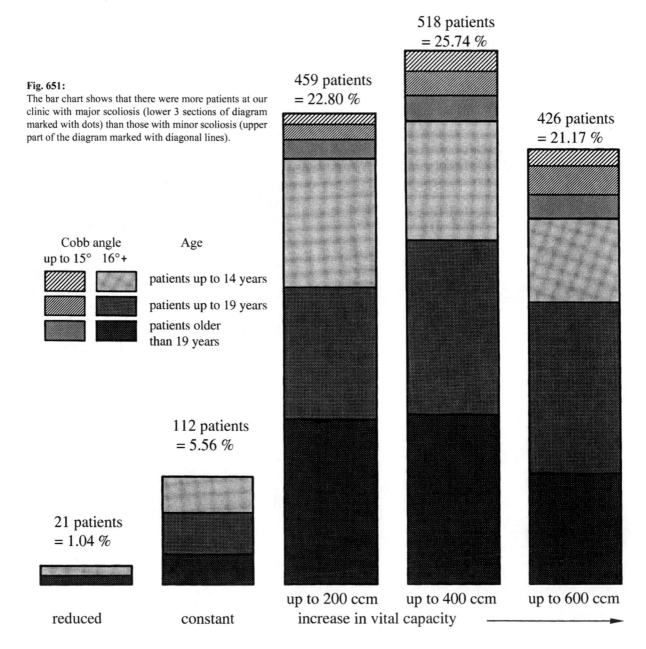

Fig. 651:
The bar chart shows that there were more patients at our clinic with major scoliosis (lower 3 sections of diagram marked with dots) than those with minor scoliosis (upper part of the diagram marked with diagonal lines).

line average: 2499 cc; average at end of treatment: 2944 cc. The average in this age group was 10.74 % (n = 124; p < 0.001) after repeated treatment. The average increase was 264 cc (baseline average 2694 cc; average at end of treatment: 2958 cc).

148 scoliotic patients at the Schroth clinic for their first course of treatment and above the age of 24 showed a smaller average increase in VC of 13.77% (p < 0.001). The average increase was 398 cc, with a baseline average of 3246 cc and end-of-treatment average of 3644 cc, and is thus significant (Fig. 652b).

Goetze (1978) evaluated a small group of teenagers, some of whom were repeating the program at the clinic, and he found an increase of 11% in VC. This is in keeping with repeat-course studies cited above.

It is clear, however, that the increase after the first course of treatment is almost twice as large as that after subsequent courses of treatment. This confirms the possibility of a long-lasting effect after the first course of treatment which is only partially lost over subsequent years.

It is clear that a course of intensive in-patient treatment at the Schroth clinic is of more value than a fitness training lasting several weeks. Although both result in an increase in cardiopulmonary capacity, neither Bjure (1969) nor Goetze (1976) were able to demonstrate an increase in VC after a fitness programme.

As a reduction in VC leads to an increase in right ventricular load in the scoliotic patient (Meister 1980), it can be assumed that a course of Schroth in-patient treatment will relieve stress on the right ventricle.

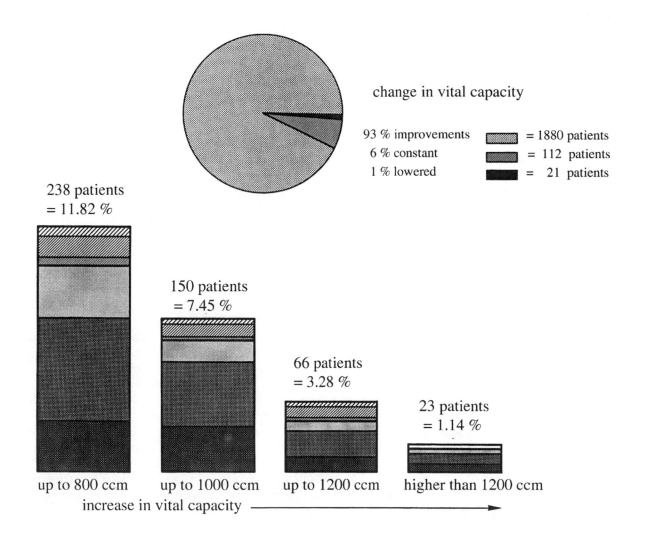

change in vital capacity

93 % improvements   = 1880 patients
6 % constant   = 112 patients
1 % lowered   = 21 patients

238 patients = 11.82 %

150 patients = 7.45 %

66 patients = 3.28 %

23 patients = 1.14 %

up to 800 ccm   up to 1000 ccm   up to 1200 ccm   higher than 1200 ccm

increase in vital capacity ⟶

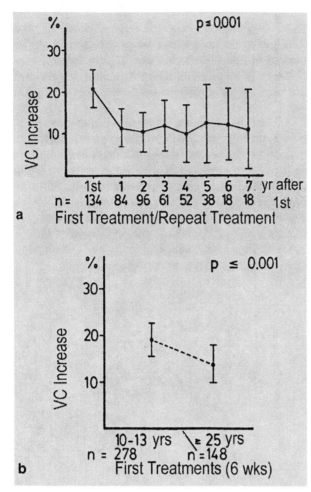

a

b

Fig. 652

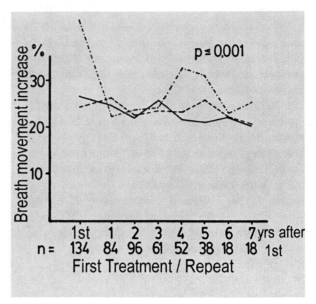

Fig. 653

2. Changes in breathing movement

An increase in breathing movement may be considered indicative of rib mobilization. Measurements are taken under the axilla, at the junction of sternum and the xyphoid process, and the waist, always by the same qualified staff member. Mistakes in circumference measurements in general are unimportant because it is not the single measurement but the difference in measurements that counts.

Weiss (1989a) reported an increase in chest expansion of between 0.5 and 7 cm. Highly significant increases exceeding 20% were found for all three measuring points, both in first-time and repeat-course patients (Fig. 653: reprint authorised by author).

Comparison of adolescent and adult patients showed no significant difference (Weiss 1989b). Average increase in breathing movement in 10– to 13-year-old patients was 29%; adults above age 25 showed an increase of 33.3%. All adolescents showed an average chest movement increase of 29.4%, and adults 31.5%.

Increases in breathing movement at waist level were significant: 45.1% in young scoliotic patients and 42.8%

in the adults. A reason may be the RAB exercises which pay special attention to the depression of the diaphragm and inclusion of the 11th and 12th rib.

Only general conclusions can be drawn from these measurements. They do not indicate an exact point at which the trunk was enlarged. Further studies were therefore conducted: see below.

3. Changes in length of exhalation phase and chest circumference in the transverse plane

Before and at the end of each course of treatment, maximum exhalation time is measured in seconds after inhaling deeply in standing position.

The long exhalation time is achieved mainly by training the diaphragm and the intercostal muscles with continuous exercises. These breathing exercises form part of each patient's personal exercise programme. A further motivation is the challenge to increase this value by one second per day. This increase does not happen continuously, of course, yet hardly a patient fails to improve exhalation time during in-patient treatment.

Even patients wearing braces are not limited. Only among patients with major scoliosis above 100° Cobb, especially older patients, is the increase small. Enlargement of the rib cage in the transverse plane is not as obvious as the exhalation-time increase. This is essentially explicable, since here additional structural changes play a significant role.

The measurements are taken laterally and ventrodorsally, once at each measuring point during maximum exhalation and inhalation.

Measuring points are:
1. Lateral axilla
2. 6th rib, lateral
3. Manubrium of sternum/T3, ventrodorsal
4. Xyphoid process/T11, ventrodorsal

Measurements taken with a pair of pelvic compasses show in centimetres the diameter of rib cage increase at the points measured.

Breathing in a diagonal direction is particularly important, from the dorsal concavity to the frontal concavity. Although possibilities of observation are limited for the patient, we do find significant increases here as well.

Table 7 shows the increase for patients up to age 40 (89% to age 20; 11% 20 to 40), and for patients aged 40 to 64 during the first course of in-patient therapy.

Table 7:

		up to 40 years	older than 40 years
		seconds	seconds
		15.16 – 35.29 = 132 %	17.00 – 30.01 = 77 %
		centimeters	centimeters
Ø	1.	1.41 – 2.03 = 44 %	0.85 – 1.65 = 17 %
Ø	2.	1.64 – 2.29 = 39 %	0.75 – 1.50 = 100 %
Ø	3.	1.18 – 1.66 = 40 %	1.10 – 1.30 = 18 %
Ø	4.	1.19 – 1.72 = 44 %	1.25 – 1.60 = 28 %

4. Changes in scoliometer values

To evaluate the effect of RAB on the scoliotic breathing pattern, we assessed 76 patients suffering from scoliosis with a scoliometer (Fig. 654) and on the scoliometer bench (Fig. 655).

It is important to hold the device with only one finger at the centre, on top of the spinous process (Fig. 656), to avoid unwanted pressure in either direction by the therapist.

At the start and end of each in-patient course, we tested exhalation-inhalation difference in scoliometer readings. The exhalation reading was taken during the non-breathing phase. Then we asked the patient to guide breath into the thoracal concavities of the trunk and, in lumbar curve cases, below the waist rib hump. We drew the patient's awareness to these areas by lightly tapping with the index finger, then noted the inhalation value.

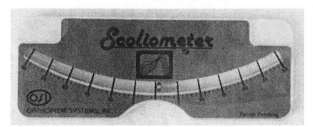

Fig. 654: Scoliometer

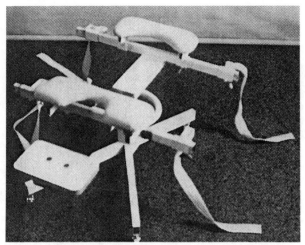

Fig. 655: Scoliometer bench.

In general, the inhalation value was lower than that for exhalation. This difference, which existed in some cases at the beginning of a course, was greater towards the end of treatment, mainly at the height of the apical vertebra: thoracic 7.98% (p < 0.001); lumbar 12.37% (p < 0.001). Thus in most cases, final inhalation values were lower than for exhalation. This was also reflected in the highly significant increase in difference between exhalation and inhalation values. We conclude that uneven trunk areas flatten during the inhalation phase using RAB.

Since pre-treatment and post-treatment examinations were made under the same standardized conditions (tapping at the concavities), it seems justified to presume that the typical scoliotic breathing pattern can be changed and that trunk deformities can be corrected at the same time.

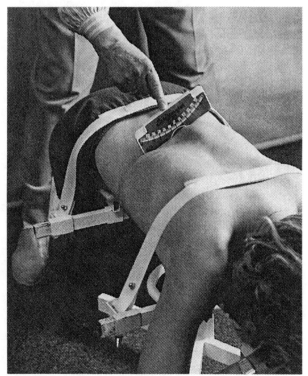

Fig. 656: See text for explanation.

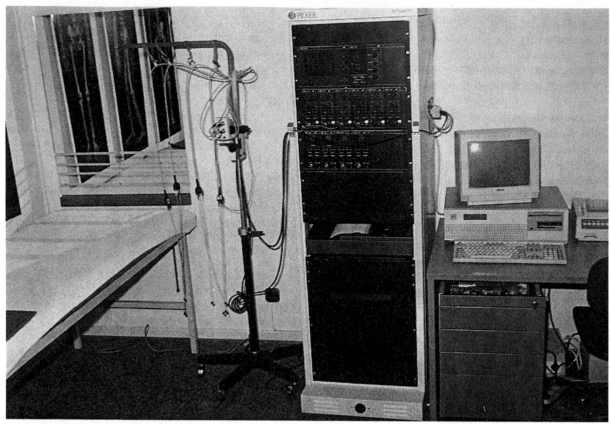

Fig. 657: Our EMG room. At the head end of the stretcher is a mirror with horizontal lines. The patient is encouraged to observe the raising of his or her trunk during the lifting experiment.

5. Electromyographic changes

In all cases of scoliosis, treatment of the musculature is the prime objective. On the one hand, specific training in posture can only be successful if the musculature is able to maintain the corrected posture for a long period (Goetze 1975). On the other, myogenic pain can only be relieved by adequate training (Hettinger 1978, Weiss 1989a). Many publications on this topic refer to muscle strengthening. The patients themselves feel much better and stronger after a course of in-patient treatment (Weiss 1989a). We are not aware of any objective assessment of changes in postural capacity after a physiotherapeutic treatment.

In general, studies have noted increased muscular activity on the outer side of the curvature increased (Basmajian and De Luca 1985, Schmitt 1985, Heine 1980, Gueth and Abbink 1980, Brussatis 1962). This seems to be an adaptive response to the greater use of the muscles on the convex side. The muscular activity can be better economised with suitable exercises. This means that increasing loads can be lifted by a smaller amount of activated motoric units (Stobody and Friedebold 1968). Consequently, a training effect can be seen in decreased electromyographic activity while applying equal strain (Basmajian and De Luca 1985, Schmitt 1985).

Artefact-free electromyograms of 259 patients were evaluated in a study by Weiss (1990). They had been obtained using a standardized study protocol developed by Schmitt (1985). The patients in the prone position lifted the trunk for one minute. Electromyographic activity was recorded by surface electrodes (Ag/Ag – C1), paravertebrally at the level of the thoracic apical vertebra and on the lumbar part of the M. erector spinae, as described by Macintosh and Bogduk (1987).

After a course of in-patient treatment, evaluation of convex-side thoracic activity showed a significant decrease of 6.79% ($p < 0.05$). There was also a decrease in convex lumbar activity of 14.2% ($p < 0.001$). The activity quotient convex-side/concave-side decreased in the thoracic segment significantly by 11.9% ($p < 0.001$) and in the lumbar segment by 7.91% ($p < 0.01$) (Fig. 658).

The results therefore show an increase in postural efficiency. We can also conclude that Schroth in-patient treatment strengthens the musculature and "economises" or exploits muscle activity better.

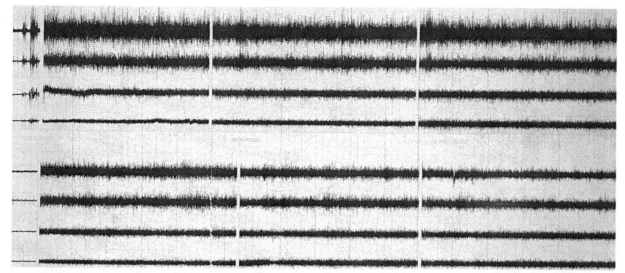

Fig. 658: EMG taken before (top four wave lines) and after (bottom four lines) a course of Schroth treatment. Electromyographic activity of the M. erector trunci on the thoracic convex side (uppermost line). The thoracic concave side (second line), lumbar convex side (third line), lumbar concave side (fourth line) during an attempt to raise the trunk in the prone position.
One can see that with the same energy input, there is a marked decrease in activity in both lumbar and thoracic musculature on the convex side. A decrease in activity of the lumbar musculature on the concave side shows much more economical use of the intrinsic lumbar parts of the M. erector spinae. This is precisely the muscle group that straightens and derotates the lumbar curvature.

6. Target muscle control with surface EMG electrodes

In 1988 and 1989, we conducted electromyographic studies with scoliotic patients to examine the effects of certain Schroth exercises more closely.

We attached silver/silver chloride surface electrodes 1.5 cm to the side of the spinous processes in the thoracic area along the M. erector trunci/M. trapezius, and in the lumbar area on the M. erector spinae in direction of the fibres, in each case at the level of the apical vertebra (Fig. 659).

The upper tracing line shows the electromyographic activity of the thoracic paravertebral musculature on the convex side. The second tracing line shows the activity on the concave side. The activity of the lumbar paravertebral musculature on the convex side is documented in the third tracing line, and the fourth line shows the lumbar concave side.

In the lumbar region, electromyographic activity comes directly from the M. erector spinae, since the parts of the surface musculature caudally from L2 mostly consist of tendons (Macintosh and Bogduk 1987).

In the thoracic region, the activity of the M. erector spinae mixes with the surface muscles (e.g., M. trapezius). According to Friedebold (1958), if the extremities are fixed (in our case, with a pole or shoulder countertraction), we can expect primarily activity from the M. erector spinae at the point mentioned. We studied the following exercises with different approaches.

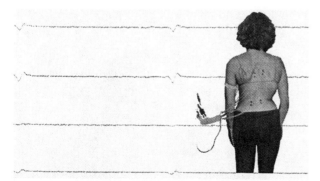

Fig. 659
Standing upright. The 18-year-old patient is held passively by the ligamentous structure. Thus no activity is noticeable in the area of the holding musculature. Usually the first and third line show increased muscle activity, which indicates that the lumbar segment on the convex side is possibly bearing the weight of the laterally overhanging thoracic part. The increased activity in the area of the rib hump may possibly be due to the effort made by these muscles to maintain the upper trunk with the head and shoulder girdle in a vertical position.

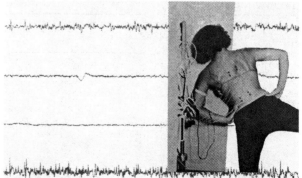

Fig. 660
Muscle cylinder exercise, standing with hands on the hips. The fourth line shows increased muscular activity in the right lumbar region, as well on the thoracic convex side. This may indicate activation of a postural reflex, which is the aim in this case.

243

7. Comparative X-rays

Three X-ray comparisons of Cobb angles show patients standing and performing an exercise. They do not quite reflect reality, since the patients could not exert full force. The X-ray apparatus wobbled when patients braced their foot or arm against it. Remarkably, these exercises even have a positive influence on older patients and scolioses above 60° (Figs. 378, 379).

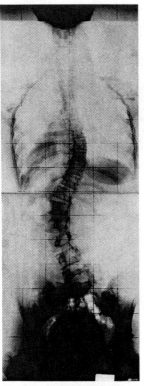 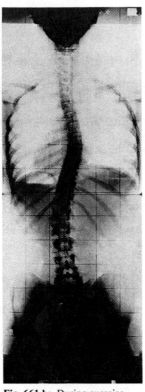 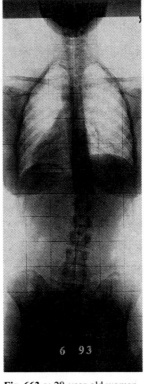 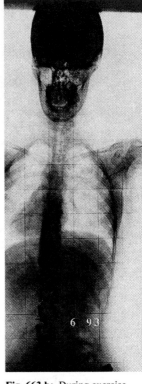

Fig. 661 a: 18-year-old girl.   **Fig. 661 b:** During exercise.   **Fig. 663 a:** 28-year-old woman.   **Fig. 663 b:** During exercise.

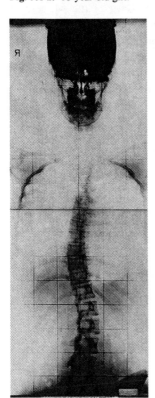 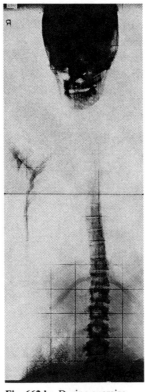 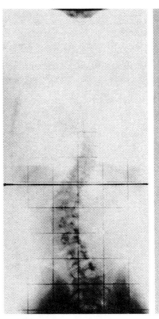

Fig. 662 a: 21-year-old woman.   **Fig. 662 b:** During exercise.

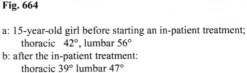

Fig. 664

a: 15-year-old girl before starting an in-patient treatment;
     thoracic 42°, lumbar 56°
b: after the in-patient treatment:
     thoracic 39° lumbar 47°

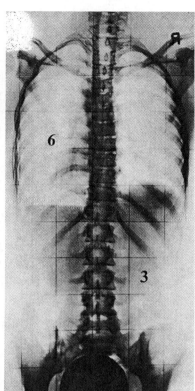

Fig. 665

a: On the left, a girl aged 12 years, 8 months, four months before a course of in-patient treatment: thoracic 13°, lumbar 15°.

b: Same girl at the age of 13 years, 4 months after inpatient treatment: thoracic 6°, lumbar 3°

The girl exercised continuously at home using exercises she learned at in-patient training.

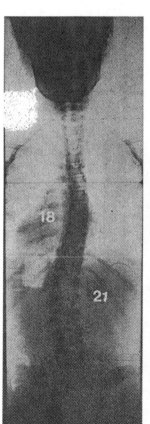
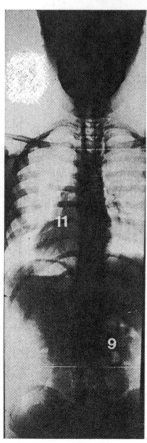
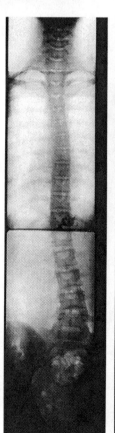
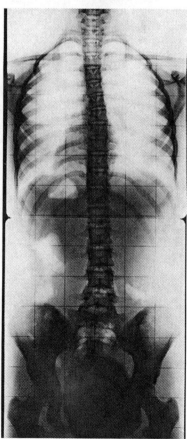

Fig. 666:

a: Girl aged 9 years and 5 months: thoracic 18°, lumbar 21°
b: At 10 years, 6 months: thoracic 11°, lumbar 9°, following 6 weeks of in-patient treatment.

Fig. 667:

a: 15-year-old girl with idiopathic scoliosis; at the beginning of Schroth treatment.
b: After 2 months of exercising with a Schroth therapist. (1½ to 2 h. sessions)

Fig. 668: Table 8, Evaluation of X-rays

No.	Age	Standing Vertebra	COBB°	Apex	on exercise	difference
1.	14	T 10	13		6	- 7
		L 4	30	L 2 / L 23	6	-24
			17		0	-17
2.	15	T 5	20		18	- 2
		T 11	44	T 8/9	28	-16
		L 3	40	T 12 / L 1	30	-10
		L 5	14		20	+ 6
			0		5	+ 5
3.	16	T 3	7		0	- 7
		T 10	15	T 8	0	-15
		L 3	17	L 1	12	- 5
			17		4	-13
4.	18	T 5	18		11	- 7
		T 11	39		22	-17
		L 4	47	L 2	18	-29
			26		7	-19
5.	20	T 3	9		6	- 3
		T 10	23		16	- 7
		L 3	34		21	-13
			20		11	- 9
6.	20	T 4	7		7	0
		T 11	23	T 8	23	0
		L 3	16	T 12	8	- 8
			6		0	- 6
7.	20	T 7	45		37	- 8
		L 1	85		57	-28
		L 4	44	T 10	30	-14
			6		10	+ 4
8.	22	C 4				
		T 5	44		35	- 9
		T 11	87		75	-12
		L 4	77		58	-19
			31		23	- 8
9.	24	T 4				
		T 12	18	T 8/9	20	+2 *)
		L 5	71	L 2/3	47	-24
		sacrum	58		35	-23
			22		11	-11
10.	27	C 5	6		22	+16 *)
		T 7	11		0	-11
		L 3	24	T 12	6	-18
			14		5	- 9
11.	28	T 11	4		2	- 2
		L 3	15		2	-13
			11		3	- 8

*) The patient held head at an angle during the exercise.

246

No.	Age	Standing Vertebra	COBB°	Apex	on exercise	difference
12.	30	T 3	13		-	-
		T 11	23	T 8	2	-21
		L 3	28	L 1	24	-4
			18		16	-2
13.	31	C 7	17		17	0
		T 9	54		46	- 8
		L 2	63		49	-14
			25		19	- 6
14.	31	T 3	6		6	0
		T 8	23		14	- 9
		L 2	30	T 12	8	-13
			13		6	- 7
15.	32	T 1	10		9	- 1
		T 5	39	T 3	31	- 8
		T 10	49	T 7/8	36	-13
		L 3	49	L 1	29	-20
			27		15	-12
16. rotational slipping L1 -L4	36	L 1	29		15	-14
		L 3	57	L 2	40	-17
			28		25	- 3
17.	37	T 3	12		12	0
		T 10	46	T 5	34	-12
		L 3	69	T 12	46	-23
			35		24	-11
18.	37	T 10	52	T 7	30	-22
		L 3	47	L 2	30	-17
			18		20	+ 2
19.	38	T 1	17		23	+ 6
		T 6	57		57	0
		L 2	66	T 10	53	-13
			26		20	+ 6
20. L 2/3 OP fused	63	T 6	20	T 8/9	?	?
		L 4	56	T 7/8	49	- 7
			52		34	-18
		sacrum	23	L 2	18	- 5

The remarkable results of such exercises are also obtainable by elderly patients with scoliosis of more than 60°.

8. Pulse measurements

During a 4-week period at our clinic in 1995, we studied pulse rate in 169 patients who had both scoliosis and malposture. The study tested the stress of Schroth exercises on their system. Subjects were male and female, chosen at random, ages 14 to 30 years. We measured pulse before, during, and after a specific Schroth exercise. The sample included first-time and repeating Schroth patients.

The following were determined:
1. Resting pulse after 5 min in supine position (average rate 71 beats/min).
2. Measurement during an intensive Schroth exercise (average 85 beats/min).
3. Measurement after 2 – 5 min in supine position (average 73 beats/min).
4. Measurement after 5 min of targeted relaxation (average 61 beats/min).

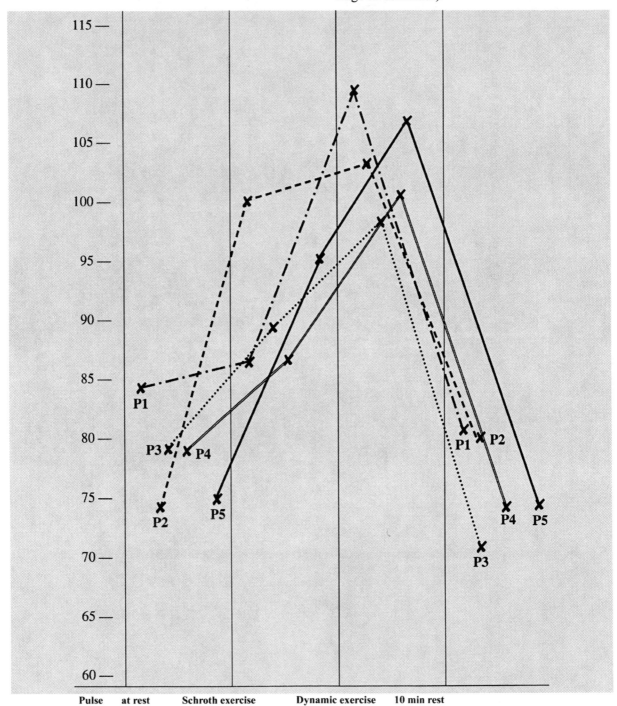

Pulse   at rest   Schroth exercise   Dynamic exercise   10 min rest

Fig. 669: Five patients: average values over a four-week period.

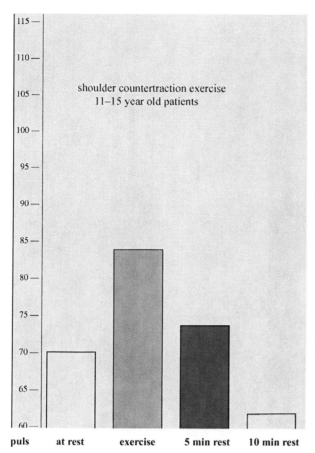

Fig. 670: Morning

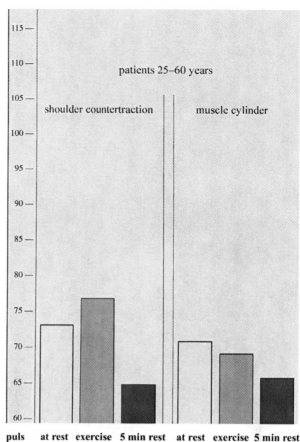

Fig. 671: Morning

The aim of the tests was to establish how the sometimes strenuous Schroth exercises influence blood pressure and pulse, and whether any would overburden the patient. The difference between resting and exercise pulse rate was not higher than 20 beats/min in any case. During the 4 weeks of testing, the patients were able to return to their starting pulse rate after a short recovery period, and even to shorten it by 8 to 12 beats/min lower than baseline resting pulse.

If we assume a resting pulse rate of 75 beats/min lowered by 15 beats/min, this means lowering the pulse by 650,000 beats/month, quite a rest for the heart. It appears therefore that the circulatory system is relaxed rather than stressed by concentration on breathing and muscle contraction. The patients agreed that a quiet and concentrated atmosphere in the group and the room during exercises is necessary. The time of day was also important: in the evening, the patients felt more stressed and nervous, while the morning they were relaxed and calm (e.g. Sunday morning). These observations were reflected in the results. The patients all agreed that they planned to do exercises at home in the morning as well.

It was also interesting to see that the mental work, which is necessary for all Schroth exercises, was motivating and helpful to increase in building the patients' power to concentrate.

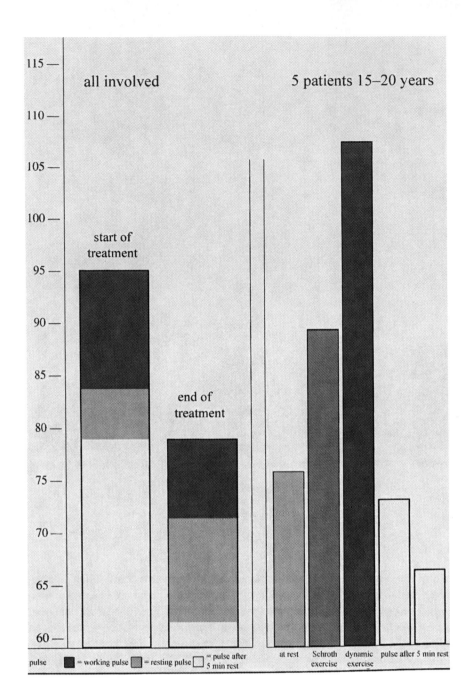

Fig. 672

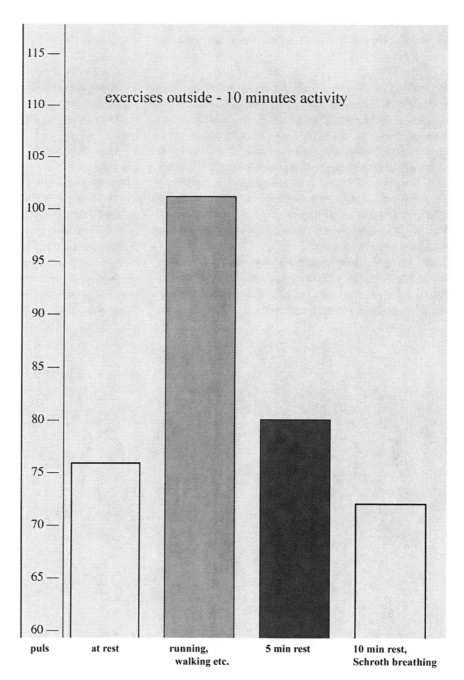

exercises outside - 10 minutes activity

puls   at rest   running,   5 min rest   10 min rest,
                   walking etc.   Schroth breathing

Fig. 673: Morning

9. Favourable side effects of the three-dimensional Schroth treatment

We have done retrospective and prospective studies to document the treatment results at our clinic. We found that even severe scoliosis could be straightened by a certain amount. Naturally, cases at the beginning of scoliosis and those with curves below 30° are easiest to influence. **Surface measurements** taken by the Formetric system which we use at the clinic showed significant reductions, mainly in lateral deviations and rotation, but also in the length of the spine.

Measurements taken with the **scoliometer** showed reductions in angle as well.

Vital capacity and **breathing movement** increased, which, in turn, has a positive influence on the load on the right side of the heart. The ECG showed an improvement in **cardiopulmonary capacity**.

Pulse measurements taken before, during and after the stressful exercises also showed greater cardiocirculatory economising. There is also a **positive influence on pain**.

We also documented an economising change in **muscular** imbalance with the electromyographic studies.

These favourable physical changes also had a positive effect on the **psychological status** of patients, as demonstrated by the 'Baseler Befindlichkeits-Skala' (Hobi's Basle Well-Being Scale) and the 'Beschwerdeliste' (Complaints List of von Zerssen).

Naturally, our **follow-up pictures** speak for themselves.

All studies are summarised in scientific detail in "Praxis der Skolioserehabilitation" (A Practical Guide to the Treatment of Scoliosis) by H-R Weiss.

PART E
General Data

I. In-patient treatment at the Katharina-Schroth-Klinik in Bad Sobernheim

The Katharina Schroth Klinik was purchased by the Asklepios GmbH on 1 August 1995. A new, modern clinic was built: the Asklepios Katharina Schroth Klinik, Korczakstrasse 2, D-55566 Bad Sobernheim, Germany.

1. Diagnosis of pathological changes using photographs and measurements

Before treatment, after two weeks, and at the end of in-patient treatment, patients are photographed from all four sides, boys in shorts, girls in bikini, always under the same lighting conditions and from the same camera angles.

The patient's height and breathing values are also determined at the beginning and at the end of treatment. Each patient undergoes a complete physical examination by one of our physicians and, if necessary, X-rays are taken.

2. Rotational-breathing exercises

These are performed in groups and individually in the morning and afternoon, outdoors, if possible. The sessions start with music and specially-formulated rhythmic exercises performed by all patients. This activates breathing and circulation. The individual groups work with a therapist for two hours in the morning and afternoon. They change gyms and equipment – wall bars, chairs, tables, beams, rings, poles, and footstools. The therapist observes the patients individually and corrects their movements. The mirrors are used during the exercises at all times for monitoring and support.

3. Massage and relaxation

Normally, the patient receives a back massage twice a week, and in special cases a connective tissue massage. Relaxation is part of the daily program and takes place in the correct individual position.

4. Rest periods

To guarantee successful treatment, there have to be scheduled periods of rest during the day. When the weather permits, the patients rest outside on the lawn or on the balcony after lunch, or in bed during inclement weather.

5. Leisure time activities

These include table tennis, arts and crafts, singing, dancing, and games.

6. Length of in-patient treatment

Generally, the first course of treatment should be at least 6 weeks long. It is not possible to acquire a new postural awareness in a shorter period of time. In severe cases, a course of 6 to 8 weeks is necessary. Repeated shorter courses can also be successful.

7. Age of patients

The Schroth method is suitable for the treatment of patients of all ages, from 7 to 70 years. It is of less importance that the bones are still "flexible". What is important is that the patient be able to follow the instructions and visualize the goal. Self motivation is also important. Children between the ages of 5 and 9 should be accompanied by a parent who can support the child when exercising at home, even if this is only with the physical aspects of the method. The method is not suitable for babies or very young children. We recommend courses of physiotherapy using the Neumann-Neurode, Vojta, or Bobath method for infants.

II. Orthopaedically-oriented daily life

The daily orthopaedic movements trained using the Schroth method (lying down, standing, sitting, walking etc.) should be continued regularly to further improve posture. Specific exercise times should be incorporated into one's daily schedule. Each day, patients should exercise for about one hour, which may be divided in two half-hour periods. Clean air is necessary, also at night. Smoking is not allowed during treatment and should be given up altogether. Before going to sleep the posture should be checked, and changed if necessary. The patient has to develop a very strong sense of correct posture, so that (as we know from our clinical experience) a patient who is in the wrong position (e.g., lying on the rib hump side), will wake up, correct the position, and go back to sleep.

It is perhaps useful to remember that many people like to sleep with back to the wall. Therefore the bed should be turned, if necessary, or the head and foot ends of the bed reversed, to promote sleeping on the concave side. Corrective cushions should, however, be placed under the lumbar convexity, so it is not exacerbated. During daytime, care should be taken to ensure when lying and reading, for example, that the body does not drop into an inappropriate curve, or when standing, that the weight is not rested on the side of the rib hump. When reading and studying while lying on the back, patients should always use prismatic lens spectacles. A great deal of effort is put into achieving an improvement, but this improvement can be destroyed in a very short time by careless posture. At school, the teacher should make it possible for the child to look straight ahead. If a child with scoliosis sits at the side and has to turn constantly, this will exacerbate the scoliosis.

Patients should take every opportunity to observe their posture in a mirror, shop windows, or using their shadow to correct their sitting, standing and walking behaviour. The exercise '**between two mirrors**' is very suitable because it enables the back to be observed without rotation. When the back appears straight in the mirror, the posture is right. Judging the posture by 'feeling' alone is sometimes not adequate. It is not enough simply to achieve an upright posture during exercises, because in well-established scoliosis, the body tends to drop back into malposture. This fact makes overcorrection necessary during exercise because the body will then return to a good middle position. Only through overcorrection can the patient change her mental postural picture, that cerebral image that had become distorted during the long development of the scoliosis. This postural correction must be performed long enough that the patient adopts it securely.

Swimming is the best exercise for the heart and the circulation. We recommend swimming 2 or 3 times a week.

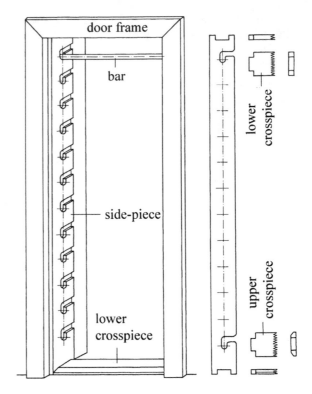

Fig. 674: Drawing showing "wall bars" using a door frame.

At home the patient should perform many different exercises **to train all muscle groups**. The **exercise aids** used at the clinic can be replaced by simple, self-made devices at home. For example, a wall bar fixed in a door frame. Suggestions for 'home-made' devices are made at the clinic.

Several audio **cassettes** are available to increase the intensity, proper goal orientation, and variety of exercising at home.

The **follow-up photos** taken at the clinic should be viewed repeatedly to make visualization easier and enable the patient to form the mental picture of the goal during each exercise. Simple mechanical exercising is not enough!

Finally, a **positive attitude** is of great importance in achieving lasting success in stabilising results.

Quite a few patients do not have room for wall bars at home. However, exercises at the wall bars are very important for stretching and strengthening, and patients should try to find room for them. Fig. 674 shows how wall bars can be fixed inside a door frame without nails or screws. The wall bars consist of 4 wooden slats which fit exactly into the frame: 2 on the sides; one above and one on the floor, beveled on both edges to prevent stumbling. There are also two to four bars. You need only four slits: one all the way across the top: one all the way down, and two at hip height. To secure the bars, you can make the notches only on one side and obliquely, so the bar can slide into the hole. You can also close the notches and lock the bars in place with a board.

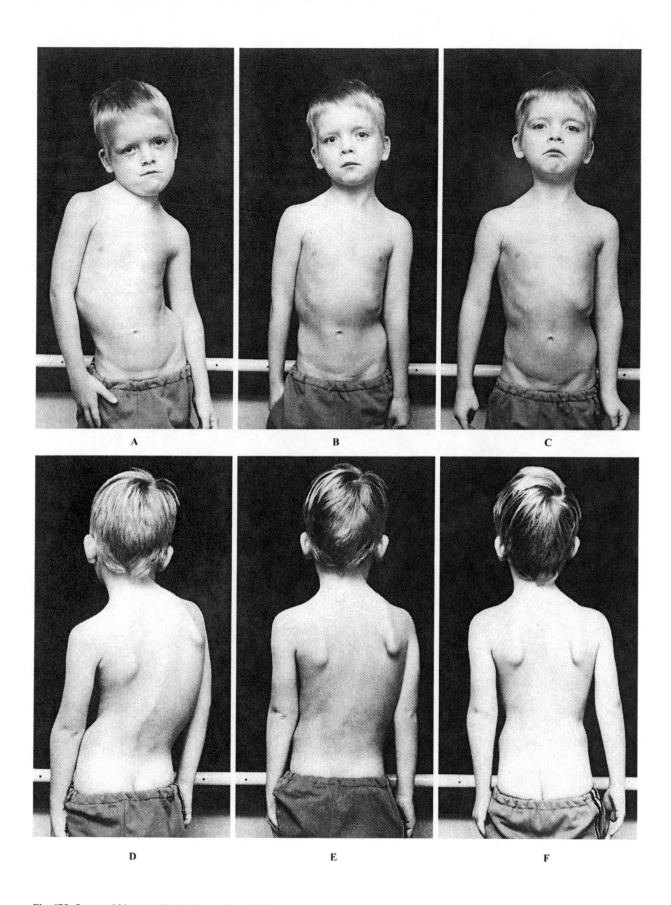

Fig. 675: 5-year-old boy: scoliosis after poliomyelitis.

A and D: At the beginning of treatment.
B and E: After three weeks.
C and F: After eight weeks of Schroth treatment.

III. Indications and contraindications

a) Indications

1. Scoliosis, kyphoscoliosis, scoliosis caused by paralysis
2. Hollow back, Scheuermann's disease (adolescent kyphosis), postural collapse
3. Contracted round back, hyperlordosis, posture-related back pain

b) Relative indications

4. Gibbus (Potts hump) after recovery from tuberculosis of the spine; residual defects of a spinal compression fracture; pre- and posttreatment after spinal surgery

c) Contraindications

Uncontrolled circulatory disorders, grave osteoporosis, tuberculosis of the lung or bones, spastic paralysis, resection of a lobe of the lung, dementia.

Appendix

Here we quote an article that Katharina Schroth wrote to support an East German patient who was not allowed to come to West Germany for political reasons. The article was later published in the 1977 edition of the journal *Physiotherapie*. This article demonstrates her love for her patients and her dedication to detail which is omnipresent in all the Schroth exercises.

Katharina Schroth emphasized repeatedly:
"Scoliosis results from a multitude of wrong movements that finally result in a rigid posture. This is why the patient first of all needs very careful observation to recognize them, and to reverse them completely with exercises – in the beginning at least in one's imagination. Treatment is like doing a jigsaw puzzle: we take piece after piece and put them together until we finally reach the upright position. Only this way can we heal the suffering. The therapist has to inject all her/his love, energy and affection for the patient into treatment and share the motivation. Each exercise has to be performed as if it were the only piece which will bring success".
This was Katharina Schroth's maxim in her youth when she treated herself. She maintained this level of dedication throughout her life. Our aim is to let this spirit live on in the clinic.

What is "rotational breathing"?

Rotational breathing means correcting defects by breathing.
Example: First, very easy exercises as an introduction:

Exercise 1.

a) Supine position. The arms are close to the sides of the body. The fingertips and elbows are pushed towards the feet – a little more with each breath.
b) At the same time, the head is pushed upwards (as a countermovement). It is also increased a little with each breath.
c) The same with inhalation – it is similarly increased in small steps.
d) At the end of this elongation, the entire body is tensed – the arms and the back, head and neck. The chin has to be lowered but not pressed upon, to elongate the back of the neck. The floor should be felt supporting the head.
e) After you feel this tension and are aware of it, this is followed by a strong elastic contraction of the entire back during exhalation. The arms, head and shoulder ridges stay on the floor. Only the back becomes a little hollow. This entire procedure is guided mentally.

f) Now the attention is turned to the phase after exhalation: Do not do anything, just observe what happens. From now on, breathing is automatic and should be very deep. The chest expands energetically – no active breathing is required. The second breathing movement expands half again as widely: it happens on its own. Afterwards, we are quite calm, and the exercise can be repeated. Even the smallest details need to be repeated over and over again. In this way, the exercise is engraved in the mind and becomes an important tool in the improvement of the body and its posture. It is most important to be aware of and feel every tiny movement. Even the straightened elbows have to become active and push step by step against the floor during these contractions of the back, as the back tenses and the chest expands.

Exercise 2.

a) With this new all-feeling awareness, we now push with the hand and the elbow on the right side – including also the shoulder ridge – and push up with the back of the neck at the same time. We inhale during these actions. We feel the right anterior chest arching forwards and the right side of the back automatically tensing itself.
b) The movement is refined and evaluated when we retain this posture during exhalation. We continue then the tensing of the back on one side (which includes widening of the front on one side) in the small, increasingly strong steps. The aim is not to reach maximum tension with one movement, but to build up slowly in a series of elastic movements.

The arms soon feel warm and stimulated. (I remember a physician saying: "You obtain the correct degree of complete tonicity. I envy your results".) It must be kept in mind that all large pectoral muscles and arm muscles are attached to the upper arm, which means that it is useful to exercise the arms in this manner.
Exercising the right side this way may then be performed on the left side as well, and is used systematically in scoliosis to arch the flat side of the chest and flatten the rib hump. It is of utmost importance to keep the head extended and to push it upwards without cramping the front of the chest and neck. This is basic rotational breathing: guided breathing that results in a correction of shape.

Exercise 3.

a) We sense the pushing of the arms again from exercise 1 above, while concentrating mainly on the upper shoulder blades, about 3 times. We are first totally relaxed, then start to use the elastic tightening to shape the upper chest and the back during exhalation.

b) Now, while pushing, we concentrate on the elbows during tightening. The back is tensed differently and the chest is opened in a different area: more in the middle. When we have learned how to reach the area of the back during exhalation, carefully and precisely, we gain complete control over the shape of our chest and back. We are able to reduce and flatten each unilateral prominence that we recognize. For example, a patient who has the rib hump on the right side in the middle might have another on the left close to the shoulder ridge. They might not be aware of it (the therapist might not detect it either), but it is important to flatten it out to look better in clothing. In such cases, we have to start the tensing of the muscles of the back all the way up to the left shoulder ridge while pushing the elbow down during exhalation. The result is a rotation of the right shoulder towards the floor. Once this degree of correction has been achieved, it is essential to use inhalation consciously to alter the shape. We pull the right shoulder down and guide the breath to the narrow front of the chest to breathe it upwards and outwards. "Feeling is everything", to quote Goethe. We now feel a wonderful warmth in the back, a soft widening of the chest, and a beautiful ventilation of the lungs when we stop exercising, a reward for all our hard work. 'Dried' and closed capillaries have opened up; inactive, overstretched tissue has started to work again. The blood flow to the skin has improved and it is rejuvenated. The reward is greater than we expect, and it is beneficial to the healing of the entire body.

c) We now concentrate especially on pushing the hands onto the floor (without ignoring the floor contact of the elbows and shoulders). As before, we 'listen' to everything that is happening. This instruction is repeated until it becomes second nature to the patient.

d) Now we concentrate in the same way on pushing the fingers onto the floor. We feel how the movement spreads up the arms, reaching areas located higher, depending on where the muscles are attached. The way the hands warm up so quickly is striking. The back has become almost hot, flooded by pulsating, healing and cleansing blood.

Using this technique, even a patient confined to bed can reduce boredom and do something useful for his or her health, even if – depending on their strength – this happens in very small steps. Many small steps result in one large step. The metabolism is stimulated and when you get up again, your body has been improved – stronger and thus more beautiful. Additionally, you have gained a physical awareness which will always remain with you.

EXERCISE 4.

These arm exercises can be performed with the arms rotated inward or outwards. This is an advantage for the orthopaedic correction of shoulder malposture. Soon each patient will be capable of performing these exercises alone and in this way will develop a feeling for them. This is an additional tool to correct and shape the body. Each patient will be a proud and happy sculptor of her/his own body.

EXERCISE 5.

In the same way, we can develop a feeling for the right and the left leg, in the normal extended position, or rotated inwards or outwards. We can combine this with controlling and correcting the hip position and the counterposition of the trunk.

a) We start by pushing the heel of the extended leg downwards. The feet are flexed, toes clenched. At the same time the back of the neck is elongated and is pushed upwards while the lungs are gently filled with air. It is advantageous to visualize the many large blood vessels coming from the back and shoulders through the neck to the middle of the head. They are being stretched and nurtured. We can also feel the back of the legs being stretched. This is especially true for the shortened parts of the flexors. They will regain their normal length and a warming blood supply will be sent to all the inactive blood vessels and lymph vessels.

b) As we push, we concentrate on the waist – the centre of the body. It will become slimmer and will also be stretched. We also feel a response from the area of the lowest ribs, at the front, back and sides. Breathing is always used at the same time and has a positive effect on the base of the lungs. The diaphragm should be consciously depressed to complete the exercise. During pushing, after reaching the best possible length, the elastic tensing of the muscles follows. In this way, we feel the gluteal muscles, the thigh and knee area, the lower legs – at the side and in the back – depending on where we direct our attention. This is also used to shape and correct the hip position in scoliosis – and each of the different movements involved can, of course, also be used separately. You will never have cold feet or legs again! The whole body pulsates with warmth.

Patients with a right convexity should tense the left buttock and the right pelvic area in particular, to influence the rotational movement of the pelvis.

This is an essential movement to complete the pushing down of the right shoulder and arm with the forward arching of the chest and the flattening of the rib hump. These are the three different parts of a countermovement.

a) The pressure of both legs, which can be termed 'pushing pressure' (heels push downwards and head upwards out of the shoulder girdle), can be used by non-scoliotics and bedridden patients as well. Applying more force, it can lead to a slight lifting of the pelvis and a strong tightening of all muscles to form a muscle mantle, not only of the leg musculature, but the buttocks and lower and upper back as well.

b) The main force of the tightening can also be shifted to the front of the thighs. Not only does this correct the shape of the deformed leg, it also lifts the upper frontal pelvic crest by activation of the inner pelvic musculature which has been largely overstretched and worn out and has led to structural collapse of the centre of the body and thus the entire body. Without this ordered tightening of the body centre, there can be no beautiful, slender straightening and formation of the body.

c) It is now easy to combine the following exercises: the elastic increasing tightening of the gluteal muscles leading to slight lifting of pelvis and the simultaneous tightening of the anterior thigh muscles and a mentally guided lifting of the upper frontal pelvic crest. One can feel muscles that did not even seem to exist before. At the end of the exercise, we breathe out – a large, full, natural exhalation which we let happen and slowly fade so there is no overstraining. The lung thus includes and forms many formerly excluded areas. It will be strengthened, enlivened, and better nurtured. There will be no more distortions.

d) This exercise can be taken a little further: We feel the lifting of the anterior pelvic crest all the way to the lumbar area which, contrary to hyperlordosis, will stay in contact with the floor. Our intestines are 'fixed' there with peritoneal folds. The ligaments are taut, the intestines move to their designated place, and the stomach is relieved. During exhalation, we can bring tension into the abdomen lightly or tighter, ordered and carefully increasing, by using the elastic tightening. This lifting and guiding has to be guided mentally, starting at the lowest point, and then moving upwards. It will result in gentle but dynamic contraction of the overstretched abdominal wall. A comfortable feeling of warmth, better blood supply, and nurturing of all inner organs is the result. This is where the celiac plexus (plexus solaris) is located. Small wonder that healthy impulses flow from there to the rest of the body, the spinal cord and the brain, especially because we do our exercises outdoors, in places with sun and fresh air to provide the right environment and impulses.

During the last phase of the exercise, monitoring the uppermost areas and sides of the thighs with the hands, we can feel how they are being shaped. This is positive for the beauty of the legs, but it also leads to the healthy muscle tone which they should have but do not. This muscle tone now develops in the way nature planned it. This will also permanently correct deviation in the waist area of the body. It is not until you try this that you experience the wonderful way strong warmth floods the entire pelvic girdle, the inside of the pelvis and the abdomen. Warmth is awakened everywhere. Sick people often have cold feet and legs and a cold pelvic area and abdomen. This can be changed energetically and is of additional benefit to the circulatory system. This technique may seem to involve a great deal of effort, but to do something right from the beginning is always the best way, although this demands a great deal of commitment on the part of the patient and the therapist.

Excerpt from the
Biologisch-Medizinisches Taschenbuch
(Bio-Medical Pocket Book, 1937),
pages 559–560:

Functional treatment of scoliosis

"Following Klapp and others, orthopaedics has long advanced from the static-mechanical concept of treating scoliosis with supportive corsets, etc., to functional treatment methods. In cases of major fixated scoliosis, physical aids remain, however, quite prominent. These methods have not yet led to satisfactory results.

Frau Schroth (Meissen, Boselweg 52), a self-made therapist, has taken it upon herself to treat scoliosis, even major, third-degree cases, with functional techniques that have been confirmed by the experience of many physicians as well.

From experiences derived from her own body, she has learned to use the shaping force of breathing to rebuild the deviations in form and improve function. This technique of 'breathing orthopaedics' uses a number of different exercises which are applied, taking into account the individual needs of each patient. She develops mainly body awareness and the self-examination of the position of the extremities and trunk in relation to each other and the general posture. Her main concern is the derotation of the vertebral bodies. This is accomplished by using breathing while the ribs assist as lever arms for the vertebrae. The technique of 'rotational breathing' is learned in minute steps and requires great commitment on the part of the patient.

The method includes the overall treatment of the constitution (diet, light, air, sun etc.), spiritual guidance and an education in self motivation. There have been good results even in cases where physician specialists could not even halt progression of the deformity. Judging by all that has become known about it, this method deserves precise scientific verification. As there are only a few physicians who know about it, we want to focus attention on it at this point. Even more so, since we can draw valuable conclusions from this treatment that can also be used for preventative treatment – in orthopaedic gymnastics at school, for example."

Professor Martin Vogel, M.D., Dresden

Excerpt from
Atemheilkunst
(Respiratory Medicine),
3rd Edition (1956), pages 543-544:

"We would like to mention the Schroth rotational breathing school. This school departed from traditional breathing treatment in health care and found a basis in the purely orthopaedic field. It uses the mechanics and function of breathing movement to eliminate scoliotic vertebral and rib deformities in a breathing-orthopaedic treatment developed by Frau Schroth, which has now demonstrated impressive successes for three decades.

The improvement of the diaphragmatic-abdominal mechanics of breathing, which is usually disturbed in a scoliotic patient, and shifting this to expanded breathing in the upper chest accomplishes an essential element in re-erecting the spinal column. In specialised procedures in the supine, prone and lateral positions with accompanying orthopaedic positioning using corrective cushions, and later with observation in mirrors, the patient learns to innervate and move isolated breathing muscles and rib segments. The patient learns a series of positive movements that fill the rib valleys caused by scoliotic deformity. This process of 'rotational breathing' lifts deformed segments that sink downwards in the scoliotic. The ribs act as long levers that derotate the vertebral bodies into a normal position. Lung segments newly developed by the increased functional capacity serve as an internal support like air-cushions, as described by Schanz. Considering how short the period of treatment is, the results really are extraordinarily good.

The author pays special attention to treatment in the open air – the influence of light, air and sun being of importance as well as a changing the patient's habits. She points out that a positive attitude has to be developed as well as a positive new breathing pattern. This has been her observation over many years of treatment."

Johannes-Ludwig Schmitt, M.D.

In conclusion: The courses of treatment in six very different cases

1. A quotation from a letter from a 43-year-old patient whose pictures are shown in Fig. 676.

"As you know, I had fantastic results during my six weeks of in-patient treatment. I feel much better because I know which posture to adopt; I also feel much more optimistic.

I asked at the health insurance office for wall bars. They refused to pay for them. Later, at an appointment with my orthopaedic doctor, I showed him my photos. He looked at me dumbfounded, was pleased with my success, and asked if he could show the photos to a fellow doctor. I agreed. I told my doctor about the wall bars, and he gave them to me as a present. I have sent my pictures to you because I want to show the other patients what can be done. During the first week in the A-group (beginners) I lost confidence often because it was really hard work.

Today, however, I know how important this education is, and that the first week is the basis for the rest of the treatment. I do my exercises daily, as often as I can." (Fig. 676)

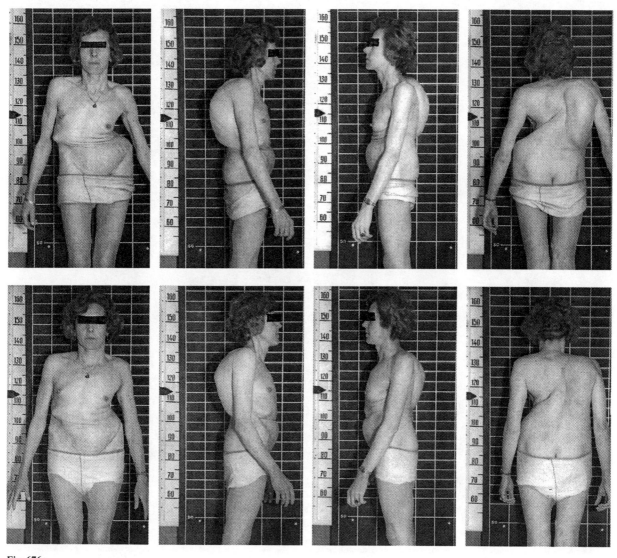

Fig. 676:
43-year-old patient with idiopathic scoliosis who had undergone spinal-fusion surgery during puberty.
The patient was nevertheless able to do our exercises, which she performed with enthusiasm.
Upper row: Beginning of treatment.
Second row: At the end of a 6-week course of in-patient treatment.

2. Report by a 65-year-old female patient

A 65-year-old female patient was asked: "Why do you return every year for two or three weeks' in-patient treatment?"
The answer:
"I have had severe scoliosis since the age of fourteen. I have always been sports-orientated despite my scoliosis. At the age of 50, I spent time at the Katharina-Schroth-Klinik in Bad Sobernheim for the first time. Since then I have been doing exercises daily according to the method of the clinic. In addition, once a week, I visit a physiotherapist who has been educated in the Schroth method. Despite all these activities, it is not possible for me to maintain the results I achieve after intensive training. This is why I go back every year.

At 60, for instance, I had a 32° scoliometer value at the start of treatment. After three weeks of training, it was down to 26°, which indicates that my spine had straightened by six degrees. Two years ago I arrived with a lung capacity of 33% and left the clinic after two weeks of training with a 37% capacity.
This time, two years later, I arrived with 43% capacity and left the clinic with 47%. I also 'grew' 2 cm as well. This indicates that the spine can straighten with the help of the strengthened musculature. The thorax widens and allows room for the lungs. It is not right to believe that, at advanced age, intensive training of the muscles and breathing cannot lead to positive results. Quality of life and performance potential are considerably increased."

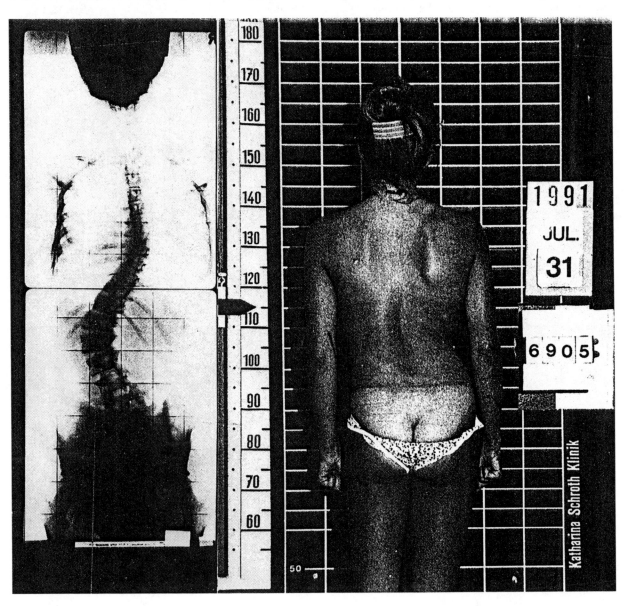

Fig. 677:
Left : X-ray of a 13-year-old girl at the beginning of Schroth treatment: thoracal 43 °, lumbar 58°, lumbosacral 25°.
Right: This patient with idiopathic scoliosis. The right hip is prominent, and there is a large convexity in the lumbar segment on the left side.

3. A course of treatment over ten years:
Schroth therapy in combination with a brace
(Figs. 677-679)

At this point I want to show the course of treatment of a female patient who for a long time was also wearing a well-fitting brace.

The patient had physical therapy from the age of six to thirteen. She started with malposture which then developed into a scoliosis. The treatment was 1-2 times a week according to the general therapeutic methods of Klapp and Niederhoeffer (German treatments).

The first x-ray control was taken at the age of 12 years and 3 months. Nine months later, before starting in-patient treatment at the Katharina-Schroth-Klinik, the X-ray control showed a progression from 28° to 43° (thoracal) and 32° to 58° (lumbar) (Fig. 677 a and b).

Diagnosis: idiopathic scoliosis, thoracic convexity on the right, lumbar convexity (very prominent) on the left and a lumbosacral curvature on the right which shifts the right hip laterally. The body statics have shifted towards the left side. The left leg seems shorter. Since the scoliosis was very progressive between the age of 12-13, a very well fitting Chéneau-brace was made during the first in-patient stay (Fig. 678 a and b) This corrected the curvatures to 13° in the thoracic segment and to 18° in the lumbar segment. During the following four years the patient wore the brace 21 to 23 hours a day, after that about 18 hours a day for a year, and towards the end of the treatment, between the ages of 18 to 23, only at night (Figs. 679 a and b). The patient was very reliable as far as the Schroth treatment was concerned. She went once a week to a Schroth therapist, she practised daily at home by herself, and joined a swimming team.

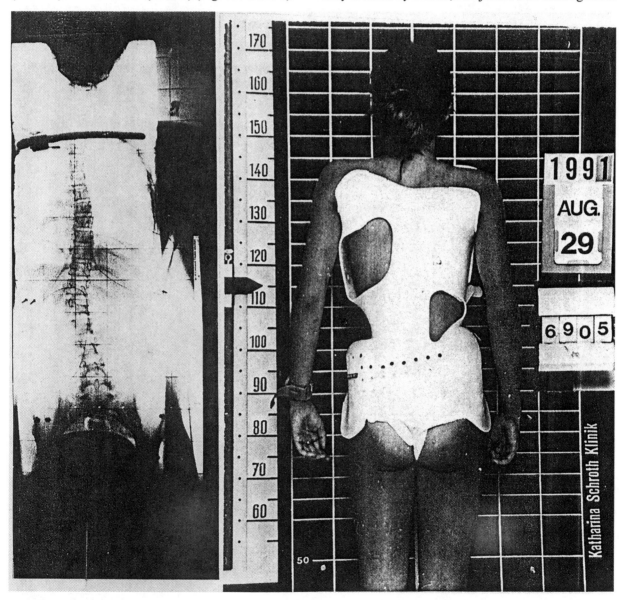

Fig. 678:
Left: X-ray of the same patient wearing a brace: Thoracal 13°, lumbal 18°.
Right: The patient wearing the brace.

Today, after completely abandoning the brace, her appearance is upright and straight. Her curvatures have been reduced to 24° thoracic and 30° lumbar.

Correction of the outward appearance leads automatically to a correction of the spine. A brace does not have to be worn in every case. In this case the patient was at the onset of maturity and this made it necessary. It was a good combination of treatment methods. The patient is mobile and glad to have invested time and money into the Schroth method. Without this treatment, her scoliosis would have progressed and she would have had to have spinal fusion surgery.

For a surgeon it is most important to reduce the Cobb angles. But Katharina Schroth tried to improve the outer appearance as well, which was and still is very important to the patients, since she never had any X-rays at hand in the beginning. The patients were also very glad when there was no more pain, which previously was produced by the sunken upper trunk, which caused friction between ribs as well as between ribs and the hip bones.

Tip: It is useful for the patient to see herself from all four sides in the mirror, even dressed. A video camera can be most helpful in this regard. Figs. 515-516 show this patient during her first in-patient treatment. Due to the considerable shifting of the pelvis, the right hip is prominent and moved upwards. The belt shows this obliquity. The right leg of the trousers seems about 5 cm shorter. After fifteen minutes of exercises the hips are almost even, the belt is almost horizontal. The right leg of the pants seems only about one centimeter shorter.

This case proves how important it is to achieve the necessary feeling for one's body, in order to attain good results. This patient was able to internalize this feeling and call it up repeatedly in her daily life, finally even without a Schroth therapist.

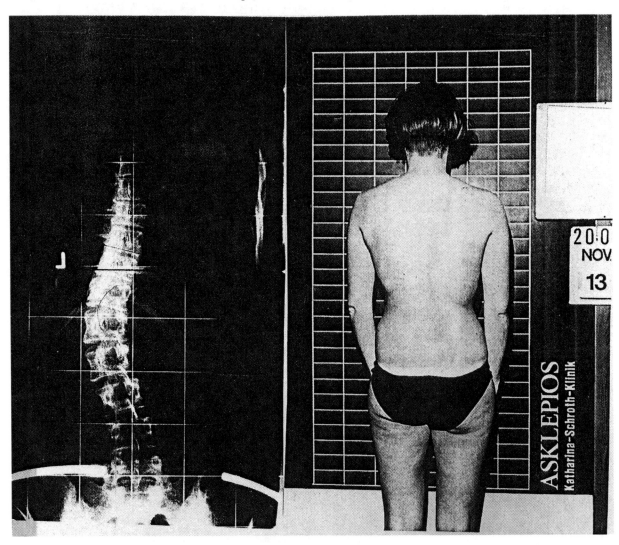

Fig. 679:
Left: X-ray of the patient in Figs. 677-678, after the 8th Schroth treatment, thoracal 24°, lumbar 30°, lumbosacral 21°.
Right: The same patient at the age of 25½ years at the end of the treatment (2006). Straight and upright posture.

4. Report by an 81-year-old patient

The following report is meant to encourage even patients with extremely severe scoliosis to continue with Schroth therapy, so as to maintain their fitness into advanced old age. I am very grateful for the following account from the 81-year-old patient Georg S., because it proves that it is anything but the norm for patients (like Mr. S.) with an extremely severe scoliosis to die at an early age. I met Mr. S. in Bad Sobernheim looking fit and happy while he was staying there for a course of treatment. His face was wreathed in smiles as he told me his story. I asked him to write it down for me so that it could be published here, and he gladly agreed to do this.

Katharina Schroth in Meissen:
My experiences in the 1930s
"When I arrived at age 17 in the beautiful town of Meissen on the banks of the river Elbe to take part in a special exercise course (the site was located on the slopes outside the town), I was not received by a kindly lady ushering me into the fine rooms of a health resort. Rather, I was welcomed by a lovely meadow with fruit trees, all in summer mood. This regular feature with nature at its centre, also remained a recurring theme. Each morning this was the place where Frau Schroth instructed an exercise group using tried and tested exercises. Each day she shared her ideas with those who were exercising, commenting very specifically and as appropriate for each individual's condition. We sensed this and understood that this was a new idea whose time was coming: breathing – oxygen – life. Everything was designed to help suffering individuals back to a normal healthy life. And so she stood with her assistants in the exercise area. We sensed that her gaze was directed towards the sun. This explains why she loved the colour yellow, a shining element, and she chose it for the clothing she wore to exercise in.

Her exercise system was forged in the crucible of practice and experience, not in the academic lecture halls of orthopaedic medicine. It is easy to imagine that she must have been constantly wrestling with all kinds of theoretical thinking and practices. She gave us some insights into her struggle. Among others, she made mention of Prof. Gebhardt who worked in Hohenlychen and expressed a positive opinion about her approach.

In high spirits I used to walk from my lodgings, in the company of my fellow members of the exercise group, and climb up the slope to devote myself single-mindedly to the exercise programme so that success would be visible, as recorded with tape measure and camera.

The Meissen experience was doubly impressive: first because of Frau Schroth and the success of her exercises, and second because of lovely Meissen itself, which provided a beautiful backdrop to our leisure time."
(Written during a course of treatment at the Asklepios-Katharina-Schroth-Klinik in the autumn of 1999).

Mr. S. remains very active. In 2003 he wrote to say that at the age of 85 he was still cycling and engaged in writing. He updated his story again in 2005:

"I'll soon be 88 years old. I'd love to come back to the clinic in Bad Sobernheim for rehabilitation, but my health insurance provider has refused to finance it. Yet I am still keeping myself very fit by cycling between May and October. I've been doing that now for 20 years.
When I was last in your old clinic I used to run up the 120 stairs from my room in the 'Huf-Haus' to the dining room 4 or 5 times every day. I managed this easily. I'm still involved in writing, an activity that I enjoy.
Every morning for 40 years now, I do my 25 pushups and other exercises for my back for 20 minutes. And in the evenings I do the same again for another 10 minutes. I take a 30 minute rest from time to time. I don't need any drugs at all for my heart. I only take calcium tablets. I live alone and follow the Waerland dietary regime, I eat a lot of uncooked foods – 80% vegetables, salad, potatoes, 'Quark' (German-style cottage cheese) with linseed oil, and 20% meat and meat products.
In 1934, as a 17-year-old, I first came to Frau Schroth in Meissen for three months. After that I kept on coming back and have remained an adherent of Schroth therapy right up to the present day. I haven't been sick in bed for one day in 50 years, and I'm also not under doctor's care or on any drugs. Despite my 88 years and my severe scoliosis, I'm still fit."

5. A letter of an 84-year-old female patient

An 84½-year-old patient recollects that, after the war had ended, we asked her how she was getting on.
"And now my hands are holding your postcard, it's almost 60 years old. How fascinating to read how things really were then. And how good to know that even though it had small beginnings, it has grown into something big
(…)
"The present-day clinic is beautiful … but I often think back to earlier times, and most specially to the many weeks spent by the Woerthersee lake (where our summer treatments took place). In the meadow where we exercised, we used a couple of poles, a firm tubular support and two small sandbags. Sitting crosslegged on a blanket we breathed and brought our spine into correct alignment. Simply recalling a relaxation and exercise session, I realise that Frau Schroth was far ahead of her time. People today talk about 'autogenic training', but back then, 65 years ago, no one was using the term. Nowadays therapists proudly refer to such concepts as wellness and autogenic training and the like. We had them long before with Frau Schroth, and it was so effective that I can still feel the benefit in my bones, just from one single session. … It was a blissful time. I can

still climb stairs without struggling for breath. And all the credit for that goes to the good Schroth system of rotational breathing."

6. A visit of a 32-year-old patient

A 32-year-old patient enthusiastically reports that when she was young she had to wear a brace for several years. After that she sewed herself a special pyjama jacket with three pockets into which she would place her Schroth correction pads at night. Because she had been used to sleeping on her back anyway due to the brace, the pyjama jacket was not a problem for her. And now, after 12 treatment-free years that have included 3 pregnancies and the usual housework, as well as a few Schroth exercises every day, her scoliosis has not worsened. Quite the opposite in fact: her rib hump is now no longer visible through her clothing, i.e. her spine has untwisted itself. Sleeping on your back is simply a question of inner attitude and not a problem at all. I have never come across a report like this before and I believe that it should be published here so that others may copy the idea.

Literature

Basmajian, J. V., De Luca, C. J.: Muscles alive: Their functions revealed by electromyography. Williams & Wilkins, 5th ed. (1985).

Bjure, J., Grimby, G., Nachemson, A.: The effect of physical training in girls with idiopathic scoliosis, Acta orthop. scand. 40(1969) 325-33.

Bottenberg, H.: Biologische Therapie des praktischen Arztes. J. F. Lehmann Verlag, München, 314.

Brussatis, F.: Elektromyographische Untersuchungen der Rücken- und Bauchmuskulatur bei idiopathischen Skoliosen. Die Wirbelsäule in Forschung und Praxis, Vol. 24, Hippokrates Verlag, Stuttgart (1962).

Caillet, R.: Scoliosis, Diagnosis and Management. F. A. Davis Company, Philadelphia (1983).

Cheneau, J., Gaubert, J.: Zur Entwicklung des Cheneau-Korsetts. Grundlagen der Biomechanik für Orthopädie-Mechaniker. Lite ratursammlung, Verlag Orthopädie Technik, Dortmund (1988).

Collis, D., Ponseti, I. V.: Long-term follow-up of patients with idiopathic scoliosis not treated surgically. J. Bone Joint Surg. Am, 51(3) (1969) 425-445.

Dickson, R. A.: The Pathogenesis of idiopathic scoliosis, Biplanar spinal asymmetrie from St. James University Hospital, Leeds. The Journal of Bone and Joint Surgery, 1. 1. 84.

Duthie, R. B.: Manifestation of musculosceletal disorders, Kap. 5. Principles of Surgery, Volume 2. Herausgegeben von Schwartz, S. I., New York, McGrave-Hill Bock Company (1969) 1532-1583.

Eder, M., Tilscher, H.: Chirotherapie, Hippokrates-Verlag, Stuttgart (1988).

Farkas, A.: Über Bedingungen und auslösende Momente bei der Skolioseentstehung (Versuch einer funktionellen Skoliosenlehre) Beilagenheft der Z. f. Orthopädische Chirurgie Bd. XLVII Verlag v. Ferdinand Enke, Stuttgart (1925).

Friedebold, G.: Die Aktivität normaler Rückenstreckmuskulatur im Elektromyogramm unter verschiedenen Haltungsbedingungen, Z. Orthop. 90 (1958)

Götze, H. G./Vogelpohl, H./Seibt, G.: Der Einfluss einer 4wöchigen krankengymnastischen Behandlung nach Schroth auf die organische Leistungsfähigkeit jugendlicher Skoliosepatienten, Z. Krankengymnastik 27 (1975) 316-321.

Götze, H. G.: Die Rehabilitation jugendlicher Skoliosepatienten. Untersuchungen zur kardiopulmonalen Leistungsfähigkeit und zum Einfluss von Krankengymnastik und Sport. Habilitationsschrift Münster (1976).

Götze, H. G.: Pathophysiologie der Atmung und kardiopulmonaler Funktionsdiagnostik bei Skoliosepatienten. Z. Krankengymnastik 30 (1978a) 228.

Götze, H. G.: Metrische Befunddokumentation pulmonaler Funktionswerte von jugendlichen und erwachsenen Skoliose patienten unter einer 4wöchigen Kurbehandlung. Z. Krankengymnastik 30 (1978b) 333.

Grumeth, F.: Bisherige Erfahrungen mit der dreidimensionalen Skoliosebehandlung nach Schroth. In Skoliose aus der Buchreihe f. Orthopädie und orthopädische Grenzgebiete, Bd. 5, Hrsg. v. Meznik, F. Böhler, Medizin.-Literarische Ver lagsgesellschaft mbH Uelzen (1982) 113-118.

Güth, V., Abbinck, S.: Vergleichende elektromyographische und kinesiologische Untersuchungen an kongenitalen und idio pathischen Skoliosen, Z. Orthop. 118 (1980) 165.

Hansen, Th.: Praktische Bewährung der Methode Schroth, Z. Orthop. u. ihre Grenzgeb., 114 (1976) 462-464.

Heine, J.: Die Lumbaiskoliose, Enke-Verlag (1980).

Heine, J., Meister, R.: Quantitative Untersuchungen der Lungenfunktion und der arteriellen Blutgase bei jugendlichen Skoliotikern mit Hilfe eines funktionsdiagnostischen Minimalprogrammes. Z. Orthop. 110 (1972) 56.

Hettinger, Th.: Trainingsgrundlagen im Rahmen der Rehabili tation. Z. Krankengymnastik 30 (1978) 339-344.

Hundt, O. E.: Möglichkeiten der krankengymnastischen Beeinflussbarkeit der Skoliose und die damit verbundenen Wirkungen auf die Herz-Kreislauf-Funktionsbereiche. Rehabilitation der Atmung, Gustav-Fischer-Verlag, Stuttgart (1975) 100-105.

Kahn, F.: Das Leben des Menschen, eine volkstümliche Anatomie, Biologie, Physiologie und Entwicklungsgeschichte des Menschen. 4 Bände. Kosmos-Gesellschaft der Naturheilkunde. Francksche Verlagsbuchhandlung, Stuttgart (1929).

Karch, J.: Klinische Zeichen der lumbosakralen Gegenkrümmung bei Skoliosepatienten und der daraus resultierende Korrekturaufbau. Z. Krankengymnastik 41 (1989) 467-468.

Klawunde, G. et al.: Neurophysiologische und lungenfunktionsdiagnostische Untersuchungen zur Wirkung von Gymnastik und manueller Therapie bei juvenilen Skoliosen. Z. Physiotherapie 40 (1988) 103-111.

Klein-Vogelbach, S.: Funktionelle Bewegungslehre. Springer-Verlag, Berlin-Heidelberg, 4. Aufl. (1983).

Klisic, P., Nikolic, Z.: Attitudes scoliotiques et scoliosis idio-pathiques: Prävention ä l'ecole. Vorgetragen auf der inter nationalen Tagung zur Prävention der Skoliose im Schulalter in Rom, Italien, 1. April 1982.

Lehnert-Schroth, Ch.: Die Behandlung der Skoliose nach dem System Schroth. Z. Krankengymnastik 9 (1975): 322.

- Die Probleme der krankengymnastischen Skoliosebehandlung. Z. Der deutsche Badebetrieb 67 (1976): 317-324.

- Grundlegende Gedanken zu den atmungs-orthopädischen Skolioseübungen nach System Schroth. Rehabilitation der Atmung, Gustav Fischer-Verlag, Stuttgart (1976): 102-105.

- Die Besonderheiten der krankengymnastischen Übungsbehandlung nach Schroth. Z. Physikalische Medizin und Rehabilitation 17 (1976) 3-8.

- Skoliosen und die verschiedenen krankengymnastischen Behandlungsmethoden. Eigenverlag Katharina-Schroth-Klinik, Sobemheim (1977-1990).

- Die Beeinflussung der Lumbosakralskoliose durch die drei dimensionale Skoliosebehandlung. In Meznik and Böhler, "Die Skoliose," Buchreihe für Orthopädie und orthopädische Grenzgebiete, vol. 5, Medizin.-Literarische Verlagsgesellschaft Uelzen (1982): 116-118.

- Dreidimensionale Skoliosebehandlung, 7th ed., Urban & Fischer, Munich and Jena (2007).

- Prävention von Haltungsschäden im Schulunterricht und beim Schulsport. Z. Sozialpädiatrie in Praxis und Klinik 8 (1986): 344-348.

- Haltungsschwäche und Haltungsschäden. Z. Sport Praxis 27 (1986): 40-42.

- Die dreidimensionale Skoliosebehandlung nach Schroth. DKZ (Deutsche Krankenpflegezeitschrift) 40 (1987): 1750-1756.

- Haltungsschäden und deren Vorbeugung im Schulunterricht. Z. Turnen und Sport (1988): 62. 1-2, and in brochures published by the Katharina-Schroth-Klinik, Sobemheim.

- Unsere Erfahrungen mit einem Verkürzungsausgleich in der Skoliosebehandlung. Z. Orthopädische Praxis (4/1991).

- Krankengymastische Behandlung von Patienten mit operativ versteifter Skoliose, Zeitschrift für Physiotherapeuten, Richard Pflaum Verlag München, 48.Jg (2/1996) S. 212-219

Lehnert-Schroth, Ch./Weiss, H.-R.: Dokumentation zur Entwicklung der dreidimensionalen Skoliose-Behandlung nach Schroth, Eigenverlag Katharina-Schroth-Klinik, Sobemheim (1989).

Lewit, K.: Manuelle Medizin, Urban und Schwarzenberg, München, 5. Aufl. (1987).

Lonstein, J. F., Carlson, J. M.: Adult scoliosis, Moes Textbook of Scoliosis and other Spinal Deformities. W. B. Saunders Company Philadelphia (1987).

Macintosh, J. E., Bogduk, N.: The morphology of the lumbar erector spinae. Spine 12 (1987): 658-68.

Meister, R.: Atemfunktion und Lungenkreislauf bei thorakaler Skoliose. Thieme-Verlag, Stuttgart (1980).

Mollon, G., Bogduk, J. C: Scoliosis structurales mineurs et kinesitherapie. Etude statistique comparative des resultats. Kinesitherapie Scient 244 (1986) 47-56.

Nachemson, A., Lonstein, J., Weinstein, S.: Report of the prevalence and natural history committee. Denver (1982).

Pitzen, P.: Kurzgefasstes Lehrbuch der orthopädischen Krankheiten. Urban u. Schwarzenberg, München-Berlin. 5. Aufl. (1950).

Rigo, M., Quera-Salva, G.: Effect of the exclusive application of physiotherapy in patients with idiopathic scoliosis. Retrospective study. Not yet published.

Rogala, E. J., Drumond, D. S., Gurr, J.: Scoliosis. Incidence and natural history. J. Bone u. Joint Surg. 60 A (1978) 173.

Scheier, H.: Prognose und Behandlung der Skoliose. Georg-Thieme-Verlag, Stuttgart (1967) 48-49.

Schlegel, K. F.: Wert und Wertlosigkeit der krankengymnastischen Behandlung der Skoliose. Wissenschaftl. Zeitschrift der Ernst-Moritz-Arndt-Universität, Greifswald, Mathematisch-Naturwissenschaftl. Reihe XX (1971) 2321-2333.

Schlegel, K. F.: Die Skoliosebehandlung nach Schroth. Z. Orthop. 114 (1976)761.

Schmidt, F. A., Kohlrausch, W.: Unser Körper. Handbuch der Anatomie, Physiologie und Hygiene der Leibesübungen, Verlag R. Voigtländer, Leipzig, 8. Aufl. (1981).

Schmidt, R. F., Thews, G.: Physiologie des Menschen. Springer-Verlag. Berlin-Heidelberg-New York.

Schmidt, W.: Die idiopathische Skoliose aus der Sicht der funktionellen Bewegungslehre (FBL) Z. Krankengymnastik 36 (1984) 2-10.

Schmitt, J. L.: Atemheilkunst. Hanns-Georg-Müller-Verlag, München und Berlin. 3. Aufl. (1956).

Schmitt, O.: Skoliosefrühbehandlung durch Elektrostimulation, Bücherei der Orthopädie Bd. 45, Enke-Verlag, Stuttgart (1985).

Schroth, K.: Die Atmungs-Kur, Leitfaden zur Lungengymnastik. Buchdruckerei Gustav Zimmermann, Hohndorf Bez. Chemnitz 1924.

- Atmungs-Orthopädie und funktionelle Behandlung der Skoliose (seitl. Rückgratverkrümmung). Volksarzt-Verlag, Essen 1930.

- Behandlung der Skoliose (Rückgratverkrümmung) durch Atmungs-Orthopädie. Z. Naturarzt 59 (1931).

- Krise in der Orthopädie. Obererzgebirgische Zeitung Buchholz/Sachsen (v. 11. 5. 1935).

- Wie helfen wir den Rückgratverkrümmten? Obererzgebirgische Zeitung Buchholz/Sachsen (v. 23. 6. 1935).

- Naturgemässe Betreuung Rückgratverkrümmter besonders im Krieg. Z. Der Heilpraktiker, Richard-Pflaum-Verlag, Mün chen (4/1943).

- Atmungs-Orthopädie Original-System Schroth. Z. Der Heilmasseur - Physiotherapie. Gebr. Bossard, Zürich/Schweiz 1955.

- Was ist Atmungs-Orthopädie? Z. Atem - Massage - Entspannung - Moderne Gymnastik (1/1963) Helfer Verlag Schwabe, Bad Homburg v.d.H., Nachdruck in Z. Physiotherapie 68 (1977) 652-654.
- Der hohlrunde Rücken in atmungs-orthopädischer Behandlung. Z. Z. für Atempflege - Massage - Entspannung
- Moderne Gymnastik, Helfer-Verlag E. Schwabe, Bad Homburg v. d. H. (4/1966) 8-9.
- Atmungs-Orthopädie Originalsystem Schroth. Z. Erfahrungsheilkunde Bd. XV (6/1966).
- Atmungs-Orthopädie Original, Schroth. Taschenbuch der Physiotherapie, Karl F. Haug-Verlag, Heidelberg 1968.68-92.
- Gefahren der Behandlung seitl. Rückgratverkrümmung. Z. Der Naturarzt 9 (7/1972) 399-400.

Scoliometer-Beschreibung: Orthopedic Systems, Inc. 1897 National Avenue, Hayward, CA 94545 (415) 785-1020.

Stobody, H., Friedebold, G.: Evaluation of the effect of isometric training in functional and organic muscles atrophy. Archiv Phys. med. rehab. (1968) 508-514.

Sobotta, J.: Deskriptive Anatomie des Menschen. J. F. Lehmanns Verlag, München 1931.

Tomaschewski, R.: Die funktionelle Behandlung der beginnen den idiopathischen Skoliose. Dissertation. Vorgelegt der med. Fakultät der Martin-Luther-Universität, Halle-Wittenberg (1987).

Vogel, M.: Funktionelle Skoliosebehandlung. Biologisch-Medizinisches Taschenbuch, Hippokrates-Verlag, Stuttgart 1937, 559-560.

Vogelpohl, H.: Dissertationsarbeit: Die Beeinflussung der kardiopulmonalen Leistungsfähigkeit von Skoliosepatienten durch intensive Krankengymnastik und leichtes Ausdauertraining. Arbeit im Auftrag der Westfälischen Wilhelm-Universität, Institut für Sportmedizin, Münster (1975).

Weinstein, S. L., Zavala, D. C, Ponseti, I. V.: Idiopathic scoliosis: Longterm follow-up and prognosis in untreated patients. J. Bone and Joint Surg. 64 (1981) 702-712.

Weiss, H.-R.: Prävention sekundärer Funktionseinschränkungen bei Skoliosepatienten im Rahmen einer mehrwöchigen Intensivbehandlung nach Schroth. Z. Physikalische Medizin, Balneologie, med. Klimatologie, 17 (1988) 306.
- Eine funktionsanalytische Betrachtung der dreidimensionalen Skoliosebehandlung nach Schroth. Z. Krankengymnastik 40 (1988) 363.
- Krankengymnastische Rehabilitation bei idiopathischer Skoliose. Z. für Allgemeinmedizin (ZFA) 64 (1988) 1027-1030.
- Schroth - Ein skoliosespezifisches Rehabilitationsprogramm. Teil 1: Theoretische Grundlagen. Teil 2: Praktische Durchführung. Therapeutiken 2 (1989) 682-694.
- Effektive Skoliosebehandlung durch Krankengymnastik. Z. Rheuma 4/5 (1989) 177-180 u. 233-237.
- Ein Modell klinischer Rehabilitation von Kindern und Jugendlichen mit idiopathischer Skoliose. Z. Orthopädische Praxis 25 (1989a): 93-97.
- Prävention und Rehabilitation von Skoliosefolgen im Erwachsenenalter. Z. Krankengymnastik 41 (1989b): 468-473.
- Krümmungsverläufe idiopathischer Skoliosen unter dem Einfluss eines krankengymnastischen Rehabilitationsprogrammes. Z. Orthopädie Praxis (10/90) 648-654.
- Influence of an in-patient exercise program on scoliotic curve. Ital J Orthop Traumatol. 1992;18(3):395-406.
- Beeinflussung skoliosebedingter Schmerzzustände durch ein krankengymnastisches Rehabilitationsprogramm. Z. Orthopädie-Praxis 26 (1990) 793-797.
- The Effect of an Exercise Program on Vital Capacity and Rib Mobility in Patients with Idiopathic Scoliosis, Spine, Vol. 16 (1/1991).
- Wirbelsäulendeformitäten Band 1, Springer, 1991; Band 2, Gustav Fischer, 1992: Band 3, Gustav Fischer 1994
- Einflüsse des Schrothschen Rehabilitationsprogrammes auf Selbstkonzepte von Skoliose-PatientInnen. Rehabilitation 33, 31-43, 1994
- Auswirkungen der Schroth'schen Dreh-Winkel-Atmung auf die dreidimensionale Verformung bei idiopathischen Thorakalskoliosen in Wirbelsäulendeformitäten (Vol 3), Gustav Fischer 87-92, 1994
- Skolioserehabilitation, Qualitätssicherung und Patientenmanagement, Thieme, 2000
- Befundgerechte Physiotherapie bei Skoliose, Munich, R. Pflaum (2001).
- Operationsinzidenz bei konservativ behandelten PatientInnen mit Skoliose. Med. Orth. Tech. 2002
- Rehabilitation of scoliosis patients with pain after surgery. Stud.Health Technol Inform. 88: 250-3 (2002).
- Incidence of curvature in idiopathic scoliosis patients treated with scoliosis-in-patient rehabilitation (SIR), an age- and sex-matched controlled study. Pediatric Rehabilitation, Jan-Mar:6(1)m 23-30, (2003).
- Incidence of surgery in conservatively treated patients with scoliosis. Pediatric Rehabilitation, Apr.-Jun.6(2):111-8. (2003).
- "Best Practice" in Conservative Scoliosis Care, Munich, Richard Pflaum Verlag, 2nd ed. (2006).

Weiss/Bickert: Veränderungen elektromyografisch objektivierbarer Parameter der Rechtsherzbelastung erwachsener Skoliosepatienten durch das stationäre Rehabilitationsprogramm nach Schroth. Orthopädische Praxis 32, 450-453, 1996

Weiss/Cherdron: Befindlichkeitsänderungen bei Skoliosepatienten in der stationären krankengymnastischen Rehabilitation, Orth. Praxis 28, 87-90, 1992

German

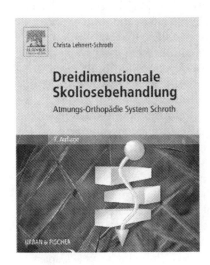

Christa Lehnert-Schroth, P.T.

Dreidimensionale Skoliosebehandlung

Atmungs-Orthopädie System Schroth

Urban & Fischer - Elsevier

ISBN : 978-3-437-44025-0
678 schwarz-weiß Abbildungen
7. Aufl. vom 16.05.2007

Dreidimensionale Skoliosebehandlung
Atmungs-Orthopädie System Schroth

Das Standardlehrbuch der dreidimensionalen Skoliosetherapie in der 7. Auflage enthält neue Übungen und Patientenbeispiele.

Das „System Schroth" hat seit Jahrzehnten einen festen Platz in der konservativen Behandlung auch ausgeprägter Skoliosen. Es korrigiert die Deformierungen der Wirbelsäule durch Extension, Detorsion und Entlordosierung. Wichtig ist dabei die aktive, individuelle Beeinflussung auch durch Muskeldehnung und Atemtherapie. Besonders berücksichtigt wird die psychische Unterstützung der Patienten.
Das Buch ermöglicht Anfängern durch seine einfache und verständliche Sprache einen schnellen Einstieg in die Methode. Durch die enge Verbindung von Theorie und Praxis finden auch fortgeschrittene PhysiotherapeutInnen auf jede Frage zur dreidimensionalen Skoliosetherapie die passende Antwort.

The standard text on three-dimensional scoliosis therapy in the 7th edition now contains new exercises and patient examples.

For decades the 'THREE-DIMENSIONAL TREATMENT FOR SCOLIOSIS' has occupied a prominent place in the conservative treatment of scoliosis – even in severe cases. The Schroth System corrects deformations through elongation, derotation, and reversal of the lordosis. Of importance is the active, individual influence through muscle elongation and breathing therapy. Psychological support of the patient gets special attention.
Beginners can get started quickly with the exercises since the book is written in a simple and understandable language. Connecting theory and practise, the book is also of interest for experienced physical therapists as it provides an appropriate answer to every question concerning the three-dimensional treatment of scoliosis.

Título de la traducción en español de la 6a- edición:

Tratamiento functional tridimensional

de la escoliosis.

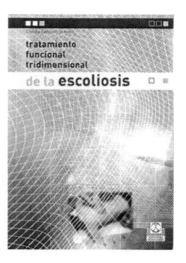

Autora: Christa Lehnert-Schroth, P.T.
ISBN 84-8019-754-4

Publicista:
Editorial Paidotribo, S.L.C/De la Energía, l9-21
08915 Barcelona, ESPAÑA
e-Mail: paidotribo@paidotribo.com

El tratamiento tridimensional para la Escoliosis
-El Sistema Respiratorio Ortopédico de Schroth-

Este libro de texto ha sido escrito especialmente manteniendo en mente a los terapistas y ha sido escrito por una practicante para uso en la práctica diaria. Se compone de seis partes. Después de varios prólogos y prefacios médicos y la descripción de la carrera professional de **Katharina Schroth** el libro está dividido en las siguientes secciones:

Parte A describe los principios teóricos sobremarcados del tratamiento por el **método Schroth** con ilustraciones que explican estos principios teóricos están tan bien descritos, que cualquier persona los puede seguir. La autora demuestra que en la escoliosis, los tres segmentos del tronco (la articulación de la pelvis, la caja toráxica y la articulación de la escápula y del hombro) están desplazadas y torcidas una en contra de la otra y es cuando se demuestra como se puede destorcer. En un capítulo aparte se describe el poder de la respiración. Se explica también la práctica de la respiración rotatoria angular desarrollada por **Katharina Schroth**.

Parte B explica la teoría demostrando por escrito con ilustraciones y usando ejemplos prácticos. Los músculos afectados por la escoliosis están descritos con bastante detalle extensamente y se demuestra como ellos pueden re-educarse cerca a lo normal por medio de ejercicio. Otro capítulo separado demuestra las diferentes formas de escoliosis y sus tratamientos especiales.

La parte C cubre una gran variedad de ejercicios utilizando barras en la pared, mesas, sillas, el piso y bandas hechas de caucho para ejercicios fuertes de resistencia o Theraband. Los espejos aquí juegan un papel muy importante porque sin ellos y sin las fotos de control, es difícil para el paciente seguir la lógica que existe detrás de estas instrucciones de tratamiento. También se describen discusiones para casos con problemas que se pueda enfrentar en la práctica de terapia. Aquí se demuestran las soluciones. Se demuestra claramente por qué el tratamiento para un „caso" particular se tiene que dar de cierta manera y no de la otra. El terapista encontrará eventualmente el ejercicio apropiado.

La parte D provee fotografías, documentación, evaluación radiológica y análisis estadísticos de los cambios en la capacidad pulmonar para mejorar la salud durante varios años.

La parte E describe la experiencia ortopédica, día por día que es lo que el paciente puede hacer en su hogar, en términos de tratar su escoliosis.

Un apéndice reproduce compresivamente instrucciones de ejercicios escritos por **Katharina Schroth** personalmente para el paciente. También hay dos extractos de libros de textos escritos por practicantes médicos alagando el valor del **método Schroth**.

Index

Printed in the United Kingdom by
Lightning Source UK Ltd., Milton Keynes
137471UK00001B/26/A